W0259825

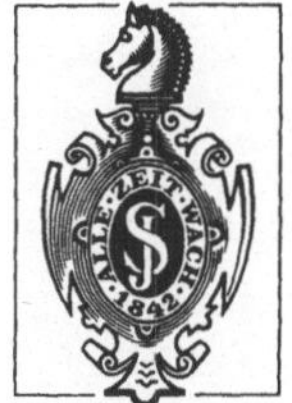
ALLE ZEIT WACH
1842

Ovarialtumoren

Herausgegeben von
Gisela Dallenbach-Hellweg

Mit 152 Abbildungen und 38 Tabellen

Springer-Verlag
Berlin Heidelberg New York 1982

Dr. med. GISELA DALLENBACH-HELLWEG
Professor für allgemeine Pathologie und pathologische Anatomie,
Leiterin der Abteilung für gynäkologische Morphologie
und morphologische Forschung der Universitäts-Frauenklinik
6800 Mannheim

Gedruckt mit Unterstützung des Ministeriums für Wissenschaft und Kunst,
Baden-Württemberg

ISBN 978-3-540-11327-0 ISBN 978-3-642-68462-3 (eBook)
DOI 10.1007/978-3-642-68462-3

CIP-Kurztitelaufnahme der Deutschen Bibliothek
Ovarialtumoren / hrsg. von Gisela Dallenbach-Hellweg. –
Berlin ; Heidelberg ; New York : Springer, 1982.

NE: Dallenbach-Hellweg, Gisela [Hrsg.]

Satz, Druck und Bindearbeiten: Konrad Triltsch, Würzburg
2129/3130-543210

Vorwort

Die Ovarialtumoren gehören heute mit zu den häufigsten Tumoren des weiblichen Genitale. Ihre morphologische Differentialdiagnostik und die sich darauf aufbauende gezielte Therapie ist aufgrund der Vielfalt dieser Tumoren ungleich viel komplizierter als in anderen Organen. Dementsprechend liegt der Schwerpunkt dieses Buches auf dem Gebiet der Histopathologie. Spezialkenntnisse insbesondere über die selteneren Formen der Ovarialtumoren hängen von großen Fallzahlen ab. Hier ist der internationale Erfahrungsaustausch von vorrangiger Bedeutung. Die derzeit weltweit anerkannte histogenetische Klassifikation der WHO erfährt anhand der Erfahrungen an drei deutschen Frauenkliniken kleine Ergänzungen und Variationen. Einige Länder, z. B. Israel verfügen über große epidemiologische Untersuchungen, deren Ergebnisse korrelierend aufgenommen sind. Zur klinischen Diagnostik wurden in den letzten Jahren modernste Untersuchungsmethoden neu eingeführt; ihre Anwendung setzt jedoch individuell anzupassende kritische Indikationsstellungen voraus. Abschließend werden die sich sehr differenziert auf der histologischen Diagnostik aufbauenden modernen Möglichkeiten einer gezielten Therapie der Ovarialtumoren ausführlich diskutiert. Hier steht die Chemotherapie im Vordergrund. Im Hinblick auf die Frage einer Hormonbehandlung kommt neuerdings auch dem Rezeptornachweis im Tumorgewebe Bedeutung zu.

Diese Zusammenstellung spricht somit gleichermaßen Pathologen, Onkologen und Gynäkologen an und will versuchen, gegenseitige Informationslücken der Fachexperten auf dem Gesamtgebiet der Problematik der Ovarialtumoren in zumutbarer Kürze zu schließen. Daher nehmen gerade die selteneren und bisher weniger bekannten Tumoren in Bild und Text einen verhältnismäßig breiten Raum ein auf Kosten der hinlänglich bekannten häufigeren Formen, bei denen Spezialfragen der Differentialdiagnostik aufgrund neuester Erkenntnisse im Vordergrund stehen. Wenn es der Abhandlung gelänge, die interdisziplinäre Zusammenarbeit einerseits, den Erfahrungsaustausch zwischen Fachpathologen über die Ländergrenzen hinweg andererseits auf diesem Gebiet zu intensivieren, so wäre ihr Hauptzweck erreicht.

Dem Springer-Verlag schulde ich aufrichtigen Dank für die Bereitschaft, den internationalen wissenschaftlichen Gedankenaustausch von Fachexperten unkonventionell diskussionsgetreu und daher problemnah in der jeweiligen Originalsprache in Buchform erscheinen zu lassen.

Heidelberg/Mannheim,
im März 1982

GISELA DALLENBACH-HELLWEG

Vorwort

Inhaltsverzeichnis

Mitarbeiterverzeichnis

Die Adressen sind am Anfang des entsprechenden Beitrages zu finden.

Einführung

Histogenetische Klassifikation

G. Dallenbach-Hellweg[1]

Die Histopathologie der Ovarialtumoren hat in den letzten 10 Jahren erhebliche Fortschritte erzielt. Diese gilt es, einem großen Kreis von Pathologen und Klinikern zu vermitteln und gemeinsam nach weiteren Verbesserungen in Diagnostik und Therapie zu suchen. Wir bemühen uns derzeit um eine gezielte, möglichst tumorspezifische Therapie. Diese hat aber eine ebenso spezifische Tumordiagnostik zur Voraussetzung. Dabei interessieren den Kliniker vor allem der Malignitätsgrad, das Stadium und die Ansprechbarkeit des Tumors auf die verschiedenen Formen der Therapie, den Morphologen darüber hinaus auch die Histogenese, ein speziell am Beispiel des Ovars äußerst kompliziertes Thema. Gerade die Kenntnis der Histogenese ermöglicht aber wesentliche Rückschlüsse auf das biologische Verhalten des Tumors, insbesondere seinen Malignitätsgrad.

An den Beginn möchte ich, sozusagen als Arbeitshypothese, zwei Klassifikationen stellen, die sich weitgehend decken: die derzeit offiziell gültige WHO-Klassifikation und die an unserer Mannheimer Klinik in gynäkopathologischer Zusammenarbeit entwickelte Klassifikation (Tabelle 1). Beide beruhen auf dem histogenetischen Prinzip. Wenn unsere Mannheimer Arbeitsgruppe hiermit kleine Abweichungen vom WHO-Schema in den Raum stellt, so aus zwei Gründen: Einerseits entsprechen diese Abweichungen bei uns gesammelten klinischen Erfahrungen, andererseits ist auch die WHO-Nomenklatur an einigen Stellen durchaus noch diskussionsoffen. Als Beispiel möchte ich nur die Muzinkarzinome herausgreifen: Wir sind ebenfalls der Ansicht, daß sie sich aus dem Zölomepithel entwickeln, allerdings aus einer für das Ovar ektopischen Differenzierung des Müller-Epithels, diskutieren aber gleichzeitig ihre Abstammung von den Keimzellen als einseitig determinierte Teratome, was der nachgewiesenen Ähnlichkeit einer Reihe dieser Tumoren mit Darmepithel entspricht. Eine Sonderstellung der Muzinkarzinome gegenüber den serös-papillären Karzinomen ergibt sich auch aus ihrem ganz anderen Altersgipfel (Tabelle 2) und ihrer viel günstigeren Prognose (Tabelle 4).

Bei Zusammenstellung aller physiologischen Strukturen des Ovars entsprechend ihrer Herkunft sowie ihrer pluripotenten oder für das Ovar abwegigen Vorstufen lassen sich die vielseitigen Tumorformen fast mühelos auf ihre Ausgangszelle zurückführen (Tabelle 3); die histogenetische Klassifikation (Tabelle 1) wird dadurch um so verständlicher.

1 Frauenklinik im Klinikum Mannheim der Universität Heidelberg, Morphologische Abteilung, D-6800 Mannheim

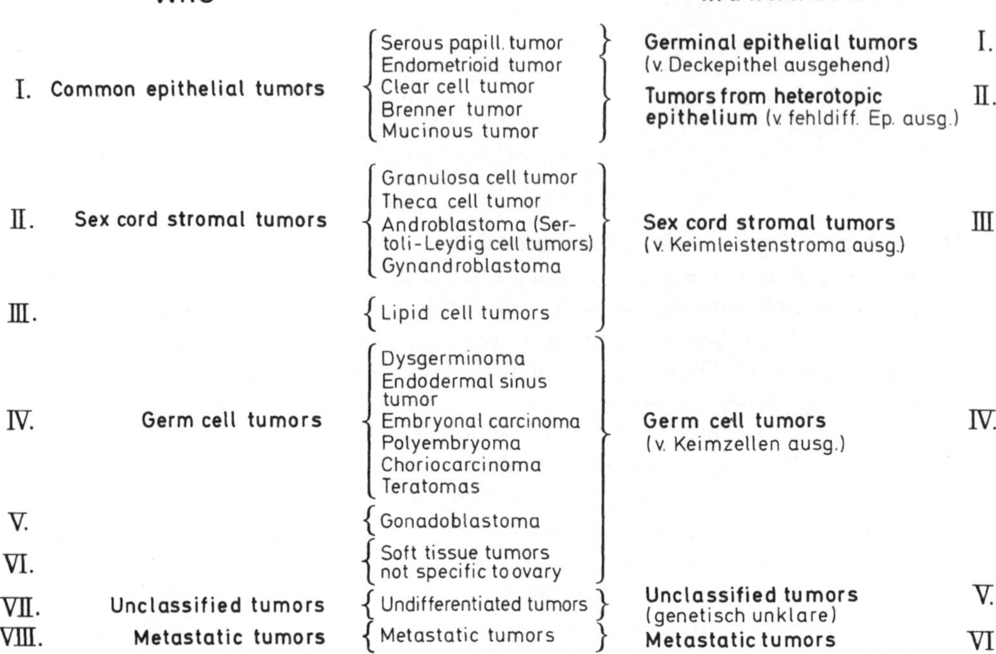

WHO		Mannheim	
I. Common epithelial tumors	Serous papill. tumor	**Germinal epithelial tumors** (v. Deckepithel ausgehend)	I.
	Endometrioid tumor Clear cell tumor Brenner tumor Mucinous tumor	**Tumors from heterotopic epithelium** (v. fehldiff. Ep. ausg.)	II.
II. Sex cord stromal tumors	Granulosa cell tumor Theca cell tumor Androblastoma (Sertoli-Leydig cell tumors) Gynandroblastoma	**Sex cord stromal tumors** (v. Keimleistenstroma ausg.)	III.
III.	Lipid cell tumors		
IV. Germ cell tumors	Dysgerminoma Endodermal sinus tumor Embryonal carcinoma Polyembryoma Choriocarcinoma Teratomas	**Germ cell tumors** (v. Keimzellen ausg.)	IV.
V.	Gonadoblastoma		
VI.	Soft tissue tumors not specific to ovary		
VII. Unclassified tumors	Undifferentiated tumors	**Unclassified tumors** (genetisch unklare)	V.
VIII. Metastatic tumors	Metastatic tumors	**Metastatic tumors**	VI.

Tabelle 1. Histogenetische Klassifikation der Ovarialtumoren nach den Richtlinien der WHO (*links*) und nach der an der Mannheimer Frauenklinik benutzten Modifikation

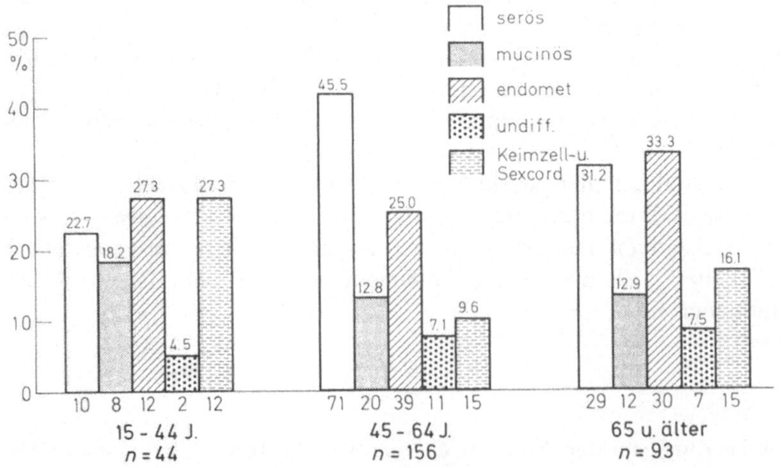

Tabelle 2. Altersmäßige Verteilung der Ovarialkarzinome eines Kollektivs der Mannheimer Frauenklinik

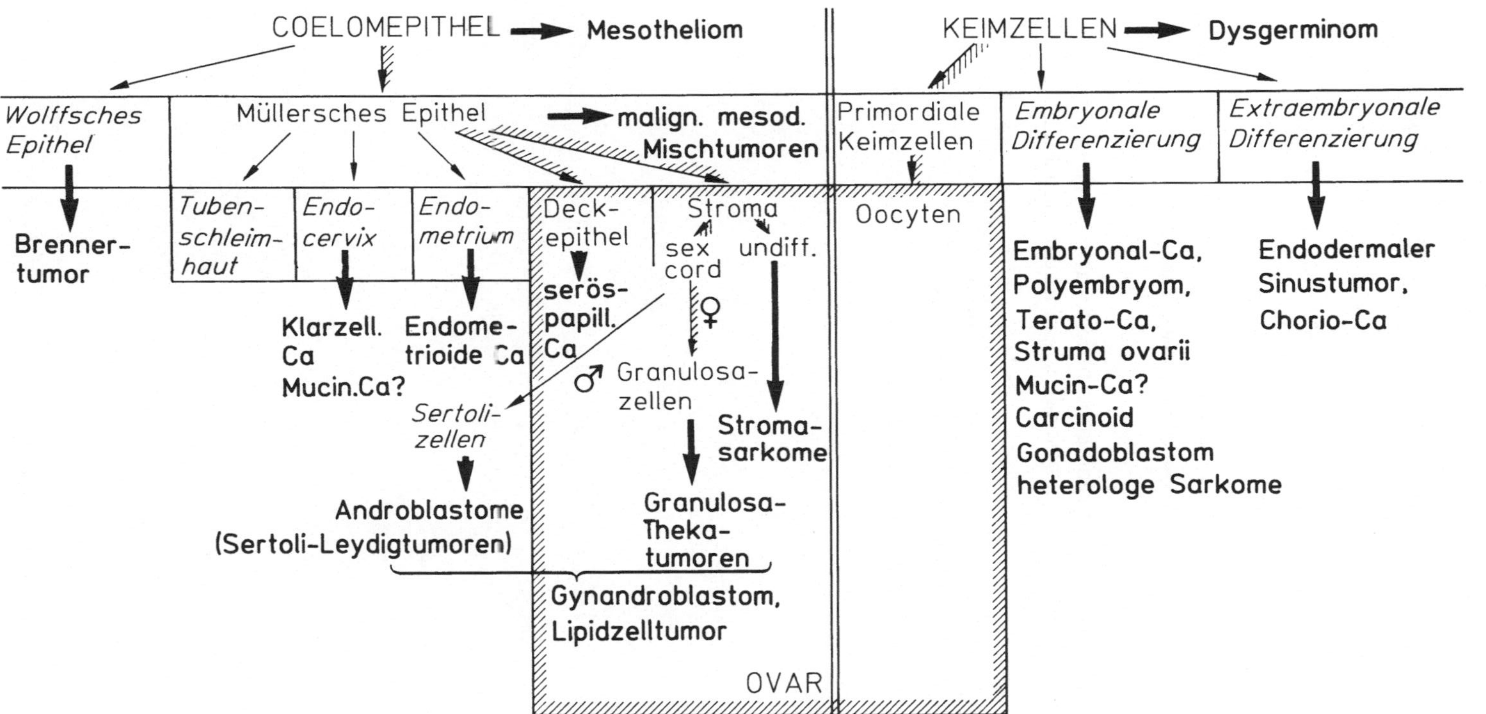

Tabelle 3. Histogenetische Ableitung der Ovarialtumoren von ihren physiologischen Ausgangszellen oder deren pluripotenten oder abwegigen Vorstufen

Histologische Diagnose	Geschätzte Überlebensraten			
	Zahl	Nach 6 Monaten [%]	Nach 2 Jahren [%]	Nach 5 Jahren [%]
Serös-papilläres Ca	110	80	35	21
Muzinöses Ca	40	92	62	41
Keimzell-Ca	19	94	65	41
Sexcord-Ca	23	86	54	41
Undifferenziertes Ca	20	60	21	10

Tabelle 4. Geschätzte Überlebensraten an diesem Kollektiv (vgl. Tabelle 2)

Wir erhoffen uns von diesem Symposion konzentrierte fachübergreifende Informationen, wobei ich zwei Fragestellungen besonders herausheben möchte:

1. Wie weit und mit welchen Kriterien läßt sich der Malignitätsgrad eines Tumors histologisch ohne Berücksichtigung des klinischen Stadiums erkennen?
2. Wie präzise läßt sich ein Borderline-Tumor diagnostizieren?

Welche Bedeutung haben bei diesen Fragen die modernen Untersuchungsmethoden?

Epidemiologie

Epidemiology of Ovarian Cancer

J. G. SCHENKER and S. M. JOSEPH[1]

Introduction

During the past decade there has been increased interest in the epidemiology of the different human cancers and the risk factors associated with them. Only limited epidemiologic data are available on ovarian cancer. Critical control studies are few, and the number of cases studied in most series are limited. Most data evaluate ovarian cancer as an entity rather than as individual ovarian tumors. This review will summarize current epidemiologic data on human ovarian cancer and on the high risk factors associated with it.

Incidence

Among the genital cancers ovarian cancer is the leading cause of death in almost every country in the world; even so, it ranks third in incidence after cancer of the cervix and corpus uteri. It is the most common genital cancer in Israel and the second commonest in Africa, as the data from Nigeria show (Fig. 1). Ovarian cancer is the third commonest cause of death in American females, following cancer of the breast and colon, and in Polish females, following cancer of the stomach and breast. It is the fourth commonest cause of death in Israeli women, following cancer of the breast, stomach, and lung, and in Japanese women, following cancer of the breast, stomach, and colon (Fig. 2).

Between 14 000 and 17 000 new cases of ovarian cancer are diagnosed every year in the United States. In the western hemisphere 1% of women over the age of 40 will develop ovarian cancer and 4% over the age of 70 will die from this malignancy.

In the western world including Israel, the incidence and mortality rate of ovarian cancer have remained relatively stable during the last decade. In the United States the mortality rates increase from 6.4 in 1930, through 6.9 in 1949, to 7.6 in 1969. In Israel the rate has been between 7.3 and 7.6 during the last 15 years. An increase in the death rate from ovarian cancer is taking place in Japan and in the underdeveloped countries. It seems that the increase in ovarian cancer observed in the western world during the previous decades and at present in the developing countries is probably due to improved diagnostic facilities and increased life expectancy.

1 Department of Obstetrics and Gynecology, Hebrew University-Hadassah Medical Center, Jerusalem, Israel

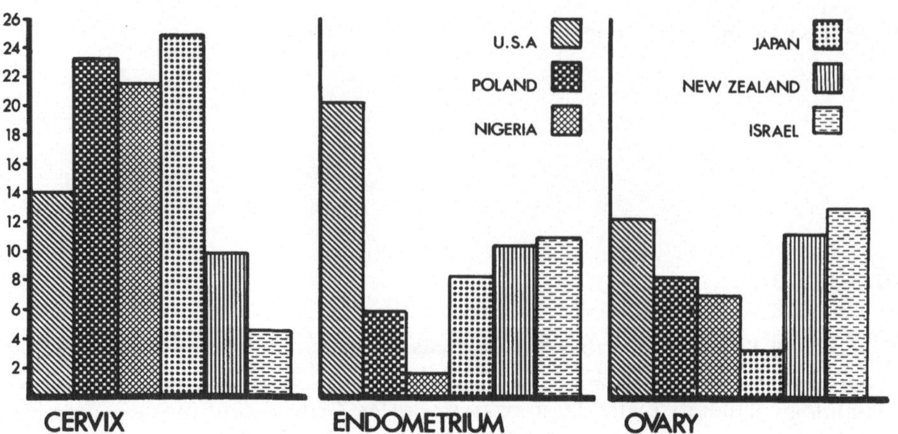

Fig. 1. Incidence of genital cancer per 100 000 women in representative countries in five continents

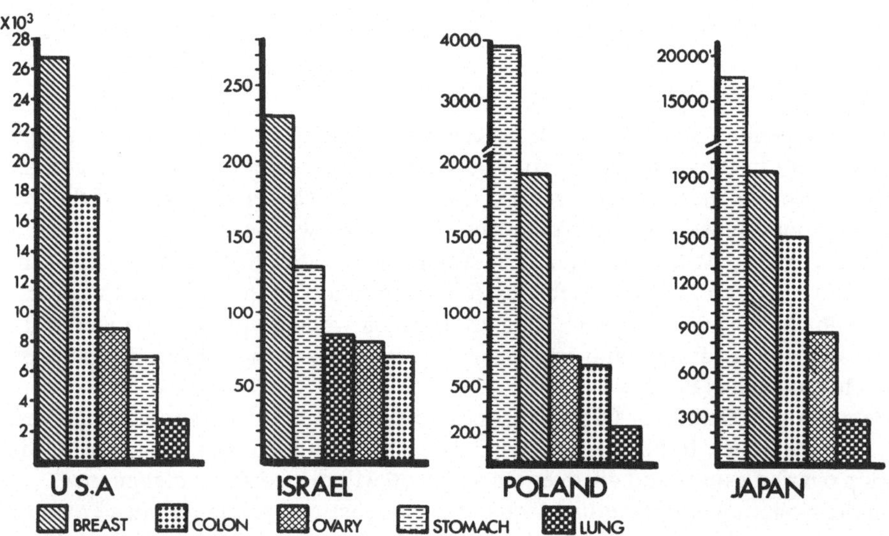

Fig. 2. Number of deaths per year in women from cancer of the ovary, breast, colon, stomach, and lung in representative countries [26]

There are wide international variations in the ovarian cancer incidence rates [22]. The highest rates are observed in Scandinavian countries and North America. Medium rates are reported from central and eastern Europe. The rates in southern Europe, South America, and Africa are relatively low. Very low incidence is observed in Asia (Fig. 3), particularly in Japan. The accuracy of cancer registration and the availability of diagnostic facilities may differ from one country to another, and this could account for some of the differences reported. However, the differences found between the various states of the United States and between Japan and western European countries, where the registration and accuracy of diagnostic facilities are probably equal, indicates a need for research into caustive factors in the environment.

High incidence rates of ovarian cancer are very similar among the developing nations according to the data from countries in five continents, e.g., Denmark, Canada, the United States, and Israel, whereas there are low rates in the developing countries, e.g., India, Nigeria, and Cuba (Fig. 4). Even in the United States higher

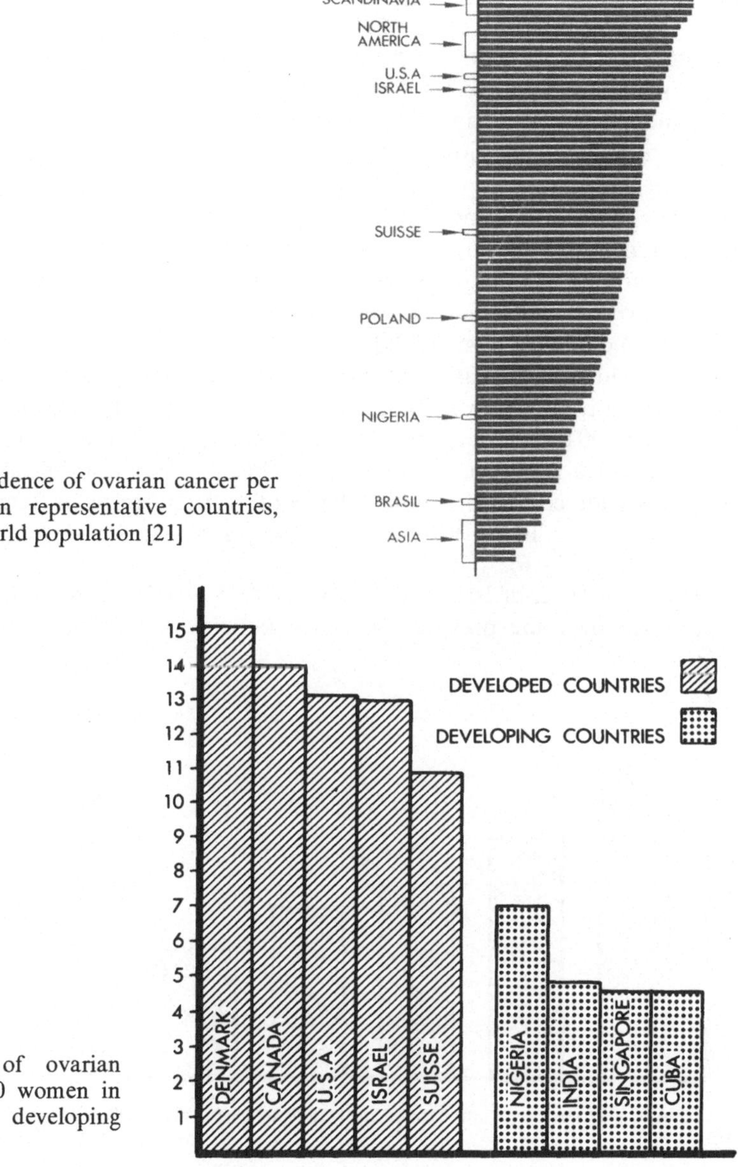

Fig. 3. Yearly incidence of ovarian cancer per 100 000 women in representative countries, standardized to world population [21]

Fig. 4. Incidence of ovarian cancer per 100 000 women in developed and developing countries

incidence rates were observed in the industrialized states on the eastern and western coasts than in the nonindustrialized states in the southern and central parts of the country [13]. It has been suggested that physical and chemical industrial pollution may be a factor contributory to the development of ovarian cancer. An exception to the general rule is highly industrialized Japan, where rates for ovarian cancers have been among the lowest recorded in the world. A control study performed in Great Britain on women working in heavy industry did not reveal that pollution might be a causative factor for the development of ovarian neoplasm [16].

Ethnic Groups

The incidence of ovarian cancer in the heterogeneous ethnic groups of the United States population studied by Weiss and Peterson [23] revealed that Japanese, Chinese, Indian, Hispanic, and black women had rates of epithelial tumors that were 19%–42% lower than those of the white women (Fig. 5). Some differences were found in the relationship of histologic components of the epithelial cancer to the race. The less common nonepithelial tumors, such as dysgerminomas, theratomas, and granulosa cell carcinomas, showed no consistent pattern and rates for each of the four groups were close to those of Whites. A United States National Council Survey revealed that black women developed epithelial ovarian tumors less commonly than did white women [24].

The incidence of malignant ovarian tumors among the white population in South Africa is almost twice that among the black population, the figures being 6.5 and 3.4 per 100 000 respectively. The incidence of ovarian cancer among the Indians in South Africa is higher than among the black population but lower than among the white. Data comparing the incidence of ovarian cancer in Blacks in the United States and in the Bantu tribe of South Africa revealed a higher incidence in the United States (Fig. 6).

The population of Israel at the end of 1978 was 3.7 million, having more than quadrupled over the previous 30 years. Official population statistics and conse-

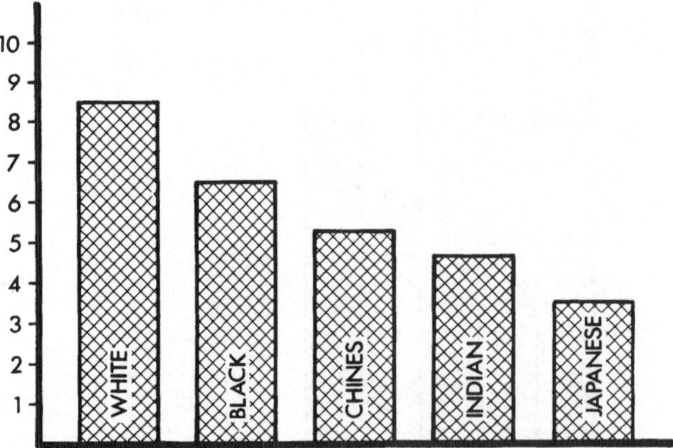

Fig. 5. Age-adjusted ovarian cancer mortality rates per 100 000 women in the United States (1950–1969)

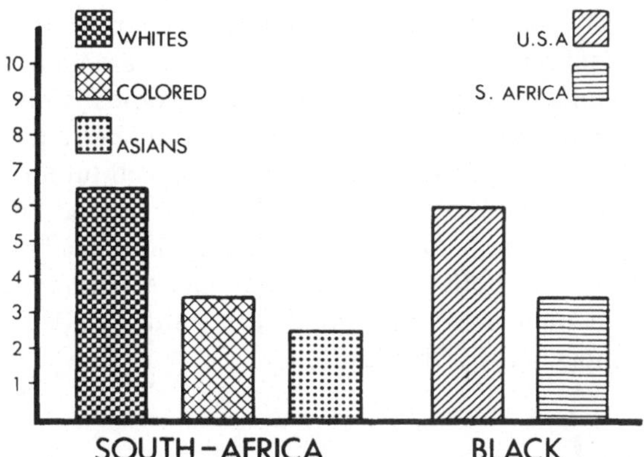

Fig. 6. Ovarian cancer mortality rates per 100 000 women (white, black, and Asian) in South Africa, and per 100 000 black women in the United States and Africa

quently also epidemiologic research divide the residents of Israel into two main groups, Jews and non-Jews, the latter being mainly Arabs of Moslem and Christian religion. The Jewish population of Israel has increased mainly by immigration from 100 different countries and therefore consists of multi-ethnic groups with diverse social and cultural backgrounds.

The Jewish population is officially subdivided by continent of birth and by country of birth. Immigrants' descendants born in Israel are uniformly described as Israeli-born. Thus, the younger age groups have a very large proportion of Israeli-born individuals, whereas in the older age-groups the immigrants are predominant. Women of European-American origin in Israel have a three times higher incidence of carcinoma of the ovary than women of Asian-African origin [20].

In New York City the Jewish population is about 2.5 million. In several studies it is reported that cancer of the ovary among the Jewish women is more common than among other religious groups. The average annual death rates for cancer of the ovary per 100 000 women aged 45 or more was 33 for Jews compared with 25 for Catholics and 28 for Protestants [17].

Several studies show that mortality from ovarian cancer has risen among immigrants from Japan to the United States and their descendants, the rates for the United States Japanese being higher than for the native Japanese but lower than for either the white or nonwhite population of the United States. Japanese immigrants provide data which suggests that environmental factors may affect the development of ovarian cancer.

Age

Ovarian cancer occurs at all ages, including infancy and childhood. There appears, however, to be a critical period near age 40 when the rate increases damatically. Data collected by Doll et al. [4] for 24 countries show that the mean age is 52. The morbidity rate in most increases until age 70, when it declines.

The data from Israel show that one-third of all the cases were in the age-group 55–64, and 75% of the patients were between 45 and 74 years [18].

The major histologic types of ovarian neoplasm occur in distinctive age ranges. Neoplasm of germ cells, mainly teratomas, dysgerminomas, etc., occurs predominantly in children and young women, while the epithelial tumors are rare before menarche but increase significantly in frequency thereafter.

The age distribution of granulosa cell tumors in our series of 170 cases in Israel shows the highest incidence between 50 and 60 years (Fig. 7). The rate of malignancies among ovarian tumors in various age groups was studied by Fatalia [5]. The number of both benign and malignant tumors rises with age. A steep increase in benign tumors is observed in the third decade and a steep increase in malignant tumors in the fifth decade.

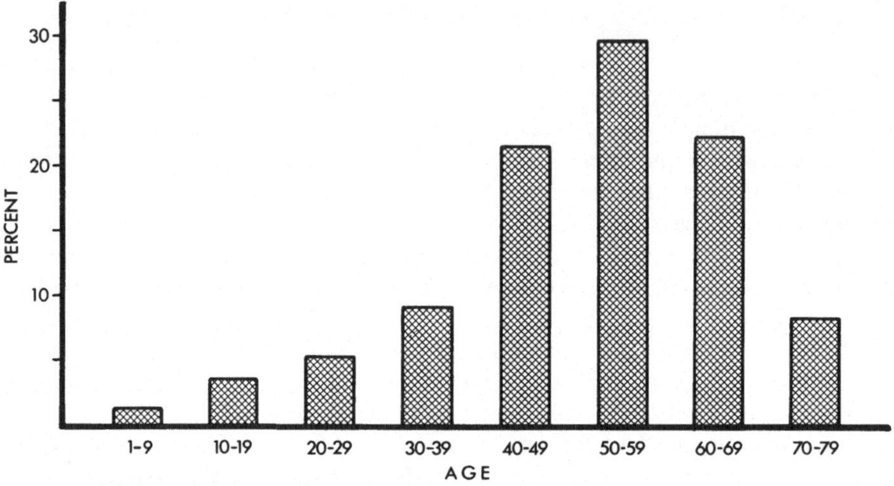

Fig. 7. Age distribution of ovarian granulosa tumors in Israel (170 cases)

A study of cases of ovarian cancer from 59 hospitals in the United States revealed that the death rates for the youngest age-range, 0–19 years, had not changed during recent decades [7]. Ovarian cancer morbidity was low in the first decade of life, but gradually rose with age. It was greatest among young Blacks, compared with a higher incidence in adult Whites. As was mentioned previously, most tumors in the young were of germ cell type, in contrast to a predominance of epithelial tumors in the elderly. Gonadal dysgenesis was the only congenital defect associated with ovarian cancer at this age.

Age of the patient is not a factor affecting the prognosis of ovarian malignancy.

Genetic and Familial Factors

Numerous studies have shown that the role of possible genetic factors in human cancer susceptibility is important. Many papers have described families in which multiple cases of cancer have occurred, including ovarian cancer. Lynch [11] reviewed 110 patients with ovarian cancer and found that 40% had a history of cancer in other members of the family. Albert and Child [1] showed more cancer cases than expected among relatives of ovarian cancer patients, predominantly cancer of the breast, uterus, and gastrointestinal tract.

Twenty-seven familial aggregates of epithelial ovarian cancer have been reported, including 92 patients affected with the disease [10]. Fraumeni et al. [6] presented six families with multiple cases of ovarian cancer, mainly serous cystadenocarcinoma.

The following factors were characteristic for the familial ovarian cancer patients: (a) ovarian tumors do not appear to differ clinically or histologically from sporadically arising tumors; (b) in most cases the age of onset of the ovarian cancer was earlier than in the nonfamilial cases, the averages being 44.7 and 53 years respectively; (c) the prognosis is less favorable; and (d) in many instances the pattern of familial occurrence suggests autosomal dominance inheritance.

Familial aggregates of mesothelial ovarian tumors have also been reported. Hereditary syndromes have been associated with an increased incidence of ovarian neoplasm. Ovarian fibromas are almost a constant feature of the basal cell nevus syndrome. Granulosa cell tumors are frequently associated with Peutz-Jeghers syndrome, which is characterized by intestinal polyposis, intraoral melamin spots, and familial incidence. Both syndromes appear to be inherited as autosomal dominants. Several studies have shown that the number of ovarian cancer patients in blood group A was higher than expected.

It is suggested that in families where aggregation of ovarian cancer exists, prophylactic oophorectomy is indicated in asymptomatic relatives, mainly after childbearing is completed. This prophylactic approach is desirable until adequate screening tests or tumor markers that detect premalignant or very early malignant ovarian lesions become available.

Information has been available concerning the familial association between cancer of the ovary and breast. Two such families were reported by Lynch et al. [12]. Women with cancer of the breast have twice the expected risk of subsequently developing a primary cancer of the ovary. Women with cancer of the ovary are three to four times as likely to develop a breast cancer as those without primary cancer.

Marital Status

Most studies show that ovarian cancer is more common in unmarried females during their reproductive and menopausal years. Age-adjusted rates of death from ovarian cancer for Whites and Blacks in the cities of the United States were higher for single than for married women, according to the Third National Cancer Survey [24]. The incidence rate of epithelial ovarian tumor was approximately 50% greater in single women than in married women. Nonepithelial tumor occurrence shows no correlation with marital status. Among the Israeli women the percentage of single women in the ovarian cancer group appears no higher than that for the general population [18]. Similar data were reported by Wynder on a group of 150 patients admitted to the Memorial Hospital in New York [27].

Menstrual History

Gynecological details studied include the menstrual history. The findings are as follows: (a) it was shown that patients with ovarian cancer tend to have an early menarche; (b) the ovarian cancer patients had significantly heavier bleeding, but the length of the menstrual cycle was similar to that of the controls; and (c) some data showed that the ovarian cancer patients had an early menopause. Women with ovarian cancer reported a history of marked irritability, general malaise, and dysmenorrhea significantly more often than did the controls.

Reproductive History

Epidemiologic studies showed that reproductive experience was to some extent related to cancer of the ovary. Women with ovarian cancer had the following characteristics:

1. A large proportion of them had never married.
2. A large proportion of them had never become pregnant.
3. There was larger proportion of married women who had never conceived than of unmarried women who had conceived.
4. There was a low mean number of pregnancies. The risk of ovarian neoplasm was greatly reduced among those who had had at least one pregnancy.
5. A large proportion had infertility problems.
6. A greater interval between marriage and the first conception.
7. First conception at an older age.
8. Controversial data concerning the frequency of conception, termination with ovarian cancer.

These characteristics would seem to indicate either that women who developed ovarian cancer had a gonadal status that also predisposed to low fertility, or that repeated pregnancies exert a protective influence against the development of ovarian cancer in susceptible women.

Socioeconomic Status

Several studies have been carried out on the occurrence of ovarian cancer at different socioeconomic levels. The data for Great Britain have shown a positive correlation between social class and mortality from ovarian cancer. In the United States the evidence was inconclusive. Among the Israeli women the highest incidence of ovarian neoplasm is found among the Jews of Ashkenazi origin, an ethnic group living of higher socioeconomic levels and enjoying better education. In considering socioeconomic status as a risk factor for the development of ovarian cancer, one should take into consideration that this cancer is probably more frequently diagnosed in the higher social classes, to whom better medical care is available.

There is no evidence of a higher incidence of obesity, hypertension, diabetes, thyroid disease, or heavy smoking in patients with ovarian cancer.

Viral Infection

Several human neoplastic diseases are currently believed to be a consequence of persistent viral infections. Case control studies of ovarian cancer patients have so far failed to reveal an association with any viral disease.

A lower frequency of clinical history of mumps has been found in patients suffering from ovarian cancer [25]. It was suggested that mumps in childhood may have a protective influence. A serologic study by Menczer et al. [15] in Israel indicates that ovarian cancer patients had a higher rate of subclinical disease and tended to present persistently lower mumps antibody titers. They interpreted their results as showing that an immunologic incompetence makes possible the development of ovarian cancer through a direct etiological role of mumps virus.

Women with ovarian neoplasm reported having had rubella between the ages of 12 and 18 more frequently than did the controls. Subjects who had had rubella between the ages of 12 and 18 were 3.9 times more likely to develop ovarian cancer than women who were infected during their early childhood years [14]. In countries where rubella vaccination is carried out in girls aged 11–14, the association between rubella viremia in the peripubertal years and the increase of ovarian cancer should be taken into consideration.

Estrogens

Exogenous female hormones can alter the risk of neoplasm development in any genital organ, for instance exposure of the uterus to diethylstibestrol (DES) can cause clear cell adenocarcinoma. There is strong evidence that exogenous estrogens given around the time of menopause have caused an increase in the risk of endometrial cancer, and the prolonged use of oral contraceptives may also be a cause of this neoplasm. Most retrospective studies have failed to show a higher proportion of ovarian cancer among women using estrogens. Only two studies, both based on a small number of cases, revealed a higher rate of ovarian cancer than expected, in patients treated with conjugated estrogens and DES [8]; it was suggested that this estrogen preparation might be particularly carcinogenic for ovaries. However, there may be a risk of development of rare histologic types such as clear cell carcinoma and endometrioid carcinoma. These types have increased in frequency during the last decade, and this may be associated with the rise in consumption of exogenous estrogens at menopause.

Chemical and Physical Carcinogens

Cancer of the ovary has not been among the neoplasms reported in women with occupational exposure to products containing anthracenes and related compounds that have resulted in cancer of the skin and other organs. Only asbestos and talc have been considered a positive cause of cancer of the human ovary. Women who have been exposed to asbestos have indicated a rate of ovarian cancer slightly higher than that expected, in addition to cancer of the lung and mesothelioma of the peritoneum and pleura [3]. It has been suggested that particles might gain access from the vaginal pool through the patent genital tract to the pelvic peritoneum. However, neoplasms of the ovaries were not observed in animal studies when other cancers, such as lung cancer and mesothelioma, were induced with asbestos. Microscopic studies failed to find asbestos particles in tissue from ovarian tumors but talc particles have been observed. Talc by itself has never been proved to be carcinogenic in animal studies.

Irradiation

X-ray radiation can induce neoplasm in the ovaries of rodents, mainly of the granuloma cell type, but the evidence so far indicates that this is unlikely in the human ovary. Association between ovarian neoplasm and exposure to x-ray radiation for induction of ovulation and for treatment of benign conditions is a controversial subject. Ovarian neoplasms have not developed in human populations exposed to levels of radiation sufficient to cause malignancies in other organs. Postirradiation sarcoma and adenocarcinoma of the uterine corpus have been reported in a significant number of patients thus exposed. Present epidemiologic data do not support a relationship between irradiation and the development of ovarian cancer.

Our data and those of others show that there is no predisposition for either the right or the left ovary to develop primary ovarian cancer; there is therefore no advantage in removing one ovary as a preventive routine in cases of laparatomy for benign conditions in late reproductive age.

Histologic Types

The classification of ovarian tumor is complicated because of various elements in the ovary which can give rise to many kinds of tumors. In 1973, WHO committee of experts published a histologic typology of ovarian tumors. However, the clinical behavior of the various histologic types indicates that ovarian cancer is not an entity but a group of diseases.

The incidence of epithelial and nonepithelial tumors differs in the various parts of the world. The relative frequency of different histologic types of tumor differs from one study to another. The most frequent tumor in all the studies is serous cyst adenocarcinoma, which accounts for approximately 35%–39%. The least common type of tumor is the anaplastic one. In Fig. 8 the distribution of histologic types is compared in three series: (a) a collaborative study by 57 institutions in various countries [9], (b) the National Cancer Survey of the United States [23], and (c) data from Israel for the years 1960–1976 [19].

1. Each category in the epithelial group shows the same general distribution regardless of age. Germ cell tumors were found predominantly in the lowest age group, while for sex cord mesenchymal neoplasm the age distribution was similar to that for epithelial tumors.

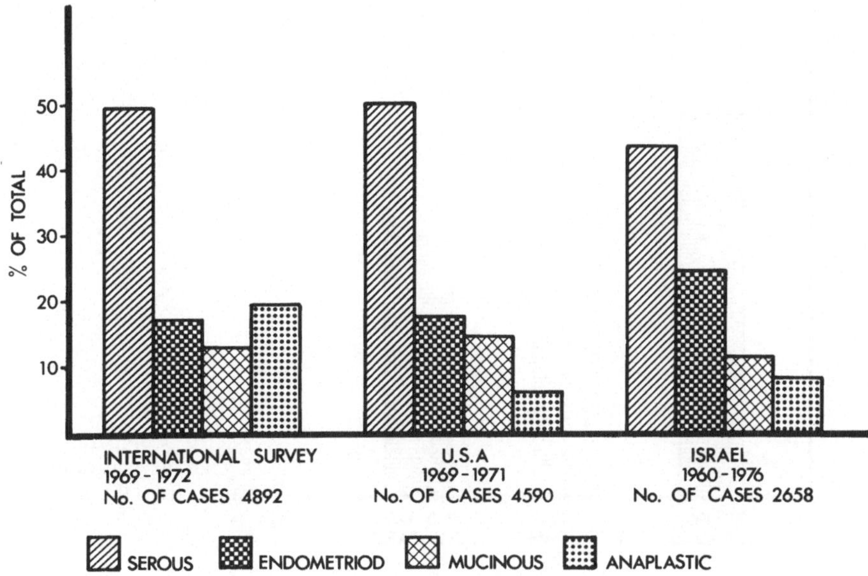

Fig. 8. Distribution of histologic types of ovarian cancer in three series

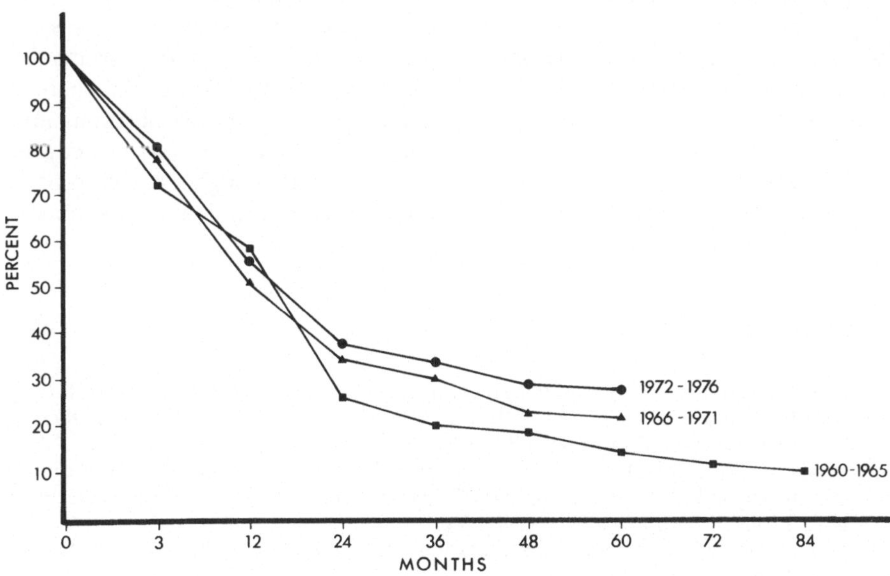

Fig. 9. Five-year survival rate of 2658 patients with ovarian cancer in Israel at three different periods

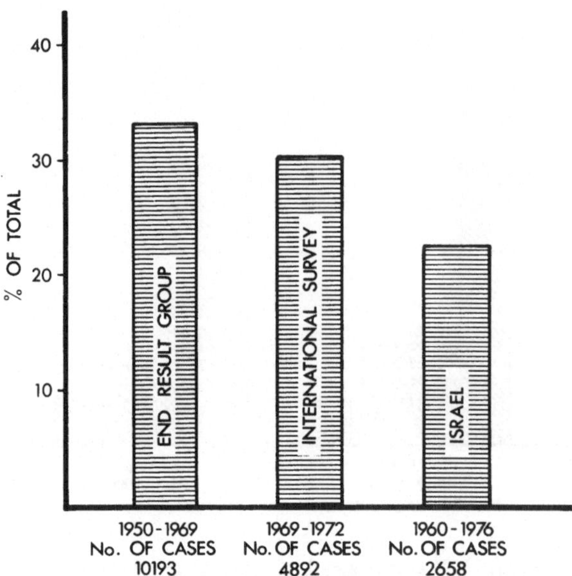

Fig. 10. Comparative data for 5-year survival rate of ovarian cancer from three series

2. The incidence of epithelial tumors was higher in the married women.
3. In the United States and Africa epithelial tumors were more common in white females than in black, while the nonepithelial tumors were more common among Blacks. In Israel there was no difference in the distribution of the histologic types among the various ethnic groups.

Overall survival rates for patients with ovarian cancer are rather low: 5-year survival rates have remained at a level of 24%–35% [5, 9, 19] over the past 20 years (Figs. 9 and 10). Of all types of ovarian carcinoma, the best prognosis was for the mucinous type, followed by the serous type, while the poorest prognosis in all three series was for undifferentiated cancer. The incidence of low potential malignancy is about 10% of all ovarian tumors, mainly in stage 1. Future investigations into the epidemiology of ovarian cancer are essential if its incidence is to be reduced by prophylactic measures. Advancement of our knowledge of high risk factors associated with ovarian neoplasm, especially with the different histologic types, may result in its more frequent early diagnosis.

References

1. Albert S, Child M (1977) Familial cancer in general population. Cancer 40:1674
2. Axtell L, Cutler S, Myers M (1972) End results in cancer. Report No. 4, Bethesda. Department of Health, Education and Welfare
3. Berg J, Baylor S (1973) The epidemiology pathology of ovarian cancer. Hum Pathol 4:537
4. Doll R, Payne P, Waterhouse J (1966) Cancer incidence in five continents. A technical report. Springer, Berlin Heidelberg New York
5. Fathalla M (1972) Factors in the causation and incidence of ovarian cancer. Obstet Gynecol Surv 27:751
6. Fraumeni J, Graundy G, Creagen E, Everson R (1975) Six families prone to ovarian cancer. Cancer 36:364

7. Fredrich P, Fraumeni J, Dalager N (1973) Ovarian cancer in the young, epidemiologic observation. Cancer 32:969
8. Hoover R, Gray S, Fraumeni J (1977) Stilbestrol and the risk of ovarian cancer. Lancet 2/8037:533
9. Kottmeir HL (1980) Annual report on results of treatment in carcinoma of uterus, vagina, and ovary. Annu Rep 17
10. Lurain J, Piver M (1979) Familial ovarian cancer. Gynecol Oncol 8:185
11. Lynch F (1976) A clinical review of 110 cases of ovarian carcinoma. Am J Obstet Gynecol 32:753
12. Lynch H (1974) Familial association of carcinoma of the breast and ovary. Surg Gynecol Obstet 138:717
13. Mason T, McKay F, Hoover R, Blot W, Fraumeni J. Atlas of cancer mortality among U.S. non whites 1950–1969. p 103
14. McGowan L, Parent L, Lendar W, Norris H (1979) The women at risk for developing ovarian cancer. Gynecol Oncol 7:325
15. Menczer J, Modan M, Ranon L, Golan A (1979) Possible role of mumps virus in the ethiology of ovarian cancer. Cancer 43:1375
16. Newhouse M, Pearson F, Fullerton J et al. (1977) A case control study of cancer of the ovary. Br J Prev Soc Med 31:148
17. Newill C (1961) Distribution of cancer mortality among ethnic subgroups of the white population of New York City. J Natl Cancer Inst 26:405
18. Schenker J, Mazzor M (1978) Cancer of the ovary in Israel. Gynecol Oncol 6:397
19. Schenker J, Mor Yosef S (in preparation) Genital Cancer in Israel
20. Schenker J, Polishuk W, Steinitz R (1968) An epidemiologic study of carcinoma of the ovary in Israel. Isr J Med Sci 4:820
21. Segi M (1977) Graphic presentation of cancer incidence by site and by area and population. (Completed from data published in "Cancer Incidence in Five Continents", vol III, pp 26)
22. Waterhouse J, Muir C, Correa P, Powell J (1976) Cancer incidence in five continents, vol 3. IRAC Scientific Publication No. 15, Lyon, France
23. Weiss N, Peterson A (1978) Racial variation in the incidence of ovarian cancer in the U.S. Am J Epidemiol 107:91
24. Weiss N, Homonchuk T, Young J (1977) Incidence of the histologic types of ovarian cancer. The U.S. Third National Cancer Survey 1969, 1971. Gynecol Oncol 5:161
25. West R (1966) Epidemiologic study of malignancies of the ovaries. Cancer 19:1001
26. WHO (1970) Mortality from malignant neoplasm 1955–1965
27. Wynder E, Dodo H, Barber H (1969) Epidemiology of cancer of the ovary. Cancer 23:352

Zur Epidemiologie der Ovarialtumoren

H.-J. Mohr und A. Sonntag [1]

Informationen über die Häufigkeit, die Häufigkeitsverteilung, die Altersverteilung sowie das Verhältnis zwischen gutartigen und bösartigen Ovarialtumoren finden sich in den Standardwerken und einschlägigen Lehrbüchern zumeist nur als unvollständige Einzelangaben und bemessen an kleineren Fallzahlen. Ausführliche Zusammenstellungen mit großen Fallzahlen hierüber bringt Miller (1937), der aus der Literatur ermittelte, daß die Rate der Ovarialtumoren zwischen 1877 und 1926 je nach Klinik sich zwischen 1,4 und 10,7% bewegte und damit einem Durchschnittssatz von 6,04% entsprach. Zur Frage des Anteils der bösartigen Geschwülste stellte Miller 16 025 Fälle von Ovarialtumoren aus dem Schrifttum, beobachtet zwischen 1880 und 1929 zusammen, von denen 2281 bösartige Geschwülste waren. Demnach betrug der Anteil der bösartigen Tumoren unter den Ovarialtumoren im Mittel 14,23%. Zur Häufigkeit des Auftretens von Ovarialtumoren, bezogen auf alle Ovarialtumoren, berichteten Knörr et al. (1972) und stellten fest, daß 20–25% seröse Zystadenome, 10–18% muzinöse Zystadenome, 15% Dermoidzysten, 1–3% Struma ovarii, 1,7% Brenner-Tumoren, 1–5% Ovarialfibrome, 1–3% Granulosazelltumoren, 1–2% Thekazelltumoren und etwa 15% primäre Ovarialkarzinome seien.

Wir gingen nun in eigenen Untersuchungen den Fragen nach, welcher Anteil im gesamten Einsendungsgut an Ovarialtumoren enthalten ist, wie groß die Raten der einzelnen gutartigen und bösartigen Geschwülste des Ovars unter den ovariektomierten Eierstöcken sind, wie deren Altersverteilung ist, ob sich Differenzen zu den Ergebnissen von Miller und Knörr et al. ergeben und Unterschiede bestehen zwischen dem Einsendungsgut von Patienten aus industriellen Ballungsgebieten und Patienten aus mehr ländlich strukturierten Gebieten.

Eigene Untersuchungen

Material und Methode

Grundlage der Studie ist das Einsendungsgut der Jahre 1969–1979. Das Untersuchungsgut wurde an Paraffinschnitten in den einschlägigen Färbungen (HE, PAS, v. Gieson, Sudan III) je nach Sachlage begutachtet, ab 1974 nach der WHO-Klassifikation „Histological Typing of Ovarian Tumours" klassifiziert und die Diagnosen

1 Pathologisches und Gewebepathologisches Institut Gelsenkirchen, D-4650 Gelsenkirchen

nach einem institutseigenen Schlüssel verschlüsselt sowie auf Magnetband gespeichert. Die Tumoren der Jahrgänge 1969–1973 wurden nach der WHO-Klassifikation nachklassifiziert. Im genannten Zeitraum wurden insgesamt 10 352 Fälle von Ovarialtumoren im weiteren Sinne untersucht und erfaßt. Dem Begriff „Ovarialtumor" in dieser Studie liegt der klinische Befund und die Operationsindikation zugrunde, unabhängig davon, ob sich der Tumor dann histologisch als Retention auf dem Boden der Funktionsstrukturen, als Endometriose oder aber als echtes Gewächs erwies.

Ergebnisse

Von den uns zugegangenen 10 352 Fällen waren 9845 (95,10%) gutartige Veränderungen und Geschwülste, und 507 (4,90%) bösartige Ovarialtumoren. Von den 9845 gutartigen Veränderungen und Geschwülsten erwiesen sich 6693 (64,65%) als Zysten auf dem Boden der Funktionsstrukturen und 3152 (30,44%) als echte gutartige Geschwülste. Somit enthält das eigene Untersuchungsgut an echten Geschwülsten des Ovars 3659 Fälle (35,34%) aller als „Ovarialtumoren" entnommenen Ovarien.

Auf diesen Gesamtanteil echter Ovarialgeschwülste entfallen 507 bösartige Tumoren, so daß von den echten Geschwulstfällen 86,15% mit einem gutartigen und 13,85% mit einem bösartigen Tumor behaftet waren.

Untersuchen wir nun zunächst das Kollektiv, bei dem ein „Ovarialtumor" klinisch vorlag, die histologische Untersuchung aber keine echte Geschwulst, sondern nur eine zystische Veränderung der Funktionsstrukturen des Ovars, eine Endometriose oder Parovarialzysten ergab, so ergibt sich folgendes Bild:

1582 Fälle wiesen Corpus-luteum-Zysten (23,63%), 3050 Follikelzysten (45,56%), 511 Parovarialzysten (7,63%) und 1555 zystische Endometriosen (23,23%) auf. Die Altersverteilung zeigt, daß diese Veränderungen von der Mitte des ersten Dezenniums bis in das hohe Alter in jeder Altersstufe vorkommen können, wobei alle diese Veränderungen im 4. Lebensjahrzehnt ihren Gipfel aufweisen und zwischen dem 2. und 5. Jahrzehnt in auffälliger Häufung in Erscheinung treten.

Bei den echten gutartigen Geschwülsten zeigt sich folgende Situation:

An der Spitze steht das seröse Ovarialzystom; hier hatten wir in unserem Untersuchungsgut 1429 Fälle (45,33% der gutartigen, 39,05% aller echten Geschwülste und 13,80% aller operierten „Ovarialtumoren"). Sie gliedern sich in 1058 solitäre und 371 multilokuläre seröse Zystome. Das Cystoma mucinosum war mit 203 solitären und 191 multilokulären und somit insgesamt mit 394 Fällen (12,50%) der gutartigen Geschwülste im Untersuchungsgut enthalten. Bezogen auf die echten Geschwülste insgesamt stellen sie einen Anteil von 10,76% und auf das Gesamtmaterial einen Anteil von 3,08% dar.

Die Ovarialfibrome und -adenofibrome machen insgesamt 353 Fälle aus. Dies bedeutet auf die gutartigen Geschwülste bezogen einen Anteil von 11,19%, auf die Zahl der echten Geschwülste einen Anteil von 9,64% und im Gesamtmaterial einen Anteil von 3,40%. Von den 353 Fällen erwiesen sich histologisch 253 als reine Fibrome (71,76%) und 100 (28,32%) als Adenofibrome. Hierbei kommen die Ovarialfibrome bereits im ersten Dezennium vor und haben zwischen dem 40. und 60. Lebensjahr ihren Häufigkeitsgipfel. Demgegenüber zeigen die Adenofibrome vereinzeltes Vorkommen im ersten und zweiten Lebensjahrzehnt, treten dann mit steigender Tendenz zwischen dem 20. und 70. Lebensjahr in Erscheinung und weisen zwischen dem 30. und 60. Lebensjahr eine deutliche Häufung mit Gipfel zwischen 40 und 50 sowie etwas flacher zwischen 70 und 80 auf.

Wir haben 76 Brenner-Tumoren, 31 Granulosazelltumoren und 4 Thekazelltumoren beobachtet. Diese Fälle bedeuten Anteile an den gutartigen Tumoren von 2,4% für die Brenner-Tumoren, 0,98% für die Granulosazelltumoren und 0,12% für die Thekazelltumoren. An den echten Geschwülsten haben die Brenner-Tumoren einen Anteil von 2,01%, die Granulosazelltumoren von 0,84% und die Thekazelltumoren von 0,10%. Die Brenner-Tumoren kommen gehäuft zwischen dem 30. und 50. und zwischen dem 60. und 80. Lebensjahr jeweils mit Gipfeln im 5. und 8. Lebensjahrzehnt vor. Die Granulosa- und Thekazelltumoren häufen sich ohne wesentliche Gipfelbildung zwischen dem 3. und dem 7. Lebensjahrzehnt.

In diese Gruppe der gutartigen Geschwülste wären noch die Dermoidzysten und die Struma ovarii einzugliedern. Dermoidzysten fanden sich in unserem Untersuchungsgut 852, Strumata ovarii 26. Die Dermoidzysten machen 27,00% der gutartigen Tumoren, 23% aller echten Geschwülste und 8,23% des Gesamtmaterials aus. Sie kommen vom 1. bis zum 9. Lebensjahrzehnt vor, werden aber zwischen dem 20. und 50. Lebensjahr gehäuft mit einem Gipfel zwischen dem 25. und 35. Lebensjahr beobachtet.

Die Struma ovarii kommt praktisch in allen Lebensaltern vor. Sie zeigt kleine Häufigkeitsgipfel im 2., 5. und 7. Lebensjahrzehnt. Die 26 Fälle bedeuten 0,82% der gutartigen Tumoren, 0,71% aller echten Geschwülste und 0,25% des gesamten Beobachtungsgutes.

Die primären Ovarialkarzinome stellen mit 465 Fällen 4,49% des gesamten Materials und 91,71% aller malignen Tumoren dar. Bezogen auf alle echten Ovarialgeschwülste bilden sie einen Anteil von 12,70%.

Die Karzinome gliedern sich in 249 seröse Zystadenokarzinome, 89 muzinöse Zystadenokarzinome, 51 endometrioide Karzinome und 76 wenig bzw. undifferenzierte, nicht weiter klassifizierbare Karzinome. Bezogen auf die Gesamtzahl der Karzinome hat das Carcinoma serosum einen Anteil von 53,54%, das Carcinoma mucinosum einen solchen von 19,13%, das endometrioide Karzinom macht 10,96% und die undifferenzierten, nicht klassifizierbaren Karzinome machen 16,34% aus. Unter allen bösartigen Tumoren bilden die serösen Karzinome eine Rate von 49,11%, die muzinösen Karzinome von 17,55%, die endometrioiden Karzinome von 10,05% und die undifferenzierten Karzinome von 14,99%. Bezieht man auf alle echten Ovarialgeschwülste, dann bilden die serösen Karzinome einen Anteil von 6,80%, die muzinösen Karzinome von 2,43%, die endometrioiden Karzinome von 1,39% und die nicht klassifizierbaren undifferenzierten Karzinome von 2.07%.

Von den Karzinomen sind besonders die Lebensalter zwischen 35 und 85 betroffen. Die Häufigkeitsgipfel liegen um das 55. Lebensjahr bei allen 4 Karzinomgruppen. Das seröse Karzinom beginnt in der Mitte des 2. Jahrzehnts in Erscheinung zu treten und nimmt zwischen dem 35. und 55. Lebensjahr stark zu. Zwischen dem 50. und dem 70. Lebensjahr treten gut 30% aller serösen Karzinome auf. Das muzinöse Karzinom und die undifferenzierten Karzinome weisen fast ähnliche Altersverhalten auf. Ein abweichendes Verhalten zeigt das endometrioide Karzinom. Es tritt bereits zwischen dem 30. und 40. Lebensjahr auf, erreicht bei 45 mit gut 30% der Fälle fast die Gipfelhöhe, nimmt bis zum 55. Lebensjahr um 2% zu, um dann ziemlich gradlinig bis zum 85. Lebensjahr auf einen Fallanteil von 2% zurückzugehen. Demgegenüber zeigen die sekundären Ovarialkarzinome 3 auffällige Altersgipfel und Häufungen im 4., 6. und 8. Lebensjahrzehnt.

Maligne Granulosazelltumoren wurden 16 (3,15% der bösartigen Tumoren und 0,43% aller echten Ovarialgeschwülste) beobachtet. Maligne Thekazelltumoren kamen 2, maligne Teratome 3, Dysgerminome 4 und mesonephrogene Tumoren 8 vor. Das macht für die malignen Thekazelltumoren 0,4%, die malignen Teratome 0,6%, die Dysgerminome 0,78% und für die mesonephrogenen Tumoren 1,57% der malignen Ovarialgeschwülste aus. Die Altersverteilung dieser Gruppe zeigt, daß die Dysgerminome nur vom 1. bis zur Mitte des 5. Lebensjahrzehntes auftreten, die malignen Granulosazelltumoren und die malignen Teratome erst im 4. bzw. 5. Lebensjahrzehnt aufzutreten beginnen und in der Mitte des 6. Lebensjahrzehnts ihre Häufigkeitsgipfel mit 50 und 67% der Fälle erreichen. Während die malignen Teratome nach der Mitte des 8. Lebensjahrzehnts nicht mehr zu beobachten waren, reicht das Vorkommen der malignen Granulosazelltumoren bis in das 9. Lebensjahrzehnt hinein. Die mesonephroiden Tumoren treten vom 3. bis zum 9. Lebensjahrzehnt auf und zeigen Häufigkeitsgipfel im 4. und 8. Lebensjahrzehnt mit jeweils 25% der Fälle.

Diskussion

Wir gingen von der Frage aus, welcher Anteil an echten Ovarialgeschwülsten – gutartig und bösartig – im gesamten Einsendungsgut der unter der Indikation „Ovarialtumor“ ektomierten Ovarien enthalten ist. Dazu ergibt sich aus unserem Untersuchungsgut, daß in den 10 352 Fällen der Jahre 1969 bis 1979 507 (4,89%) bösartige Ovarialgeschwülste und 3152 (30,44%) gutartige Ovarialtumoren enthalten gewesen sind, d.h. sich ein Gesamtanteil an echten Geschwülsten von 3659 Fällen (35,33%) ergibt. Die übrigen 64,67% der Fälle hatten zwar tumorartige gutartige Veränderungen, waren aber nicht von echten Geschwülsten im engeren Sinne betroffen.

Unter den 3659 (35,33%) echten Ovarialtumoren fanden sich folgende Geschwülste nach der Häufigkeit geordnet in folgenden Raten:

Seröse Ovarialzystome: 39,05%
Dermoidzysten: 23,00%
Muzinöse Ovarialzystome: 10,67%
Ovarialfibrome und Adenofibrome: 9,64%
Brenner-Tumoren: 2,01%
Granulosazelltumoren: 0,84%
Struma ovarii: 0,71%
Thekazelltumoren: 0,10%

Carcinoma serosum: 6,80%
Carcinoma mucinosum: 2,43%
Undifferenzierte Karzinome: 2,07%
Endometrioide Karzinome: 1,39%
Maligne Granulosazelltumoren: 0,43%

Maligne mesonephrogene Tumoren: 0,21%
Dysgerminome: 0,10%
Maligne Teratome: 0,08%
Maligne Thekazelltumoren: 0,05%

Es erhebt sich nun die Frage, ob zwischen den Zusammenstellungen von Miller und unseren Daten Differenzen festzustellen sind. Miller stellte aus der Literatur 16 025 Fälle zusammen, die in den Jahren zwischen 1880 und 1929 beobachtet worden sind. Unter den 16 025 Fällen fanden sich 2281 bösartige Tumoren (14,23%), 13 744 Fälle (85,77%) hatten gutartige Tumoren. Im eigenen Material von 10 352 Fällen von 1969 bis 1979 sind unter 3659 Geschwulstfällen 507 bösartige Tumoren enthalten. Dies entspricht einer Rate an bösartigen Geschwülsten von 13,85%. Somit ergibt sich zwischen dem Untersuchungsgut von Miller und von uns eine Differenz von 0,38%. Daraus sollte bei aller Zurückhaltung und Vorbehalten gefolgert werden dürfen, daß eine wesentliche Veränderung der Rate der bösartigen Ovarialgeschwülste unter den Ovarialtumoren insgesamt nicht feststellbar und nicht eingetreten ist.

Auch zur Altersverteilung der Geschwülste decken sich unsere Ergebnisse mit den von Miller zusammengestellten Angaben.

Von den von Knörr et al. (1972) gemachten Häufigkeitsangaben weichen unsere Daten doch teilweise deutlich ab. Dies gilt besonders für das Cystadenoma serosum, für das Knörr 20–25% angibt, der Anteil dieses Tumors aber in unserem Material bei 39,05% liegt. Bei den muzinösen Zystadenomen decken sich die Daten. Demgegenüber machen in unserem Material die Dermoidzysten 23%, bei Knörr nur ca. 15% aus. Die Karzinomrate beträgt bei uns 12,69%, während sie Knörr mit ungefähr 15% angibt.

Abschließend haben wir noch die Frage geprüft, ob sich Unterschiede in der Karzinomrate und in der Altersverteilung zwischen städtischer Bevölkerung im Ballungsgebiet Ruhr und ländlicher Bevölkerung im Münster- und Sauerland feststellen lassen. Hier zeigen die Daten keine wesentlichen Differenzen im Hinblick auf die Altersverteilung. Unter den Karzinomen steht auch hier das Carcinoma serosum an der Spitze, gefolgt vom Carcinoma muzinosum und dem endometrioiden Karzinom. Bei der ländlichen Bevölkerung fällt auf, daß das undifferenzierte Karzinom weniger vorkommt als bei der Stadtbevölkerung. Ob diese Beobachtung Relevanz besitzt, bedarf der weiteren Untersuchung.

Zusammenfassung

Es wird über 10 352 Fälle von „Ovarialtumoren" aus den Jahren 1969 bis 1979 berichtet. In diesem Untersuchungsgut sind 507 bösartige Ovarialgeschwülste (4,89%), 3152 (30,44%) gutartige Ovarialgeschwülste und 6693 Fälle (64,65%) mit tumorartigen, aber nicht den echten Ovarialgeschwülsten zuzuordnenden Veränderungen enthalten gewesen. Die Tumorraten und die Altersverteilungen werden diskutiert. Der häufigste Ovarialtumor ist das seröse Zystadenom (39,05%), gefolgt von den Dermoidzysten (23%) und den muzinösen Zystadenomen (10,76%). Der Karzinom-anteil am Gesamtmaterial beträgt 12,69%, darunter 6,80% seröse Karzinome, 2,43% muzinöse Karzinome, 2,07% undifferenzierte Karzinome und 1,39% endometrioide Karzinome.

Literatur

1. Becker V (1974) Geschwülste des Ovarium. In: Doerr W (Hrsg) Organpathologie, Bd II. Thieme, Stuttgart, S 7–102–113
2. Czernobilsky B (1977) Primary epithelial tumors of the ovary. In: Blaustein A (ed) Pathology of the female genital tract. Springer, Berlin Heidelberg New York, S 453–504
3. Hughesdon PE, Symmers WS (1978) Gynaecological pathology of the ovaries. In: Systemic pathology, vol 4. Churchill Livingstone, Edinburgh London New York, pp 1600–1651
4. Janovski NA (1972) Histologie und Einteilung der Ovarialtumoren. In: Schwalm M, Döderlein G, Wulf K-H (Hrsg) Klinik der Frauenheilkunde und Geburtshilfe, Bd 8. Urban & Schwarzenberg, München Wien Baltimore, S 651–714
5. Knörr K, Beller FK, Lauritzen D (Hrsg) (1972) Die gutartigen und bösartigen Neubildungen des Ovars. Springer, Berlin Heidelberg New York (Lehrbuch der Gynäkologie, S 367–395)
6. Miller J (1937) Die Krankheiten des Eierstockes. In: Henke F, Lubarsch O (Hrsg) Weibliche Geschlechtsorgane. Springer, Berlin, (Handbuch der speziellen pathologischen Anatomie und Histologie, Bd VII/3, S 221–224, 302–303)
7. Novak ER, Woodrieff JD (1974) Novak's gynecologic and obstetric pathology. Saunders, Philadelphia London Toronto
8. Scully RE (1977) Sex cord-stromal tumors. In: Blaustein A (ed) Pathology of the femal genital tract. Springer, Berlin Heidelberg New York, pp 505–526
9. Serov SF, Scully RE, Sobin LH (1973) Histological typing of ovarian tumours. WHO, Genf
10. Talerman A (1977) Germ cell tumors of the ovary. In: Blaustein A (ed) Pathology of the femal genital tract. Springer, Berlin Heidelberg New York, pp 527–585
11. Teilum G (1976) Special tumors of ovary and testis. Munksgaard, Kopenhagen
12. Willis RA (1967) Pathology of tumors. Epithelial and related tumours of the ovary. Butterworth, London

Klinische Symptomatik

Klinische Diagnostik von Ovarialtumoren

W. GEIGER[1]

Etwa 90% der Zeit werden wir in diesen Tagen des Symposiums damit verbringen, etwas über die Vielfältigkeit der Histologie der Ovarialtumoren zu hören. Wie ein Filigranwerk mutet allein schon die Liste der Einteilung der Ovarialtumoren an. Der Histologe ist hier in seiner Arbeit mit einem Goldschmied zu vergleichen im Gegensatz zum Kliniker, der eher an der Stelle des Goldgräbers steht, welcher mehr vom Zufall, denn von gezielter Schürfarbeit abhängig darauf vertraut, gelegentlich fündig zu werden. Und die Methoden des Klinikers sind auch vergleichsweise grob. Im wesentlichen ist er darauf angewiesen, daß er bei der gynäkologischen Untersuchung eine Resistenz im Unterbauch feststellt, die sich durch Größe und Konsistenz deutlich von dem unterscheidet, was er normalerweise erwartet hätte. Noch 1979 resümierte Johnson auf einem Symposion über Diagnostik und Therapie des Ovarialkarzinoms, daß „auf dem Gebiet der Frühdiagnostik der Durchbruch generell noch nicht erfolgt und die Frühdiagnose des Ovarialkarzinoms schwierig und unbefriedigend sei".

Das Problem liegt nicht etwa in einer hohen Dunkelziffer des Ovarialkarzinoms, nein, die Diagnose wird fast immer schon ante mortem gestellt. Das Problem liegt darin, daß die Diagnose meist zu spät gestellt wird. Nach Popkin (1979) und Watring et al. (1979) weisen 60–70% der Patientinnen bei der Erkennung des Ovarialkarzinoms bereits das Stadium III–IV auf. Dementsprechend triste ist die Überlebenschance nach der Diagnose. Sie beträgt für alle Altersstufen zusammen 1,4 Jahre bei einem Todesaltermedian von 63,7 Jahren (Barber 1979). Wie vor 20 Jahren ist die 5-Jahres-Überlebensrate insgesamt nicht höher als 20–25% (Watring et al. 1979). Daß sie für das Stadium I bei 80% liegt, unterstreicht die Notwendigkeit, nach Methoden zur Frühdiagnose zu suchen.

Bis jetzt ist das Ovarialkarzinom deshalb so schwer zu fassen, weil wir

1. keine empfindliche Methode zur frühzeitigen Erfassung, also keine Screening-Methode haben,
2. das Ovarialkarzinom keine typischen Frühsymptome macht, und
3. keine eindeutige „Risikogruppe" für das Ovarialkarzinom zu erkennen ist.

Um gleich mit dem letzten Punkt zu beginnen, so läßt sich aus epidermiologischen Untersuchungen zwar ableiten, daß gewisse Umstände wie Zyklusstörungen im Sinne der Follikelpersistenz und der hypergonadotrope Zustand das Risiko erhöhen, andererseits die Einnahme von Ovulationshemmern und Multiparität, also

1 Universitäts-Frauenklinik Köln, D-5000 Köln

Zustände der ovariellen Ruhe, das Risiko vermindern; aber einen Typus wie die hypertone, übergewichtige, kinderlose Diabetikerin, die für das Endometriumkarzinom prädestiniert ist, gibt es für das Ovarialkarzinom nicht. Eine Besonderheit stellt allenfalls die Gonadendysgenesie mit XY-Genotyp dar, die eine hohe Inzidenz an Gonadoblastomen und schließlich an Dysgerminomen aufweist. Letztlich ist hier noch das seltene Peutz-Jeghers-Syndrom zu nennen, welches oft mit Ovarialtumoren vergesellschaftet ist.

Zur Frage der Frühsymptome verlautbarte kürzlich aus der American Cancer Society, daß chronische gastrointestinale Beschwerden, für die sich vordergründig keine Ursachen finden lassen, der klinischen Manifestation des Ovarialkarzinoms fast immer vorausgingen. Dieser Komplex sei aber den wenigsten Ärzten als ovarspezifisch bekannt. Auch Barber meint, daß schon die frühe Manifestation des Kar-

Tabelle 1. Die Symptomatik des Ovarialkarzinoms. ($n=570$) (Nach Engeler 1974)

	[%]
Erhöhte Senkung (> 10 mm)	92
Bauchschmerzen	86
Zunahme des Bauchumfanges	78
Gewichtsverlust	44
Miktionsstörungen	38
Appetitlosigkeit	27
Obstipation oder Diarrhö	24
Erbrechen, Übelkeit	21
Müdigkeit	18
Resistenz im Abdomen	16
Menometrorrhagie (0–6 Monate)	16
Gewichtszunahme	5
Keine Symptome	2

Tabelle 2. Symptoms in patients with ovarian cancer. (Nach Rutledge et al. 1976)

Symptom	Taylor's patients (%)	Schueller's patients (%)
Abdominal distension	43 (35.0)	185 (36.0)
Chronic low abdominal pain	29 (24.0)	160 (31.0)
Postmenopausal bleeding	15 (12.0)	41 (8.0)
Acute low abdominal pain	12 (10.0)	14 (3.0)
Metrorrhagia	5 (4.0)	42 (8.0)
Inguinal node enlargement	4 (3.0)	6 (1.0)
Menorrhagia	4 (3.0)	3 (0.6)
Weight loss	2 (2.0)	32 (6.0)
Menometrorrhagia	2 (2.0)	0
None	2 (2.0)	17 (3.0)
Rectal fullness	1 (1.0)	9 (2.0)
Rectal bleeding	1 (1.0)	2 (0.4)
Unknown	2 (2.0)	5 (1.0)
Total	122	516

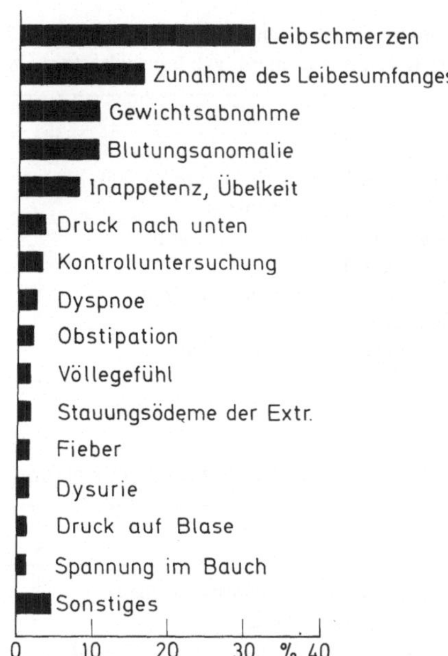

Abb. 1. Symptome, welche die Patientinnen bei Ovarialkarzinom zum Arzt geführt haben. (Nach Schultze et al.)

zinoms innerhalb des Ovars „unbestimmte Unterbauchbeschwerden wie Dyspepsie und Flatulenz" bedingte, die zwar nicht spezifisch seien, aber doch so häufig aufträten, daß Frauen mit diesen Symptomen schon zu einer Risikogruppe zu rechnen seien (Barber 1978, 1979).

Die Aufschlüsselung der Symptome von Patientinnen mit Ovarialkarzinom durch Engeler (1974) zeigt Tabelle 1. Auch hier steht die gastrointestinale Symptomatik mit Bauchschmerzen, Zunahme des Bauchumfanges, Appetitlosigkeit, Obstipation bzw. Diarrhoe und Übelkeit bis Erbrechen ganz im Vordergrund, jedoch betrifft diese Symptomatik vorwiegend fortgeschrittene Stadien. Rutledge verglich die Symptomatik bei Ovarialkarzinomen von zwei verschiedenen Zentren und fand überwiegend unspezifische abdominale Symptome, allerdings auch häufig genitale Blutungsstörungen (Tabelle 2). Dem Alter der Patientinnen entsprechend handelt es sich hierbei vorwiegend um postmenopausale Blutungen (Rutledge et al. 1976). Schulze befaßte sich mit den Symptomen, welche die Patientinnen mit Ovarialkarzinom zum Arzt geführt haben, und wiederum finden sich Leibschmerzen und Zunahme des Leibesumfanges, Gewichtsabnahme und Inappetenz an der Spitze (Abb. 1). Blutungsanomalien sind mit 15% hier relativ häufig.

Wir haben selbst ein Kollektiv von 373 Patientinnen, bei denen Ovarialtumoren histologisch befunden worden waren, daraufhin untersucht. Es handelt sich hier nicht um 373 Ovarialkarzinome, sondern um alle Arten von Ovarialtumoren. Die Tabelle 3 über die klinische Symptomatik zeigt, daß 38% der Frauen Schmerzen im Abdomen und 26% Zyklusstörungen aufwiesen. Die Fälle mit Blutungen nach der Menopause betrafen zur Hälfte Ovarialkarzinome, während die prämenopausalen Zyklusstörungen zu 60% mit „funktionellen Zysten" vergesellschaftet waren. Auffallend häufig fanden sich auch urologische Beschwerden wie Harninkontinenz und Pollakisurie, die sowohl durch mechanische Irritationen wie auch einfach altersbedingt als Folge eines Descensus uteri et vaginae zu erklären sind.

Tabelle 3. Klinische Symptomatik bei 373 Patientinnen der UFK Köln mit histologisch gesichertem Ovarialtumor

	[%]
Palpabler Tumor im Adnexbereich	85
Schmerzen im Abdomen	39
Zyklus-(Blutungs-)Störungen	26
Fluor genitalis	12
Zunahme des Bauchumfanges	6
Rückenschmerzen	5
Blutungen in der Postmenopause	3

Tabelle 4. Ovarialtumor als Zufallsbefund

	[%]
Verdacht auf Uterus myomatosus	22,3
Sterilitätsdiagnostik	8,8
Gynäkologische Vorsorgeuntersuchung	3,2
Andere Primärerkrankungen	3,2
Schwangerschaft	2,9

... Und es gibt doch ein Frühsymptom, allerdings nur für einen kleinen Teil der Ovarialtumoren! Die postmenopausale Blutung, die mit einem hohen Proliferationsgrad im Scheidenepithel vergesellschaftet ist, kann als Frühsymptom eines östrogenproduzierenden Tumors gelten. Der Östrogeneffekt kann sich schon zeigen, bevor der Tumor palpabel ist. So entgehen nach Labhart (1971) 60% der hormonproduzierenden autonomen Ovarialtumoren der Palpation. Zur weiteren Diagnostik ist dann unbedingt die Bestimmung des 17-β-Östradiols sowie der Gonadotropine FSH und LH geboten. Ist der Östradiolspiegel hoch und der FSH- und LH-Spiegel niedrig, so ist eine Laparoskopie und evtl. eine Ovarektomie gerechtfertigt. Ähnliches gilt für das Arrhenoblastom: Auffällige Virilisierungserscheinungen und hohe Testosteronspiegel im Blut sind zumindest Anlaß für eine weitere spezifische Diagnostik, die zwischen einem erworbenen AGS und einem testosteronproduzierenden Ovarialtumor zu differenzieren hat.

Bei weitem nicht alle unsere Patientinnen wiesen Symptome auf, die primär auf einen Ovarialtumor verdächtig waren. So bestand bei 22% zunächst ausschließlich der Verdacht auf Uterus myomatosus. 9% befanden sich in der Sterilitätsabklärung und 3,2% kamen zur gynäkologischen Vorsorgeuntersuchung ohne irgendwelche Beschwerden. Das weitaus wichtigste Mittel, das zur Diagnose führte, war die gynäkologische Untersuchung, also die bimanuelle Palpation (Tabelle 4).

Die Diagnostik steht und fällt also mit der Exaktheit und differentialdiagnostischen Überlegung bei der Befunderhebung.

Eine wesentliche Vorbedingung für eine exakte Palpation ist ein weiches Abdomen ohne „alimentäre Tumoren", also eine leere Harnblase und ein leeres Rektum bzw. Sigma. Mit anderen Worten, die Patientin muß gut abgeführt sein. Ich habe bei zweifelhaftem Befund wiederholt Patientinnen zwei Tage später wieder einbestellt und ihnen einen Abführtag auferlegt. Diese Maßnahme erspart oft die Narkoseuntersuchung.

Für die differentialdiagnostische Überlegung bei der Palpation ist der Funktionszustand des Ovars ganz wesentlich. Bei Frauen nach der Menopause sind atrophische Ovarien zu erwarten, die sich meist der Palpation entziehen. Schon eine für das geschlechtsreife Alter noch normale Größe von 2mal 2mal 4 cm ist hinreichend verdächtig, um eine weitere Abklärung zu veranlassen.

Barber (1978) spricht in diesem Zusammenhang von einem „postmenopausal palpabel ovary syndrome", das er als wertvolles diagnostisches Mittel bei der Früherkennung des Ovarialkarzinoms bezeichnet. Es bedeutet ganz einfach, daß das, was als normale Ovargröße bei der prämenopausalen Frau interpretiert werden könnte, für die postmenopausale Frau einen Ovarialtumor darstellt.

Barber plädiert gleichzeitig für eine großzügige chirurgische Diagnostik, da nur so die hohe Letalität gesenkt werden könne. Es ist unrealistisch zu warten, bis ein Tumor von 5 cm Durchmesser zu tasten ist, und dann noch eine Heilung zu erhoffen.

Ähnliches gilt für die Frau, die Ovulationshemmer einnimmt. Bei ihr ruhen die Ovarien zumindest, so daß es zu keiner Follikelausreifung kommt. Dies gilt nicht für die Minipille! Ganz im Gegenteil findet man hierunter laut einer finnischen Studie sogar gehäuft funktionelle Zysten als Ausdruck einer hormonellen Imbalance (Ylikorkala 1977).

Einen Tumor bis zu 2 cm Größe im geschlechtsreifen Alter der Frau zu erkennen, ist nahezu unmöglich, da auch ein sprungreifer Follikel diese Größe erreicht. Das häufigste Problem in dieser Altersphase ist dann auch die Differentialdiagnose zwischen einem Blastom und den sog. funktionellen Zysten. Wie häufig der Kliniker mit diesem Problem konfrontiert wird, zeigt schon die Verteilung der histologischen Diagnosen unseres Kollektivs aus den letzten 2 Jahren (Tabelle 5).

Tabelle 5. Histologische Diagnosen bei 373 konsekutiv erfaßten Fällen mit Ovarialtumor an der UFK Köln

	[%]
Einfache Ovarialzysten	17,7
Endometriosezysten	16,9
Luteinzysten	15,5
Ovarialkarzinome	11,0
Teratome (Dermoidzysten)	10,5
Zystome (benigne)	9,1
Kortikalisfibrose (PCO-Syndrom)	4,0
Fibrome	3,7
Keimepithelzysten (sonstige)	2,7
Parovarialzysten	2,7
Tuboovarialabszesse	1,9
Thekomatose und Fibrothekom	1,6
Hydatiden	0,8
Fibroleiomyome	0,5
Sonstiges	0,9

Die sog. funktionellen Zysten, nämlich Follikelzysten oder einfache Ovarialzysten, Luteinzysten und Endometriumzysten machen schon 50% der Tumoren in dieser Tabelle aus, wobei natürlich alle diejenigen nicht aufgeführt sind, die nur klinisch beobachtet und nicht einer histologischen Diagnostik zugeführt worden sind.

Ob eine funktionelle Zyste schließlich operiert wird oder nicht, hängt von der Größe und Konstanz des Befundes ab. Zysten von 4–5 cm Durchmesser, die nach Ovulationshemmereinnahme über 3 Wochen nicht kleiner oder wenigstens schlaffer werden oder nach zweimonatiger Ovulationshemmereinnahme noch vorhanden sind, werden operativ entfernt, da sie dann offenbar schon die funktionelle Abhängigkeit verloren haben und klinisch nicht von Blastomen mit autonomem Wachstum zu unterscheiden sind.

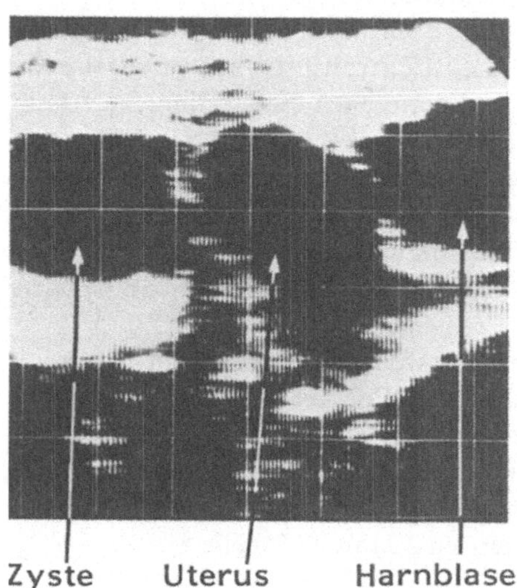

Abb. 2. Echographische Darstellung einer Ovarialzyste, des Uterus und der Harnblase (nach Stein 1977)

Ein ziemlich sicherer Hinweis auf eine Follikelzyste ist das Bestehenbleiben von spinnbarem Zervixschleim über eine Woche und länger. Die Größenänderung der Zyste kann natürlich nur immer vom gleichen Untersucher festgestellt werden, zur Objektivierung des Befundes bietet sich die Echographie an.

In der Echographie oder Ultraschalldiagnostik steht uns eine Methode zur Verfügung, deren Vorteile die Unschädlichkeit, die problemlose Anwendung ohne Belästigung der Patientin und die schnelle Verfügbarkeit des Ergebnisses sind. Die Domäne der Echographie ist die Darstellung von Grenzflächen zwischen Weichteilorganen und von Strukturen innerhalb von Organen, also insbesondere von Tumoren, die mit Röntgenkontrastmitteln nicht darstellbar sind. Mit dieser Methode lassen sich im Rahmen der Tumordiagnostik Lokalisationen, Größe, Form, Beziehung zur Umgebung, Oberflächenbeschaffenheit, Beweglichkeit, Verformbarkeit und evtl. noch Konsistenz beschreiben. Die Abb. 2 zeigt als Beispiel zwei zystische Tumoren, nämlich Harnblase und Ovarialzyste im Vergleich zu einem soliden Tumor, nämlich dem Uterus. Mehr als viele Worte zeigt dieses Bild die Möglichkeiten, aber auch die Grenzen dieser Methode.

Nach Lawson u. Albarelli (1977) und Ferrucci (1979) besitzt die Echographie eine Treffsicherheit von 82 bzw. 91%, wenn es um die Feststellung der Größe, Lokalisation und Konsistenz von gynäkologischen Tumoren geht. Kratochwil et al. (1978) berichten über eine zu 86% richtige Vorhersage der Tumorart. Kabayashi (1976) analysierte die echographischen Ergebnisse zweier medizinischer Zentren in New York, die über Lokalisation, Größe und Tumorart Aussagen machten, und fand 30% bzw. 25% falsche Vorhersagen bei insgesamt 406 Ovarialtumoren (Tabelle 6). Schlensker (Schlensker u. Beckers 1980) verglich die klinische und echographische Vorhersage mit dem tatsächlichen Operationsbefund bei Adnextumoren (Tabelle 7). Die echographische Vorhersage war dabei zu 80% richtig, zu 16% teilweise richtig und zu 4% falsch. Verglichen mit der klinischen Diagnose ergibt sich dabei eine

Tabelle 6. Echographische Vorhersage der Tumorart bei 406 Ovarialtumoren. (Nach Kabayashi 1976)

Suny DMC		Chiba Univ.	
No.	"mistaken"	No.	"mistaken"
223	66 (30%)	183	46 (25%)

Tabelle 7. Vergleich der echographischen und klinischen Treffsicherheit bei der Diagnostik von Adnextumoren. (Nach Schlensker 1980)

	Richtig	Teilweise	Falsch
US	80%	16%	4%
Klinisch	73%	21%	6%

geringe Überlegenheit der Echographie. Einschränkend ist aber zu bemerken, daß der Echograph sich grundsätzlich schon auf die Verdachtsdiagnose des Klinikers stützen kann und daß die Methode erst bei einer Tumorgröße von etwa 4 cm verläßliche Ergebnisse liefert (Karlson u. Persson 1979). So wurde in unserem Kollektiv von 373 Ovarialtumoren die Echographie nur in 141 Fällen, also bei knapp 40% der Fälle eingesetzt, weil in 60% offenbar keine Verbesserung der Diagnose erwartet wurde. Es besteht kein Zweifel daran, daß die Ultraschalluntersuchung dazu beiträgt, die klinische Diagnose aufgrund der Palpation zu verbessern und zu bestätigen. Sie ist aber kein Ersatz für die Laparotomie oder Biopsie bei einem verdächtigen Tumor, sondern muß stets als Ergänzungsmethode zur Differenzierung und Sicherung einer klinischen Diagnose gesehen werden. Sie trägt bei zu einer etwas früheren Diagnosestellung, ist aber sicher keine Früherkennungsmethode bei Ovarialtumoren.

In unmittelbarer Konkurrenz zur Echographie tritt in letzter Zeit die Computertomographie. Mit ihr ist es möglich, überlagerungsfrei Querschnittsbilder mit hoher Kontrastauflösung darzustellen. Durch Organmarkierungen und Kontrastmittelgabe läßt sich die Organdifferenzierung und Orientierung noch erhöhen, gleichzeitig stellen diese Maßnahmen aber auch eine erhebliche Belästigung, wenn nicht sogar Gefährdung der Patientin dar, so daß ihre Anwendung nur bei sicherer Indikation, also bei nachgewiesenen Vorteilen der Methode gegenüber anderen Methoden gerechtfertigt ist.

Gerade hier ist vielleicht die Bemerkung erlaubt, daß oft zu viel Machbares gemacht wird, ohne nach dem eindeutigen Nutzen für den Patienten zu fragen. Insbesondere bei jungen Frauen und bei Verdacht auf funktionelle Zysten scheint mir die damit verbundene Strahlenbelastung nicht gerechtfertigt. Anders sieht es aus, wenn die Ausdehnung eines gesicherten Ovarialkarzinoms oder der Lymphknotenbefall

Tabelle 8. Treffsicherheit des Tumornachweises durch Computertomographie (CT) und Echographie (US). (Nach Walsh et al. 1978)

	n	positiv	Falsch negativ	Falsch positiv
CT	24	15	3	0
US	24	17	3	0

nachgewiesen werden soll. Es soll nicht verschwiegen werden, daß schon die Unterscheidung zwischen einem Uterus myomatosus und einem soliden Ovarialtumor nicht immer ohne weiteres möglich ist, da Strukturen gleicher Dichte nicht voneinander unterschieden werden können. Hier ist die Computertomographie eindeutig der Echographie unterlegen. Walsh et al. (1978) verglichen die beiden Methoden bei 24 Patientinnen mit Tumoren im kleinen Becken (Tabelle 8). Sie fanden die Treffsicherheit beider Methoden etwa gleich. Von den 6 Ovarialtumoren in diesem Kollektiv wurden mit der Computertomographie nur 2, mit der Echographie 4 erkannt. In unserem Kollektiv wurde die Computertomographie 17mal angewendet, davon bei 8 Ovarialkarzinomen, von denen 6 erkannt wurden. Welchen Stellenwert die Computertomographie gegenüber der Echographie letztlich einnehmen wird, kann noch nicht abschließend beantwortet werden (Steinbrich u. Friedmann 1981).

Eine weitere radiologische Methode, die Lymphangiographie, ist sehr aufwendig und für die Patientin strapaziös. Nach Watring et al. (1979) beträgt der diagnostische Irrtum durch die Interpretation allein schon 27% für die positive und 20% für die negative Befundung. Der Nachweis von Lymphknotenmetastasen wäre für die Frühfälle zwar sehr wesentlich, denn immerhin fanden Knapp u. Friedmann (1974) im Stadium I schon in 19% einen positiven Lymphknotenbefall, bei der gegebenen Unsicherheit der Diagnostik ist das Verfahren aber nicht vorbehaltlos zu empfehlen. Für spätere Stadien ist der Nachweis positiver Lymphknoten nicht sehr relevant. Musumici et al. (1977) fanden auffallenderweise auch im Stadium IV nur bei 53% der Patientinnen einen Befall der Lymphknoten. Sie konnten jedoch eine unterschiedliche Metastasierungsrate je nach histologischem Bild zeigen. So metastasierten die undifferenzierten Ovarialkarzinome durchschnittlich zu 50%, die mesonephroiden Karzinome dagegen nur zu 14%.

Die für das Kollumkarzinom so segensreiche Methode zur Zytologie hat für die Früherfassung des Ovarialkarzinoms keine Bedeutung. Da Karzinomzellen erst ab dem Stadium Ic intraperitoneal nachzuweisen sind, kann auch eine Douglas-Punktion evtl. auch mit Douglas-Spülung, wie sie Käser empfiehlt (Käser et al. 1973), die Frühfälle nicht erfassen. Große Untersuchungsserien von Graham et al. (1967), McGowan et al. (1966) und Funkhouser et al. (1975) haben dies bestätigt. Vielmehr ist die Zytologie geeignet, die Ausbreitung des Tumors festzustellen, z. B. die makroskopisch noch nicht sichtbare intraperitoneale Aussaat oder die Dignität eines Pleuraergusses. Für die Feinnadelbiopsie ergeben sich nach Soost (1980) folgende Indikationen:

1. Rezidivverdacht nach schon behandeltem Karzinom,
2. schlechter, eine Laparotomie verbietender, Allgemeinzustand,
3. Differentialdiagnose von autonomen und funktionellen Zysten.

Als Zugangsweg für die Entnahme von zytologischen, aber auch histologischen Proben bietet sich heute die Laparoskopie an.

Diese Methode ist auf einem technischen Stand, der ihre Anwendung nur noch in Ausnahmefällen verbietet. Wegen des großen Informationsgewinnes wird ihr großzügiger Einsatz heute fast allgemein befürwortet (Frangenheim et al. 1975; Popkin 1979).

Sichere Indikationen für die Laparoskopie sind:

1. Existenz und Differentialdiagnose eines persistierenden Unterbauchtumors,
2. Klassifizierung eines Karzinoms,
3. Feststellung des Therapieerfolges bzw. Feststellung eines Rezidivs.

Bei der Anwendung der Laparoskopie geht es nicht so sehr darum, eine endgültige Diagnose zu stellen oder auf jeden Fall Material zur histologischen Untersuchung zu beschaffen, nein, es soll nur die Art eines Tumors im Abdomen festgestellt werden, um über ja oder nein zur Laparotomie entscheiden zu können. Aus diesem Grund soll die Laparoskopie zur Tumorabklärung immer in Laparotomiebereitschaft stattfinden. Wir bereiten die Patientin grundsätzlich auf eine Operation vor, sagen aber, daß wir vorher mittels Bauchspiegelung noch nachsehen, ob die Operation auch unbedingt nötig ist. Auf diese Weise konnten wir sicher vielen Patientinnen eine Laparotomie ersparen, ohne auch nur eine einzige Laparatomie durch die Laparoskopie zu verhindern. Es ist auch eine irrige Meinung, daß die Laparoskopie nur ein Ersatz für die Laparotomie ist, was die Inspektion betrifft. Nur mit der Lupenbrille wäre z. B. die Inspektion der Ovarien der Sicht durch das Laparoskop vergleichbar. Trotzdem haben wir in unserem gesamten histologischen Kollektiv die Laparoskopie nur 130mal, d. h. in 35% der Fälle zur Diagnostik eingesetzt, bei den Ovarialkarzinomen sogar nur in 25%, weil die Notwendigkeit zur Laparotomie eben vorher schon feststand. Andererseits zeigt die Aufschlüsselung der Konsequenzen, die aus der Laparoskopie gezogen wurden, daß die Laparotomie nur in einem Drittel der Fälle erforderlich war, in einem weiteren Drittel mußte überhaupt keine nachfolgende Diagnostik oder Therapie mehr durchgeführt werden und in 17% wurde eine Zystenpunktion oder Probeexzision laparoskopisch gemacht. Über die Laparotomie selbst ist nicht mehr zu sagen, als daß sie immer dann erfolgen muß, wenn die bisherige Diagnostik ein Blastom nicht sicher ausgeschlossen hat.

Zuletzt will ich mich noch einem vielversprechenden, wenn nicht sogar einem erfreulichen Kapitel zuwenden. Es ist das Kapitel der Tumormarker und Tumorimmunologie.

Seit der ersten Mitteilung von Gold u. Friedmann (1965) über ein karzinoembryonales Antigen, welches sowohl im Kollumkarzinom als auch im embryonalen Verdauungstrakt nachzuweisen war, hat sich die Anzahl der tumorassoziierten Antigene erheblich vermehrt. Es handelt sich vorwiegend um Proteine, die in der frühen Embryonalzeit von den noch omnipotenten Zellen normalerweise gebildet werden, und so verwundert es nicht, daß sich hierunter so bekannte Namen wie humanes Choriongonadotropin (HCG), AFP, fetales Hämoglobin, β_2-Makroglobulin und Enzyme wie Ribonuclease, Lactatdehydrogenase und andere befinden. Diese Substanzen sind zwar alle nicht streng tumorspezifisch, ihr positiver Nachweis oder eindeutig über der Norm liegende Serumspiegel liefern aber immerhin Hinweise auf das Vorliegen eines Karzinoms. Durch den gleichzeitigen Nachweis mehrerer dieser Antigene kann die Trefferquote deutlich erhöht werden, wie dies Sarjadi et al. (1980) z.B. für die 5 Antigene β_2-Makrogolobuline CEA, HBF, LDH und Immunkomplex zeigen konnten (Tabelle 9). Bei einer Entdeckungswahrscheinlichkeit von 21% für das einzelne Antigen errechnete er eine solche von 79% für alle 5 Antigene. Die Unspezifität und die geringe Empfindlichkeit der Tests limitieren jedoch ihren Wert. Ausnahmen sind vielleicht die HCG-produzierenden embryonalen Tumoren und die entodermalen Sinustumoren, welche in etwa 50% erhöhte α-Foetoproteinspiegel im Serum aufweisen (Neville 1980).

Das zukunftsträchtigste Gebiet der Tumordiagnostik liegt aber sicher im Bereich der Immunologie. Die bereits vorliegenden Ergebnisse sind vielversprechend (Ueda et al. 1977).

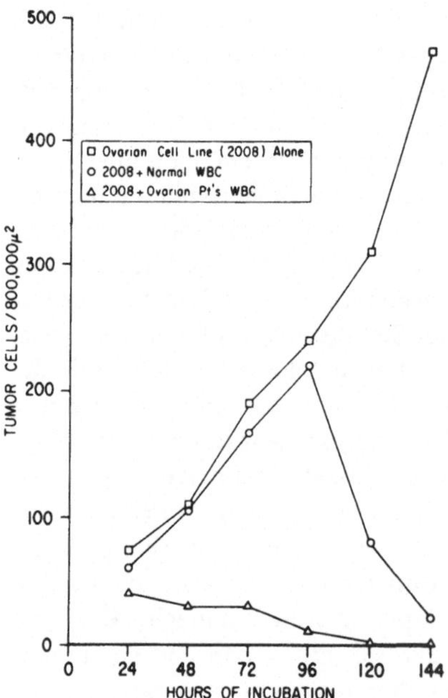

Abb. 3. Mit Lymphozyten co-kultivierte Adenokarzinomzellinie einer Patientin mit serös-papillärem Ovarialkarzinom im Stadium III im Vergleich zu Lymphozyten einer gesunden Frau

Tabelle 9. Multiparametric Tumor Marker Assessment Ovarian Cancer. (Nach Sarjadi et al. 1980)

β_2M	CEA	HbF	LDH	ImCp
21%	21%	21%	47%	26%
39%		68%		
	39%		63%	
	79%			
		79%		

Di Saia (1975) demonstrierte eindrucksvoll das Verhalten von verschiedenen Leukozyten gegenüber einer Tumorzellkultur (Abb. 3).

Der Durchbruch ist aber von der Isolierung weitgehend tumorspezifischer Antigene zu erwarten, wie sie auch von Di Saia (1975) schon demonstriert wurden (Abb. 4). Es ist auch schon gelungen, spezifische Antikörper gegen diese Antigene zu erzeugen, das Problem liegt momentan darin, die Antigene im Serum von Ovarialkarzinomträgerinnen nachzuweisen. Ein Team des Department of Pathophysiology of the Wuhan-College (1978) konnte zwar in 63 Serumproben von Ovarialkarzinompatientinnen 42mal (66%) den Nachweis eines Tumorantigens führen, wegen der mangelnden Spezifität empfahl aber auch diese Gruppe weniger die routinemäßige Anwendung, als die Intensivierung der Forschung auf diesem Gebiet. So will ich denn ganz hoffnungsvoll mit einem Zitat von Barber schließen, welches lautet: „Die Möglichkeit für eine serologische Diagnose des Ovarialkarzinoms ist ermuti-

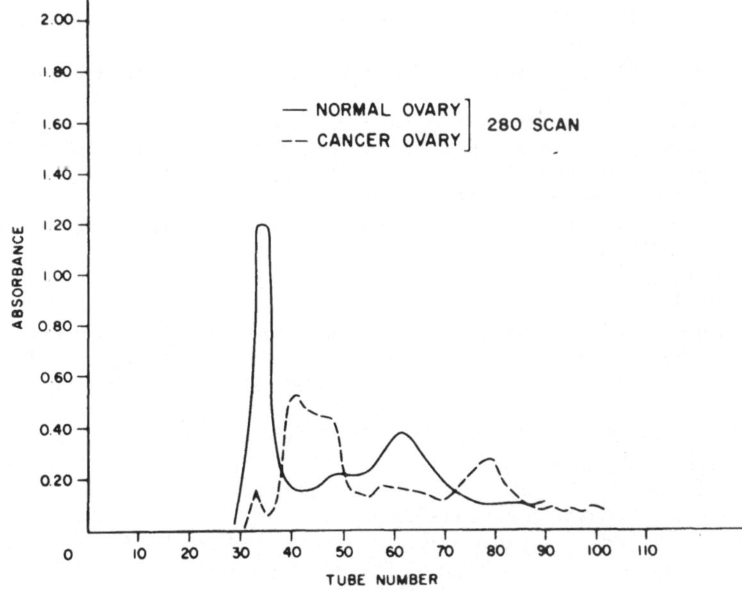

Abb. 4. Proteinprofil eines Adenokarzinoms des Ovars im Vergleich zu einem ähnlichen Profil eines normalen Ovars

gend. Diese neuen Fortschritte lassen hoffen, daß sich der langgesuchte Bluttest zur Diagnose des Ovarialkarzinoms auf dem Weg der Realisierung befindet."

Bis zu dieser Realisierung aber bleibt als wichtigste Maßnahme nur die Empfehlung an alle Frauen, die gynäkologische Vorsorgeuntersuchung regelmäßig in Anspruch zu nehmen und nicht zu vergessen, vorher einen Abführtag einzulegen.

Literatur

Barber HRK (1978) Ovarian carcinoma-etiology, diagnosis and treatment, Masson, New York

Barber HRK (1979) Ovarian cancer, Part I. CA 29:341–351

Barber HRK, Joachim HL, Dorsett BH (1975) Common antigenic component in ovarian carcinomas. In: De Watteville H (ed) Diagnosis and treatment of ovarian neoplastic alterations. Amsterdam, pp 107–121

Department of Pathophysiology of the Wuhan Medical College (1978) Possibility of immundiagnosis in ovarian cancer. Gynecol Obstet Invest 9:98–108

Di Saia PJ (1975) Antigen-ovarian-cancer. In: De Watteville H (ed) Diagnosis and treatment of ovarian neoplastic alterations. Excerpta Medica, Amsterdam, pp 99–106

Engeler V (1974) Ovarialkarzinom. Fortschr Geburtshilfe Gynaekol 53:1–116

Ferrucci JT (1979) Body ultrasonography, N Engl J Med 300:590

Frangenheim H, Hauber KP, Kleindienst W (1975) Range and limits of laparoscopic diagnosis of ovarian disease and functional ovarian disturbances. In: De Watteville H (ed) Diagnosis and treatment of ovarian neoplastic alterations. Excerpta Medica, Amsterdam, p 89

Funkhouser JW, Hunter KK, Thompson NJ (1975) The diagnostic value of cul-de-sac aspiration in the detection of ovarian carcinoma. Acta Cytol (Baltimore) 19:538–541

Gold P, Friedmann SO (1965) J Exp Med 121:467

Graham JB, Graham RM, Schueller EF (1964) Preclinical detection of ovarian cancer. Cancer 17:1414–1432

Kabayashi M (1976) Use of diagnostik ultrasound in throphoblastic neoplasma and ovarian tumors. Cancer Suppl 38:441–452

Käser O, Ilkle FA, Hirsch HA (1973) Atlas der gynäkologischen Operationen. Thieme, Stuttgart, S 54–55

Karlsson S, Persson PH (1979) Angiography, ultrasound and fine-needle aspiration biopsie in the evaluation of gynecologic tumors. Acta Radiol [Diagn] (Stockh) 20:779–788

Knapp RC, Friedmann EA (1974) Aortic lymph node metastases in early ovarian cancer. Am J Obstet Gynecol 119:1013

Kratochwil A, Altmann G, Wollmann G (1978) Ultraschalldiagnostik von Adnextumoren. Wien Klin Wochenschr 90:569–575

Labhart A (1971) Klinik der inneren Sekretion, 2. Aufl. Springer, Berlin Heidelberg New York

Lawson TL, Albarelli JN (1977) Diagnosis of gynecologic pelvic masses by gray scale ultrasonography. Analysis of specifity and accuracy. Am J Roentgenol 128:1003

McGowan L, Stein DB, Müller W (1966) Cul-de-Sac aspiration for diagnostic cytologic study, Am J Obstet Gynecol 96:413–417

Musumici R, Banfi A, Bolis G et al. (1977) Lymphangiography in patients with ovarian epithelial cancer. Cancer 40:1444–1449

Neville AM (1980) Products of gynecological neoplasma: Clinical and pathological applications. Arch Gynecol 229:311–323

Popkin DR (1979) Early diagnosis of ovarian cancer, Can Med Assoc J 120:1106–1108

Rutledge R, Boronow RC, Wharton JT (1976) Gynecologic oncology. John Wiley, New York

Sarjadi S, Daunter B, Mackay E, Magon H, Khoo SK (1980) A multiparametrie approach to tumor markers detectable in serum in patients with carcinoma of the ovary or uterine cervix. Gynecol Oncol 10:113–124

Schlensker KH, Beckers H (1980) The use of ultrasound in the diagnosis of pelvic pathology. Arch Gynecol 229:91–105

Schultze H, Weise W (1971) Über die Häufigkeit, Symptomatologie und Therapie der Ovarialkarzinome. Zentralbl Gynaekol 42:1417–1480

Soost HJ (1980) Fortbildungstagung über Ovarial-Carcinome, München 1980 (Referat). Selecta 37:3228

Stein WW (1977) Ultraschall in der gynäkologischen Tumordiagnostik. Gynaekol Prax 1:653–659

Steinbrich W, Friedmann G (1981) Computertomographie des kleinen Beckens, normale und pathologische Anatomie, Indikationen, Ergebnisse. ROEFO 134:115–122

Ueda K, Toyokawa M, Nakamori H et al. (1977) Immun-diagnosis of ovarian cancer by the aid of cell-mediated immunologic techniques. Osaka City Med J 23:73–84

Walsh JW, Rosenfield AT, Jaffee CC, Schwartz PE, Simone J, Dembner AG, Taylor KJ (1978) Phospective comparison of ultrasound and computed tomography in the evaluation of gynecologic pelvic masses. AGR 131:955–960

Watring WG, Edinger DD, Anderson B (1979) Screening and diagnosis in ovarian cancer. Clin Obstet Gynecol 22:745–757

Ylikorkala O (1977) Lancet 8021:1101

Morphologie

Germ Cell Tumors of the Ovary

A. TALERMAN[1]

Introduction

Germ cell tumors constitute the second largest group of ovarian neoplasms after the epithelial tumors, and comprise approximately 20% of all ovarian neoplasms. This incidence of germ cell tumors of the ovary is observed in Europe and North America, but the incidence is higher in Asia and Africa where epithelial tumors of the ovary are less common. Germ cell tumors are encountered at all ages from early infancy to very old age, but tend to be most common from the first to the sixth decade. On the other hand 60% of ovarian neoplasms in children and adolescents are of germ cell origin and one-third of these are malignant.

The establishment of the different distinctive types of germ cell tumors as specific entities and the recognition of the germ cell origin of this group of neoplasms are relatively recent developments.

The most widely held view concerning the histogenesis of germ cell neoplasms is that propounded by Teilum [47]. Figure 1 illustrates the histogenesis and interrelationship of germ cell neoplasms [47]. Dysgerminoma (seminoma) is considered to be a primitive germ cell neoplasm, which has not acquired the potential for further differentiation. Embryonal carcinoma is regarded as a conceptual as well as a morphological entity, and represents a germ cell neoplasm composed of totipotential or multipotential cells, which are capable of further differentiation. This differentiation can take place in an embryonal or somatic direction, resulting in teratomatous neoplasms of various degrees of maturity, or in an extraembryonal direction along two pathways, either vitelline differentiating towards endodermal sinus (yolk sac) tumor, or trophoblastic differentiating towards a choriocarcinoma. The process of differentiation of embryonal carcinoma is considered to be dynamic, and tumors may therefore be composed of, or contain, various elements at different stages of differentation. According to this view [47] the embryonal carcinoma is considered the most primitive germ cell tumor capable of further differentiation. The endodermal sinus (yolk sac) tumor and choriocarcinoma are considered to be well-differentiated, although highly malignant, germ cell neoplasms.

The considerable progress concerning the histogenetic aspects of germ cell neoplasms which has been achieved over the last three decades has also helped to produce a more acceptable classification. The formulation of a classification of ovarian

---

1 Department of Pathology and Obstetrics and Gynecology, University of Chicago, 5841 South Maryland Avenue, Chicago, Il 60637, USA

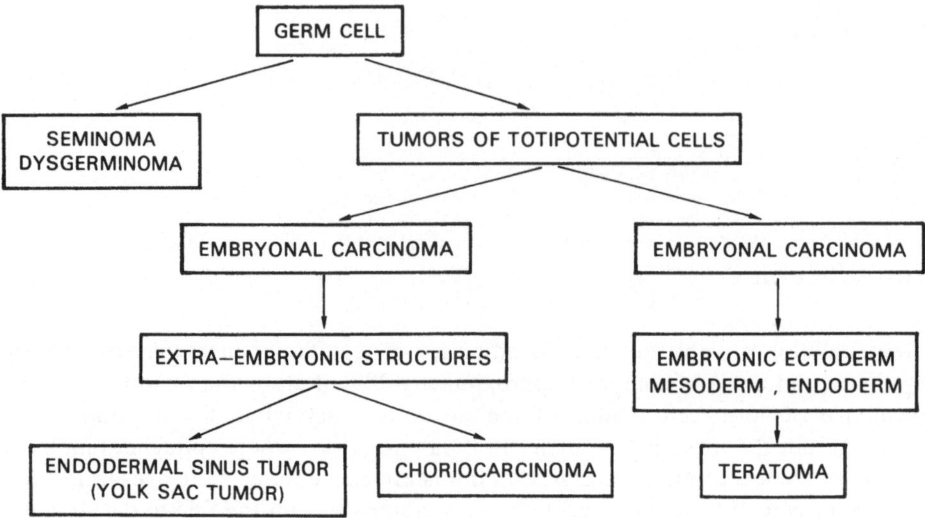

Fig. 1. The histogenesis and interrelationship of germ cell neoplasms. Adapted from Teilum [47]

neoplasms by the World Health Organization ovarian tumor panel in 1973 [33] was a very important milestone in this field, and it can be stated that this classification [33] has received very wide acceptance and acclaim.

This classification [33] divides germ cell neoplasms of the ovary as follows:

1. Dysgerminoma
2. Endodermal sinus tumor (yolk sac tumor)
3. Embryonal carcinoma
4. Polyembryoma
5. Choriocarcinoma
6. Teratomas
   a) Immature (solid, cystic or both)
   b) Mature
      i Solid
      ii Cystic
         Mature cystic teratoma (dermoid cyst)
         Mature cystic teratoma (dermoid cyst) with malignant transformation
   c) Monodermal or highly specialized
      i Struma ovarii
      ii Carcinoid
      iii Struma ovarii and carcinoid
      iv Others
7. Mixed forms (tumors composed of types 1 through 6 in any possible combination)

Tumors belonging to groups 1–5 and immature teratomas are malignant, have similar age incidence, occurring from birth till the menopause with a peak during the second and third decades, and are the most common malignant ovarian neoplasms in this age-group. They are usually unilateral and tend to spread by lymphatic and hematogenous routes, and less frequently by local and intracoelomic extension. Although they often occur in pure form, not infrequently they are composed of a number of neoplastic germ cell elements forming a mixed germ cell tumor.

In no other group of gonadal neoplasms is the homology between the various types more apparent than in the case of germ cell tumors, of which all the histologic types occurring in the ovary are represented in the testis, with the exception of spermatocytic seminoma, which occurs only in the testis. On the other hand there are considerable differences between ovarian and testicular germ cell tumors. Only 20% of ovarian neoplasms are of germ cell origin, while in the testis more than 90% belong to this category. While 90% of germ cell tumors of the ovary are benign and are mature cystic teratomas (dermoid cysts), nearly all testicular germ cell tumors are malignant, the only exceptions being mature teratomas occurring during infancy and early childhood.

Dysgerminoma

Dysgerminoma is the most common malignant germ cell neoplasm of the ovary and one of the most common malignant ovarian neoplasms of childhood, adolescence, and early adult life. In spite of this it is considered to be an uncommon ovarian neoplasm. It accounts for 1%–2% of ovarian neoplasms and for 3%–5% of ovarian malignancies.

Although dysgerminoma has been reported at all ages from infancy to old age, the majority of cases occur during adolescence and early adult life, most cases occurring during the second and third decades, and 80% of patients are under the age of 30 years [38]. Dysgerminoma was first described in 1911 by Chenot [5], who noted its marked resemblance to the testicular seminoma. The term "dysgerminoma" was introduced by Meyer [19]. Dysgerminoma has been encontered in all parts of the world and in all races.

Although Meyer [19] emphasized the frequent occurrence of dysgerminoma in subjects with various forms of sexual maldevelopment, it is now considered that only 5%–10% of dysgerminomas occur in such subjects and that the great majority of dysgerminomas are encountered in normally developed young females [32, 38]. It should be noted in this context that dysgerminoma is the most common malignant ovarian neoplasm occurring during pregnancy and one of the three most commonly encountered ovarian neoplasms occurring in pregnant women, the others being cystadenoma and mature cystic teratoma.

The most common presentation of patients with dysgerminoma is the presence of abdominal enlargement caused by a lower abdominal mass. The tumor may be found incidentally or during investigation of primary amenorrhea, when it may be associated with gonadoblastoma. Endocrine and menstrual abnormalities are uncommon as a presenting symptom but may occur due to the presence of syncytiotrophoblastic giant cells or foci of choriocarcinoma, or to luteinization of the stroma.

Dysgerminoma is usually unilateral, but is bilateral in 10%–15% of cases, thus differing from other malignant germ cell tumors of childhood, adolescence, and re-

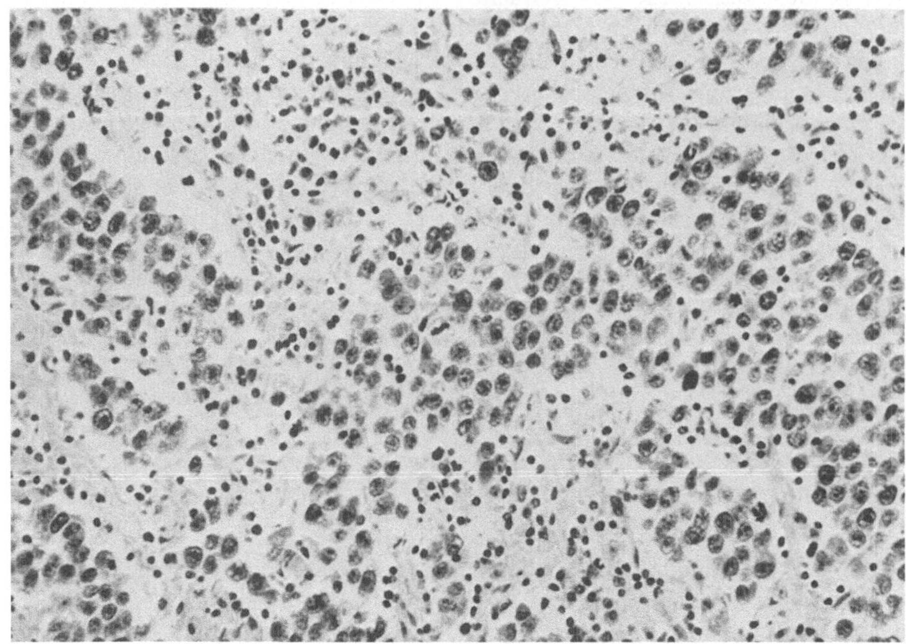

Fig. 2. Typical appearences of dysgerminoma. The tumor is composed of aggregates of uniform cells surrounded by connective tissue stroma containing lymphocytes. HE, × 160

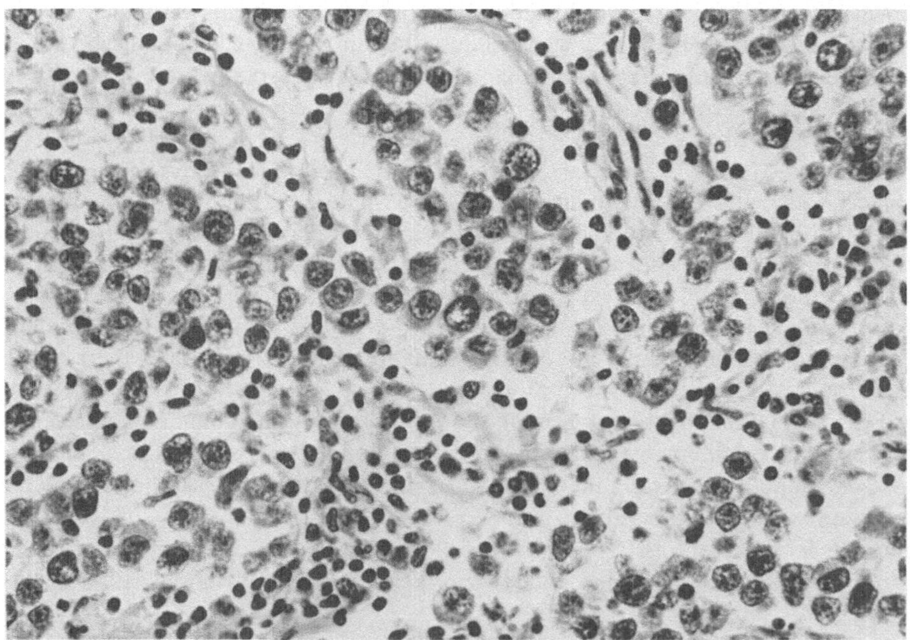

Fig. 3. Dysgerminoma showing the cellular and nuclear appearances. HE, ×380

productive age, which are only very rarely bilateral. Most series show increased incidence in the right ovary [38].

Pure dysgerminomas are solid, rapidly growing tumors, which are round, oval or lobulated with a smooth glistening capsule. They vary in size from small to very large. On cross section the tumor is solid, varies in consistency from firm and rubbery to soft, and in color from gray-pink to yellow-tan. The amount of fibrous tissue present within the tumor determines its consistency. The tumors containing a large amount of fibrous tissue tend to be firm or hard, while cellular tumors are softer. Hemorrhagic and necrotic areas are common in large tumors.

Microscopically dysgerminoma is composed of collections, aggregates, islands, or strands of large uniform cells, surrounded by connective tissue stroma containing lymphocytes (Fig. 2).

The amount of connective tissue stroma varies from delicate fibrovascular septa to large fibrous bands. The amount of connective tissue tends to determine the appearance of the tumor, but it should be noted that the amount of connective tissue and the number of lymphocytes as well as the presence and intensity of granulomatous reaction vary from one part of a tumor to another, presenting different appearances. The tumor cells are round or oval, measuring 15–25 μm. The cells contain ample amount of pale, slightly granular eosinophilic cytoplasm and a large, centrally located vesicular nucleus with one or two prominent nucleoli (Fig. 3). Mitotic activity is usually discernible, and varies from slight to brisk. The cytoplasm of the tumor cells contains glycogen which can be demonstrated by the PAS reaction, lipid which can be demonstrated by fat stains in frozen material, and alkaline phosphatase which is present beneath the cytoplasmic rim. The tumor cells show marked similarly to the primordial germ cells. This is also observed ultrastructurally and by densitometry. The tumor cells contain double the amount of DNA present in somatic cells [1].

Approximately 6%–8% of dysgerminomas contain multinucleated giant cells, which vary in appearance from basophilic giant cells containing a few nuclei to large vacuolated masses of cytoplasm containing numerous dark pyknotic nuclei or masses of chromatin, and resembling syncytiotrophoblastic giant cells (Fig. 4). These multinucleated giant cells have been shown conclusively to be capable of producing human chorionic gonadotropin (HCG) as well as its beta subunit (Beta-HCG). These giant cells must be differentiated from foreign body and Langhans' giant cells, which are frequently present in dysgerminomas and are associated with the granulomatous reaction usually seen in these tumors. Cytotrophoblastic cells have not been observed in association with the syncytiotrophoblastic giant cells. The HCG and beta-HCG which are synthesized by the tumor can be used as tumor markers in these cases. Serial determinations of these substances in the patient's serum can be used for monitoring the progress of the disease in the same way that they are used in patients with gestational or non-gestational choriocarcinoma, because the syncytiotrophoblast is the component of the tumor which synthesizes these substances. Although these dysgerminomas produce HCG, there is no evidence that patients with these tumors which contain syncytiotrophoblastic giant cells have a worse prognosis.

Dysgerminoma is frequently combined with other neoplastic germ cell elements [17, 42] (Fig. 5). In view of this the tumor must be very carefully sampled and exam-

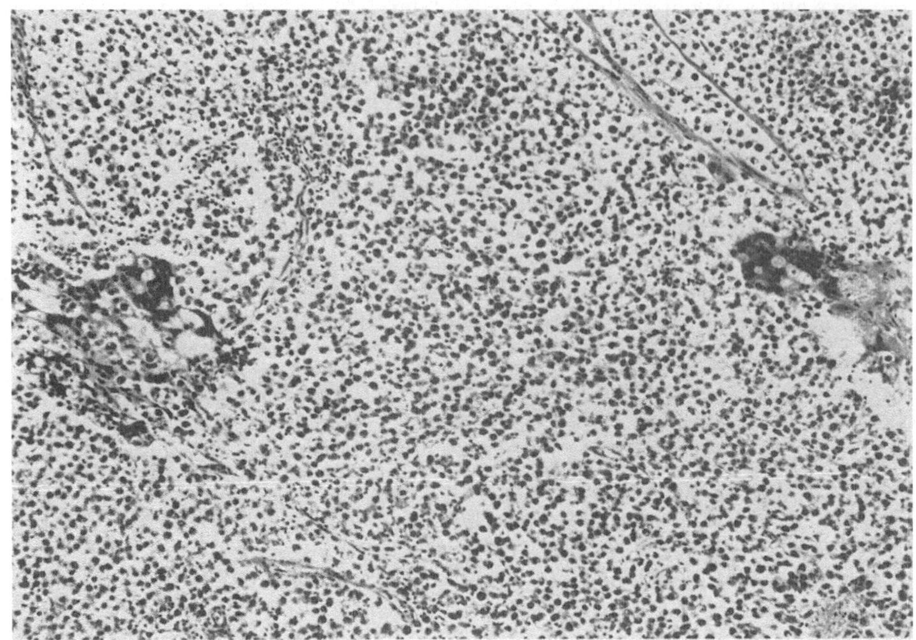

Fig. 4. Dysgerminoma containing syncytiotrophoblastic giant cells. HE, ×60

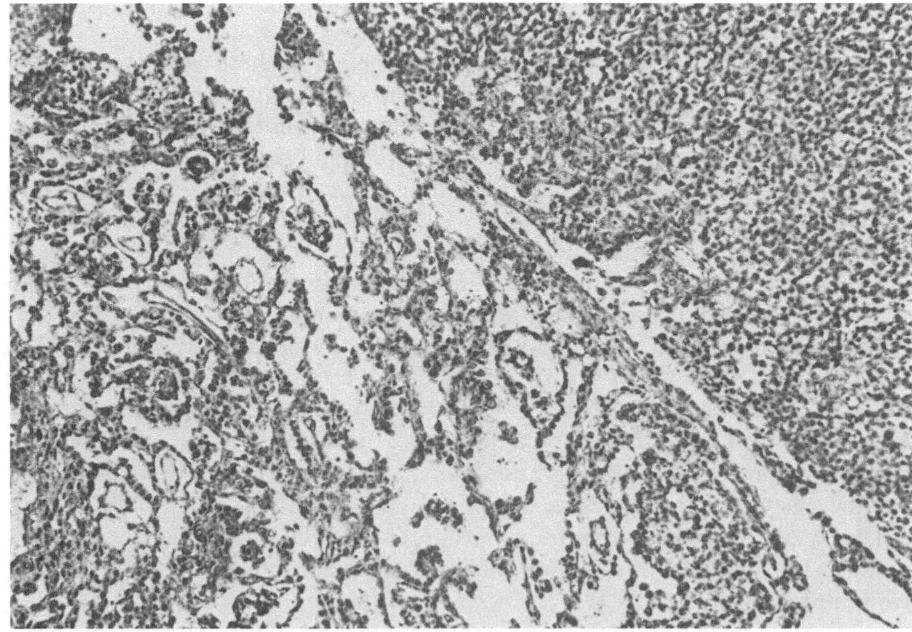

Fig. 5. Dysgerminoma (*right*) combined with endodermal sinus tumor (*left*). HE, ×60

ined in order to exclude the presence of other neoplastic germ cell elements, which alters the treatment and prognosis [17, 42].

Dysgerminoma metastasizes first via the lymphatics to the parailiac and para-aortic lymph nodes. From there further spread takes place to the mediastinal and supraclavicular lymph nodes. Hematogenous spread occurs much later and affects the lungs, liver, bones, and other organs [38]. Because of the spread of the tumor via the lymphatics, lymphangiography is an important and valuable diagnostic procedure and should be performed in all cases. Although metastases are usually composed of dysgerminoma, in approximately 10%–15% of cases the metastases do not reflect the appearances of the primary tumor and contain other neoplastic germ cell elements.

As dysgerminoma most frequently occurs in children and young women in whom preservation of fertility is desirable, and as the tumor is unilateral in 85%–90% of cases, when the tumor is small and mobile and there is no involvement of the contralateral ovary shown on biopsy, the treatment is excision of the tumor or the affected adnexa, and careful follow-up of the patient [32, 38]. It has been shown that the 5-year survival in these cases is 90%–95%, although such therapy is complicated by a 20%–25% recurrence rate, which is no worse than in cases where both adnexa as well as the uterus are excised. Due to marked radiosensitivity of dysgerminoma the recurrent disease can be treated by radiotherapy with very good results [1, 2, 42]. Therefore, this conservative therapeutic approach is highly recommended in such cases. When the tumor involves the contralateral ovary, or preservation of fertility is not desired, bilateral salpingooophorectomy and hysterectomy are performed and are followed by administration of radiation therapy to the lymph nodes draining the adnexa. As most metastases and recurrences are observed within the first 2 years following surgery, absence of disease for 2½–3 years following surgery can be considered synonymous with cure. It should again be emphasized that very careful and judicious sampling of the tumor must be carried out initially to determine wheter the tumor is in fact a pure dysgerminoma, or whether it is a mixed germ cell tumor including other elements. Due to more careful and better sampling the incidence of dysgerminomas admixed with other neoplastic germ cell elements has been found to be higher than in the past [42], and this may explain why in the past a greater number of dysgerminomas did not respond to radiotherapy and were associated with poor prognosis.

Endodermal Sinus Tumor

Endodermal sinus (yolk sac) tumor is the second most common malignant ovarian germ cell neoplasm after dysgerminoma. Although it was once considered to be very rare, more than 200 cases have been recorded, and while its exact incidence is not known it is now diagnosed more frequently.

Endodermal sinus tumor became established as a specific histopathologic entity through the exhaustive studies of Teilum stretching over more than two decades [44–47]. Teilum [47, 48] considered endodermal sinus tumor to be a germ cell tumor which has originated and differentiated from embryonal carcinoma (a tumor of multipotential malignant germ cells capable of further differentiation) along the ex-

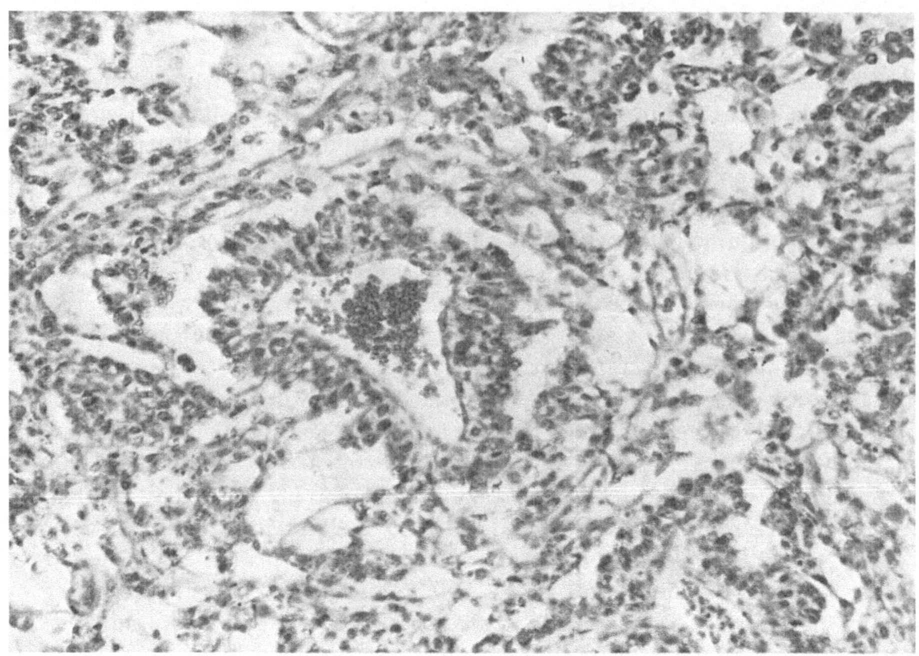

Fig. 6. Perivascular formation (Schiller-Duval body) considered a hallmark of endodermal sinus tumor. HE, ×235

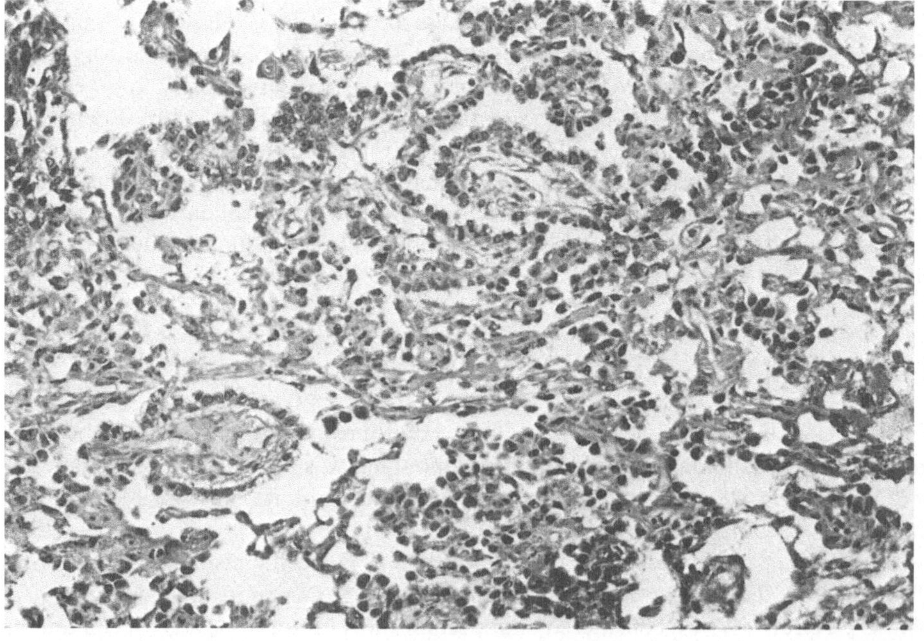

Fig. 7. Endodermal sinus tumor showing papillary pattern. Perivascular formations are also seen. HE, ×150

Table 1. Serum AFP and ovarian germ cell tumors

	No. of cases	Serum AFP
Active disease		
Mixed germ cell tumors containing endodermal sinus tumors	24	Raised
Pure endodermal sinus tumors	9	Raised
Dysgerminoma	16	Normal
Teratoma (mature and immature)	1*	Raised
Teratoma (immature and mature)	5	Normal
Teratoma (immature and mature) with dysgerminoma	4	Normal
Mature cystic teratoma (dermoid cyst)	6	Normal
Inactive disease		
Dysgerminoma	6	Normal
Teratoma (immature and mature)	1	

* Specimen was not studied adequately

traembryonal pathway of differentiation towards yolk sac or vitelline structures (Fig. 1). Although the terminology and histogenesis of this entity were a matter of debate and controversy for many decades, Teilum's [47, 48] views regarding its histogenesis are generally accepted nowadays. Recent studies which have demonstrated conclusively that endodermal sinus tumor is capable of alpha-fetoprotein (AFP) synthesis [13, 41, 43, 49, 51, 52], which also takes place in the normal yolk sac [10], have given further support to Teilum's [47, 48] views concerning the histogenesis of endodermal sinus tumor. Table 1 shows serum AFP levels in a series of germ cell tumors [40].

Endodermal sinus tumor, like dysgerminoma, is observed most frequently in the second and third decades of life, followed by the first and fourth in this order, and is very rare in the fifth and exceedingly rare after the menopause [15, 38, 48]. The patients usually present with abdominal enlargement or pain. The tumor is rapidly growing, and is usually of considerable size when encountered [15, 38, 48].

Endodermal sinus tumor is unilateral in the great majority of cases, and in most cases where bilateral tumors are encountered one of the tumors is metastatic. The tumor is round or oval and has a smooth or lobulated surface. It may be attached to, or invading, the surrounding structures. On cross section it is solid gray white with hemorrhagic and necrotic areas, and the surface is somewhat slimy or mucoid. Histologically endodermal sinus tumor shows a number of patterns which are usually seen in combination, although one or two patterns may predominate. The different histologic patterns seen in different tumors, as well as in different parts of the same tumor, have contributed materially to the difficulties in recognizing and diagnosing this neoplasm.

The histologic appearances of endodermal sinus tumor have been described in detail [38, 47, 48]. Although the endodermal sinus pattern with the typical perivascular formations (Schiller-Duval bodies) (Fig. 6) considered a hallmark of this tumor is seen in the great majority of ovarian endodermal sinus tumors, it may be far from being predominant and is not a necessary prerequisite for making the diagnosis. The other typical patterns, the papillary (Fig. 7), glandular-alveolar (Fig. 8), mi-

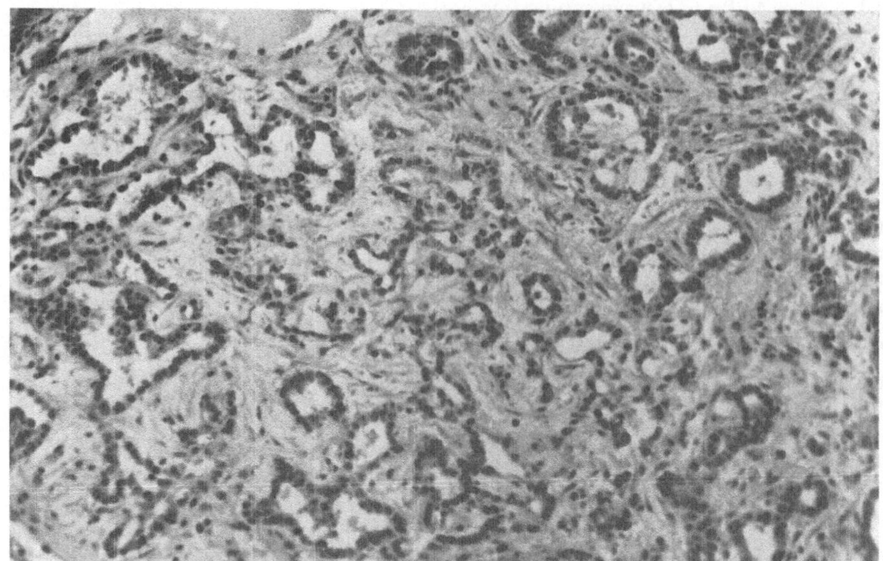

Fig. 8. Endodermal sinus tumor showing glandular-alveolar pattern. HE, ×150

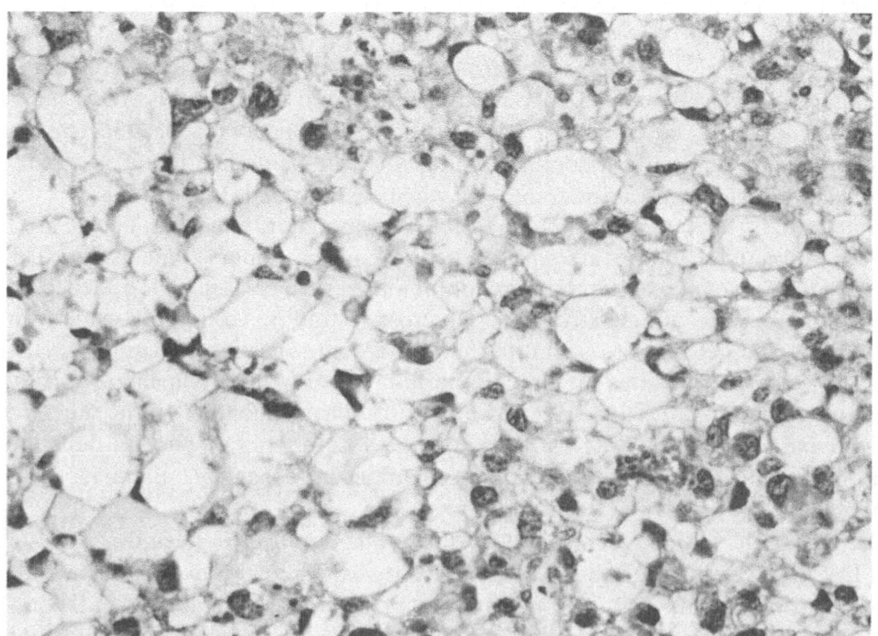

Fig. 9. Endodermal sinus tumor showing microcystic pattern. HE, ×460

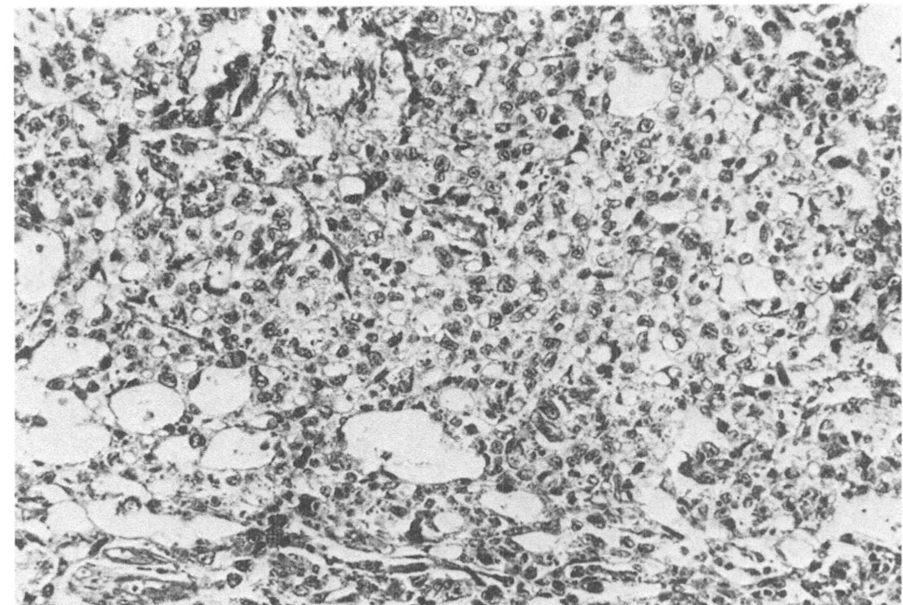

Fig. 10. Endodermal sinus tumor showing solid pattern with some cysts and microcysts. HE, ×360

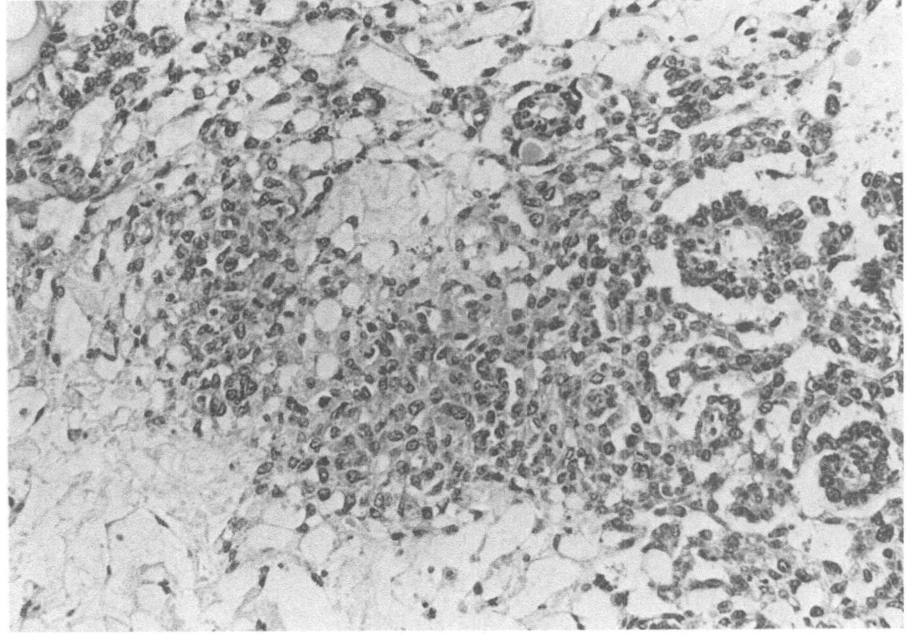

Fig. 11. Endodermal sinus tumor showing myxomatous pattern (*left*). Perivascular formations are also seen (*right*). HE, ×360

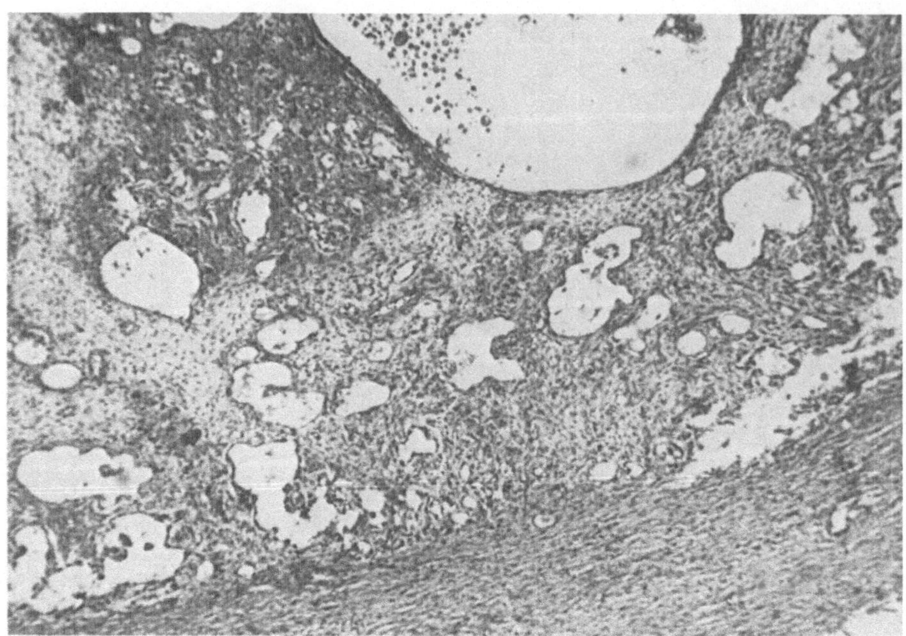

Fig. 12. Endodermal sinus tumor showing polyvesicular vitelline pattern. HE, ×60

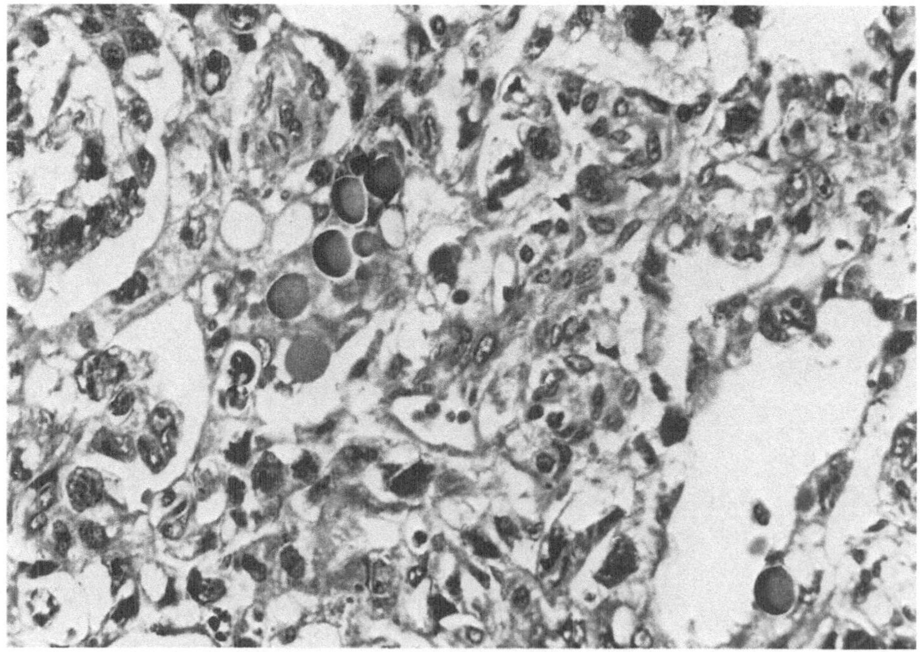

Fig. 13. Small round hyaline globules present within endodermal sinus tumor. HE, ×460

crocystic (Fig. 9), solid (Fig. 10), myxomatous (Fig. 11), cystic, and polyvesicular vitelline (Fig. 12), are usually seen in combination in many of the tumors. Small, round hyaline globules (Fig. 13), which are PAS-positive and resistant to diastase digestion, are seen in many of the tumors, both inside the cytoplasm of the tumor cells and outside them. In some areas there is also an increased amount of extracellular fluid which is pale eosinophilic. Both the globules and the fluid, especially the former, have been found by immunofluorescence and immunoperoxidase techniques to contain AFP, as well as alpha-1-antitrypsin and other proteinaceous products [52], which are also synthesized by the normal human yolk sac [9]. Endodermal sinus tumor, in common with other germ cell tumors, may be combined with other neoplastic germ cell elements and the combination with mature cystic teratoma, dysgerminoma, and embryonal carcinoma is not infrequent.

Endodermal sinus tumor is a highly malignant neoplasm which grows rapidly, invades locally the surrounding structures, and metastasizes early via the lymphatics to the regional lymph nodes and also by the hematogenous route to the lungs, liver, and other organs. Metastases are commonly present at the time of presentation. Endodermal sinus tumor is radioresistant, and not so very long ago the prognosis was dismal [47, 48]. Only very occasional patients with small tumors localized to the ovary survived. During the last decade administration of chemotherapy, originally vincristine, actinomycin D, and cyclophosphamide (VAC), and more recently cis- plati-

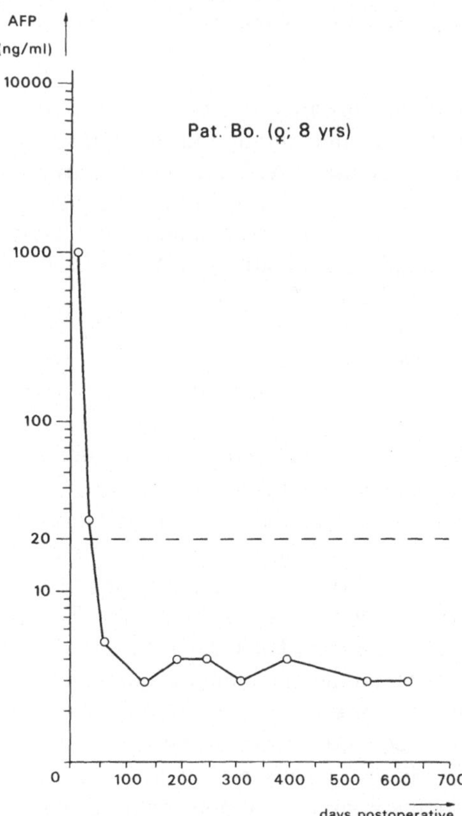

Fig. 14. Serial AFP determinations in an 8-year-old girl with endodermal sinus tumor admixed with immature teratoma. The patient is well and disease-free 4 years after surgery. The serum AFP remains normal

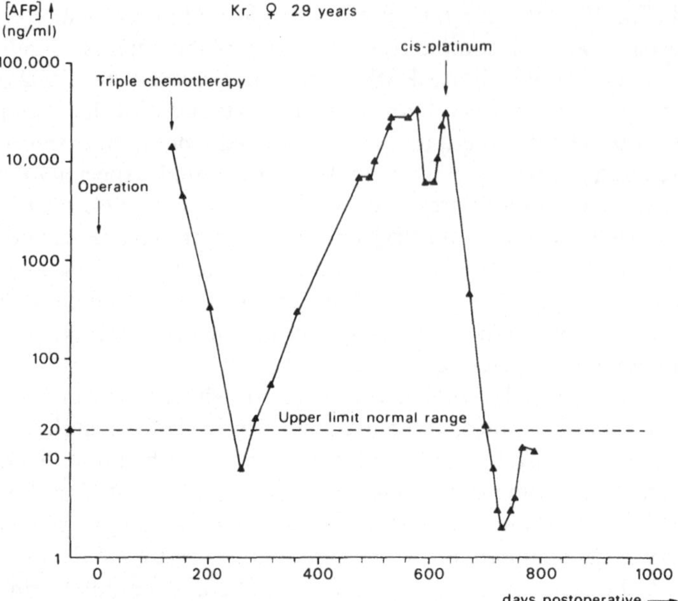

Fig. 15. Serial serum AFP determinations in a 29-year-old woman with pure endodermal sinus tumor with metastases. The levels of serum AFP correlated well with disease activity and response to various forms of chemotherapy

num, bleomycin, and vinblastine [7], completely revolutionized the treatment of endodermal sinus tumor and the number of surviving patients has increased dramatically. The use of AFP as a tumor marker has also helped to increase survival. Therefore nowadays after the primary treatment, which is unilateral salpingo-oophorectomy if there is no involvement of the contralateral adnexa, the disease is monitored by serial determinations of AFP and the patient is treated with triple chemotherapy (Figs. 14 and 15).

Embryonal Carcinoma

As already stated, embryonal carcinoma is regarded as both a conceptual and morphologic entity and as the least differentiated germ cell neoplasm capable of further differentiation [6, 47, 48]. It occurs only very rarely in the ovary in pure form, but is more common in combination, especially with endodermal sinus tumor [38]. The term "embryonal carcinoma" has been used, especially by American authors, to describe endodermal sinus tumor. This is considered incorrect and these two neoplasms are regarded as separate and distinct entities [16, 38].

Embryonal carcinoma is encountered in the same age-group as endodermal sinus tumor. It is unilateral in the great majority of cases. The tumors are large, solid, and frequently associated with hemorrhage and necrosis [16, 38].

Microscopically embryonal carcinoma is composed of aggregates of epithelial-like medium to large polygonal or ovoid cells, containing an ample amount of pale

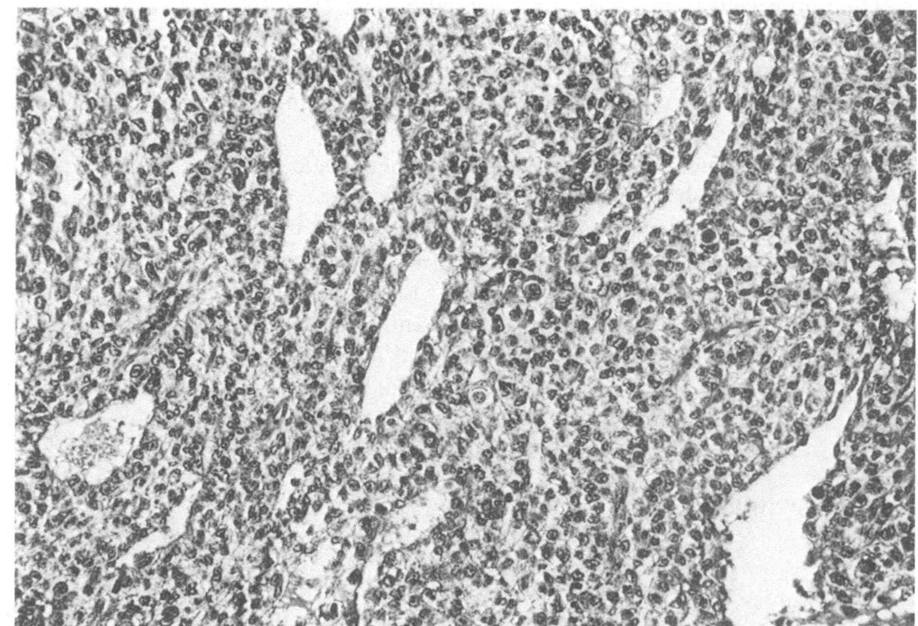

Fig. 16. Embryonal carcinoma composed of aggregates of epithelial-like polygonal cells forming a solid pattern and lining occasional clefts or spaces. HE, ×235

eosinophilic granular or clear cytoplasm with poorly discernible cytoplasmic borders (Fig. 16). The nuclei are large and vesicular, vary in shape, and have a fine nuclear membrane or may be hyperchromatic. They usually contain more than one nucleolus. Mitotic activity is brisk, and cellular and nuclear pleomorphism is frequently observed [16, 38].

Table 2. Serum HCG and β-HCG in ovarian germ cell tumors

Ovarian tumors	No. of cases	Serum HCG and β-HCG
Active disease		
Mixed germ cell tumors containing choriocarcinoma	4	Raised
Mixed germ cell tumor containing endodermal sinus tumors	14	Normal
Pure endodermal sinus tumors	7	Normal
Dysgerminoma	11	Normal
Dysgerminoma	1*	Raised
Teratoma (immature and mature)	3	Normal
Teratoma (immature and mature) and dysgerminoma	4	Normal
Mature cystic teratoma (dermoid cyst)	6	Normal
Inactive disease		
Dysgerminoma	3	Normal
Teratoma (mature and immature)	1	Normal

* Specimen was not studied adequately

The tumor cells form a solid or syncytial pattern (Fig. 16), or may line clefts or spaces, as well as forming papillae giving the tumor a certain resemblance to an adenocarcinoma. Very primitive mesenchymal tissue may be present in conjunction with the epithelial-like component. Isolated syncytiotrophoblastic giant cells may be seen and cause elevation of serum HCG and beta-HCG. As stated above, embryonal carcinoma is usually combined with other neoplastic germ cell elements and in the ovary is only rarely seen in the pure state [38].

Sometimes raised serum AFP is present due to the fact that partial differentiation into endodermal sinus tumor has begun to take place, but more frequently due to the fact that the tumors is combined with endodermal sinus tumor.

Embryonal carcinoma is a highly malignant germ cell tumor. It is unilateral in the great majority of cases, invades locally, and metastasizes early in a similar way to endodermal sinus tumor. The treatment is the same as for endodermal sinus tumor.

Polyembryoma

Polyembryoma is a germ cell neoplasm composed entirely of embryoid bodies resembling morphologically normal presomite embryos, which never develop beyond the 18-day stage. Polyembryoma in pure form has not been encountered in the ovary, and in the few cases on record the polyembryoma has been combined with other

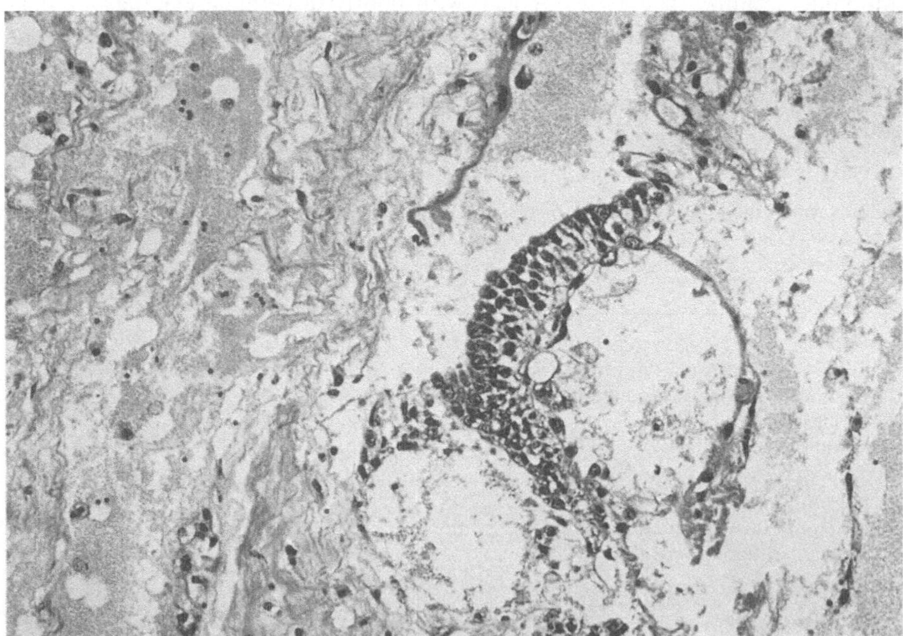

Fig. 17. Embryoid body containing embryonic disc in the center and yolk sac on the *right*. Amniotic cavity is discernible with difficulty on the *left*. HE, ×235

neoplastic germ cell elements, such as immature and mature teratoma, endodermal sinus tumor, and embryonal carcinoma [38]. Even the presence of occasional embryoid bodies in a ovarian germ cell tumor is rare.

Microscopically polyembryoma is composed of embryoid bodies, which when well formed are composed of an embryonic disc located in the center between the amniotic cavity and the yolk sac (Fig. 17). Less well-formed or atypical embryoid bodies may contain an embryonic disc and two or more yolk sacs with a single amniotic cavity, or vice versa. The embryoid bodies may vary in size and show bizarre appearences. They are surrounded by myxomatous tissue or primitive mesenchyma. Teratomatous structures in various stages of differentiation, as well as syncytiotrophoblastic giant cells, are seen in the vicinity. Polyembryoma is a highly malignant germ cell tumor and it behaves and is treated in the same way as endodermal sinus tumor and embryonal carcinoma.

Choriocarcinoma

Although the majority of choriocarcinomas are of the gestational type, only the nongestational choriocarcinoma will be discussed here. Nongestational choriocarcinoma is a germ cell neoplasm and may be found in all sites where germ cell neoplasms are encountered, such as the ovary, testis, mediastinum, and pineal region. Nongestational choriocarcinoma is histologically indistinguishable from the gestational type. Although at one time doubt was cast on the existence of nongestational choriocarcinoma of the ovary in subjects other than premenarchal children, it has been shown conclusively that the nongestational choriocarcinoma does occur in older children, adolescents, and young females in the third and fourth decades. Therefore, nongestational choriocarcinoma has similar age incidence to the other malignant germ cell neoplasms of the ovary described above. It must always be carefully differentiated from its gestational counterpart. The fact that nongestational choriocarcinoma is usually associated with other neoplastic germ cell elements helps to confirm the diagnosis.

Pure nongestational choriocarcinoma of the ovary is very rare, but the presence of choriocarcinoma as one of the elements comprising a mixed germ cell tumor is nowadays observed more frequently than previously due to the more extensive and judicious sampling of the tumors, and more than 50 such cases have been reported [32, 38].

Choriocarcinoma can only be diagnosed if both syncytiotrophoblast and cytotrophoblast are present within the tumor. Collections or individual syncytiotrophoblastic giant cells, which are present within a number of germ cell tumors, are not regarded as choriocarcinoma and do not merit this designation. The most common presentation of the patient with nongestational choriocarcinoma is similar to that observed in patients with other malignant germ cell neoplasms described above. In addition isosexual precocious puberty may be observed in premenarchal children, while in adults menorrhagia, menometrorrhagia, and signs of ectopic pregnancy may occur. Nongestational choriocarcinoma, like its gestational counterpart, produces large amounts of HCG.

Macroscopically the tumor is large, rapidly growing, and nearly always hemorrhagic. Although it is almost always unilateral, there may be metastases in the contralateral ovary. Microscopically the tumor is composed of centrally located cytotrophoblast in the form of medium-sized polygonal round or oval cells with distinct cellular borders and centrally located small round or hyperchromatic nuclei, or large vesicular nuclei containing nucleoli. Mitotic activity is brisk. These cells are surrounded by syncytiotrophoblastic cells which are large or very large and irregular in shape, and contain basophilic, often vacuolated cytoplasm. These cells contain

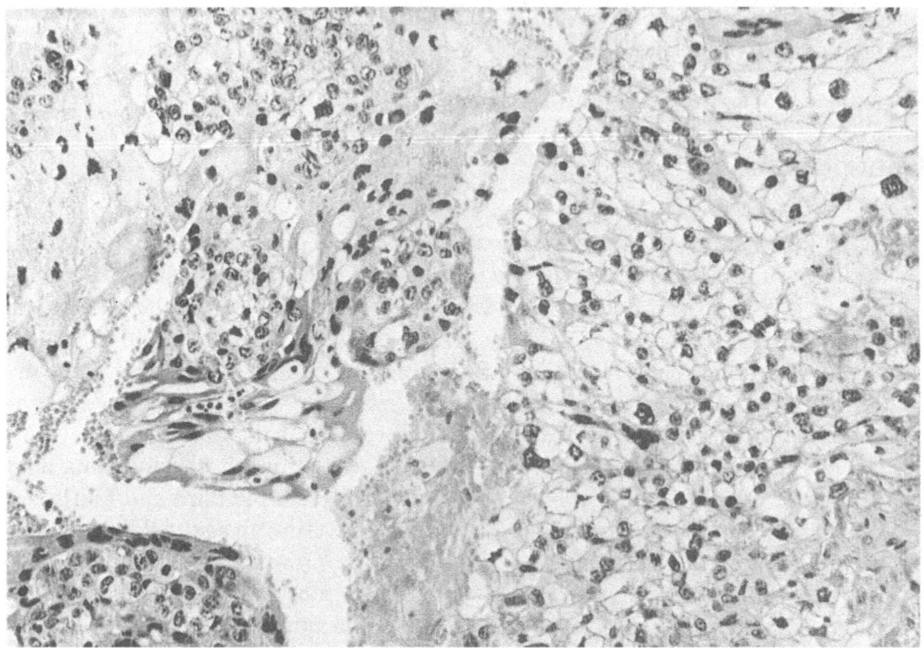

Fig. 18. Choriocarcinoma composed of cytotrophoblast and large vacuolated syncytiotrophoblast (*left of center*). HE, ×360

many hyperchromatic nuclei, which vary in size and shape, or irregular dark masses of chromatin (Fig. 18). The amounts of syncytiotrophoblast and cytotrophoblast vary. Choriocarcinoma secretes HCG, and raised serum HCG is present only in patients with tumors containing choriocarcinoma or syncytiotrophoblastic giant cells. Thus HCG and beta-HCG are very useful tumor markers in patients with tumors containing choriocarcinoma and syncytiotrophoblastic giant cells.

More recently pregnancy-specific beta globulin (SP_1) has been found to be produced by trophoblastic tissue, has been found to be a useful tumor marker in patients with trophoblastic neoplasia, and can be used in conjunction with HCG or beta-HCG estimations.

Teratoma

Teratomas are defined as germ cell tumors composed of derivatives of the three primitive germ layers: ectoderm, mesoderm, and endoderm. They may exhibit varying dègrees of maturity and are derived from embryonal carcinoma by a process of differentiation through the embryonic or somatic pathway (Fig. 1).

In the ovary the overwhelming majority (99%) of teratomas are mature, exhibit cystic pattern, and are classified as mature cystic teratomas or dermoid cysts. Because all the tissues are mature, the neoplasm is benign. Mature cystic teratomas have been recognized for a long time and have been described in detail elsewhere [4, 8, 20, 23, 32, 38]. In view of this they will be discussed only briefly here.

Mature cystic teratomas have a much wider age incidence than the malignant germ cell neoplasms described above, and are encountered from infancy to old age. The majority are observed in the first six decades of life. Mature cystic teratomas are usually unilateral, but in 15%–20% of cases they are bilateral, and in a number of cases they may coexist with a malignant germ cell tumor in the contralateral ovary.

The tumors vary in size from microscopic to very large. They are composed of derivatives of the three primitive germ layers. All the tissues present are fully mature (Fig. 19). Occasionally mature cystic teratoma may be associated with mature neural (glial) implants in the peritoneal cavity (Fig. 20). As the implants are fully mature they are benign, and there is no need for further treatment, beyond the excision of the affected adnexa [25].

Mature Solid Teratoma

Mature solid teratoma is a vary rare ovarian neoplasm, as the majority of solid teratomas of the ovary contain immature elements. A very careful search for immature elements must be made and their presence very carefully excluded before a diagnosis of mature solid teratoma can be made. The tumor is composed of derivatives of the three primitive germ layers, which are fully mature. Cystic areas are often admixed with the solid ones.

Mature solid teratoma has the same age incidence as other germ cell tumors of the ovary. It is a benign tumor and should be treated as such by excision of the affected adnexa.

Immature Teratoma

Immature teratoma shares many features with other malignant germ cell neoplasms of the ovary, such as age incidence, presentation, unilaterality, large size, malignant biologic behavior, combination with other neoplastic germ cell elements, rapid growth, and rapid spread via the lymphatic and hematogenous routes. It comprises less than 1% of ovarian teratomas.

Immature teratoma is unilateral, but may coexist with mature cystic teratoma in the contralateral ovary. It occurs most frequently during the first two decades of life and is almost unknown after the menopause. Macroscopically the tumors are usu-

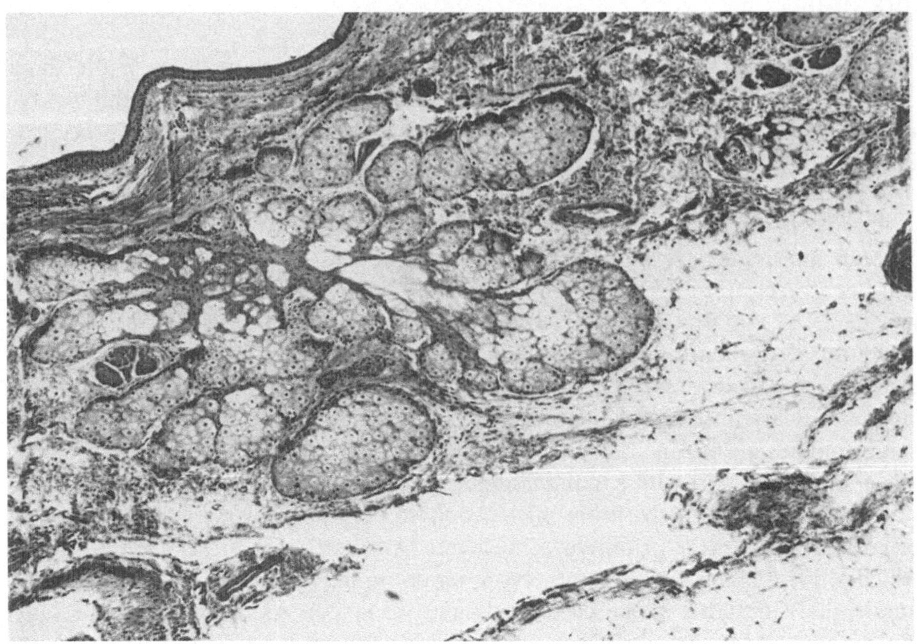

Fig. 19. Mature cystic teratoma. HE, ×60

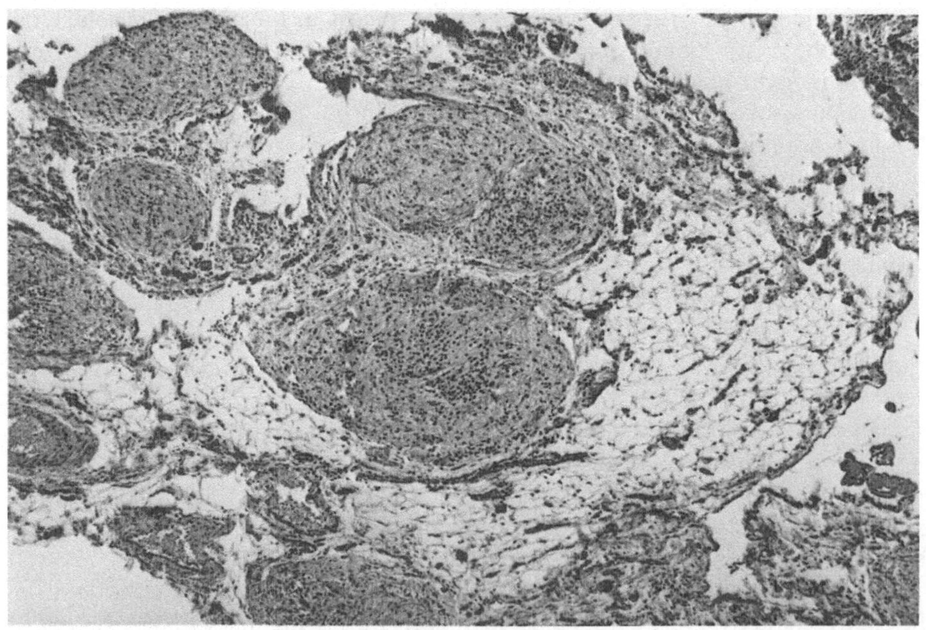

Fig. 20. Mature neural (glial) implants in the peritoneum. HE, ×75

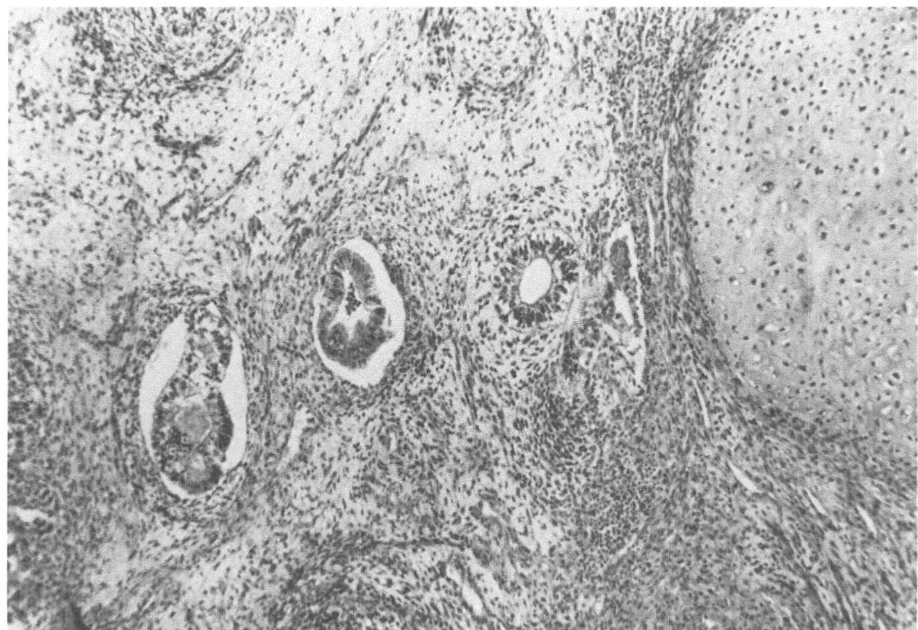

Fig. 21. Immature solid teratoma of the ovary. Note glandular tissue in the *centre* and immature cartilage (*right*). HE, ×75

ally large, round or oval, and solid, although they may contain cystic areas. Microscopically the tumors are composed of a variety of immature tissues derived from the three primitive germ layers (Fig. 21). Mature elements are frequently combined or admixed with the immature elements. In view of this great care must be taken in examining the tumor, so as not to miss the presence of the immature elements. It is the presence of the immature elements which radically alters the prognosis and their presence is synonymous with malignancy. Occasionally small foci of extraembryonal tissue like small foci of endodermal sinus tumor or individual or collections of syncytiotrophoblastic giant cells, as well as occasional embryoid bodies, may be present. Immature teratoma may be combined with other neoplastic germ cell elements forming a mixed germ cell neoplasm.

It has been shown over the years that there is good correlation between the maturity of the tumor and prognosis in patients with immature teratoma. A grading system has been proposed by Thurlbeck and Scully [50] which has been found to be very useful for prognostic purposes. This grading is as follows:

Grade 0: All tissues mature; no mitotic activity

Grade 1: Minor foci of abnormally cellular or embryonal tissue mixed with mature elements; slight mitotic activity

Grade 2: Moderate quantities of embryonal tissue mixed with mature elements; moderate mitotic activity

Grade 3: Large quantities of embryonal tissue present; high mitotic activity.

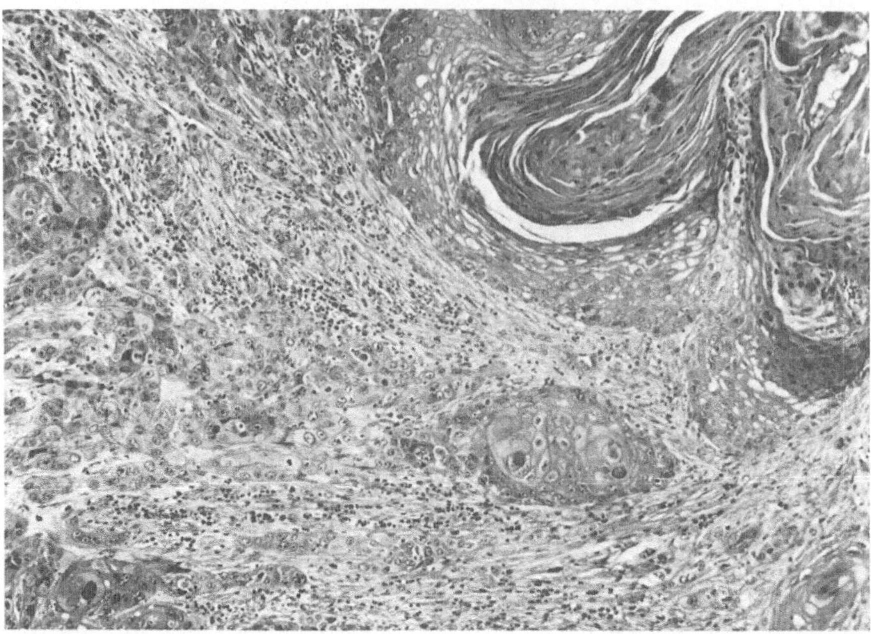

Fig. 22. Mature cystic teratoma with malignant transformation into squamous cell carcinoma. HE, ×90

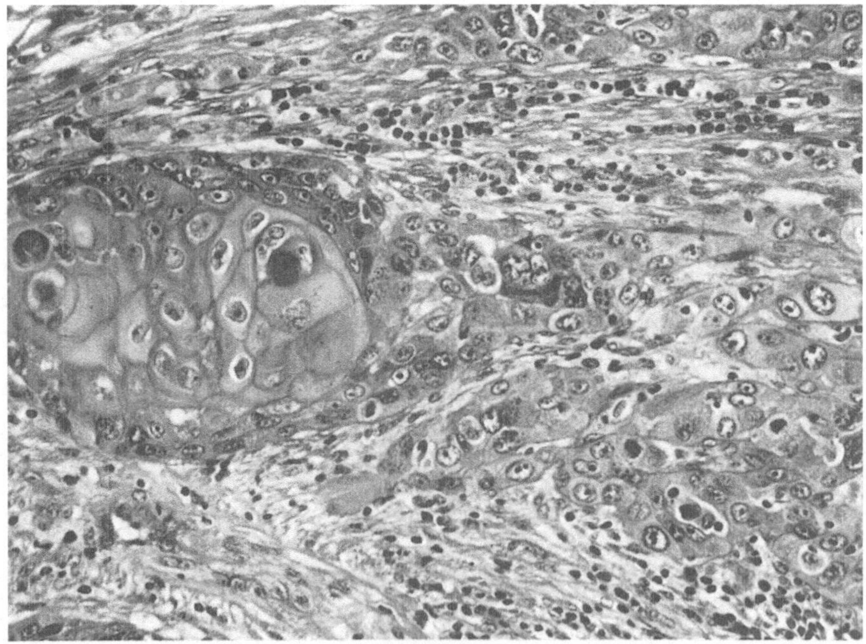

Fig. 23. Higher magnification of Fig. 22 showing well-differentiated squamous cell carcinoma. HE, ×380

The treatment of patients with this tumor is like that recommended for other malignant germ cell neoplasms. If there is no involvement of the contralateral ovary and the tumor is mobile and not attached to the surrounding structures, the treatment is one-sided adnexectomy. As immature teratoma metastasizes via the lymphatic and hematogenous routes and as it is not sensitive to radiotherapy, combination chemotherapy involving either (a) vincristine, actinomycin D, and cyclophosphamide or (b) vinblastine, cis-platinum, and bleomycin [7] is administered. The institution of this form of chemotherapy has altered the very poor prognosis in cases of immature teratomas of grades 2 and 3.

Mature Cystic Teratoma (Dermoid Cyst) with Malignant Transformation

Malignant transformation is an uncommon complication of mature cystic teratoma and although some reports state that it occurs in up to 4% of cases [21] its incidence is probably less than 1%. The age incidence of patients with this complication has been reported to range from 19 to 88 years, but patients are usually postmenopausal [21, 22].

The presenting symptoms are similar to those observed in patients with other malignant germ cell tumors or ovarian tumors in general, namely abdominal enlargement which may or may not be associated with abdominal pain. Loss of weight and other systemic symptoms may be present.

The tumors are unilateral, but may be associated with metastases in the contralateral ovary or may coexist with mature cystic teratoma in the contralateral ovary. The tumor is usually large and if there is no penetration of the ovarian surface it may be indistinguishable from a large mature cystic teratoma. When penetration occurs the tumor is lobulated or nodular and there is invasion of the surrounding structures. There may be extensive involvement of the peritoneal cavity by tumor deposits.

Microscopically the tumor usually shows its original histologic appearences at least in some areas, as well as malignant transformation of one of its components, usually squamous epithelium, which forms squamous cell carcinoma (Fig. 22). The tumor is usually well differentiated (Fig. 23).

Squamous cell carcinoma is the malignant component in 75%–80% of mature cystic teratomas (dermoid cysts) with malignant transformation, but any other component of the tumor may undergo malignant change, including glandular epithelium, thyroid tissue, and mesenchymal tissue. The malignant element invades and destroys the other parts of the tumor, penetrates through the surface, and invades the surrounding structures.

Mature cystic teratoma with malignant transformation behaves differently from other malignant germ cell neoplasms as it does not spread via the lymphatic and hematogenous routes, but spreads by direct extension and by intracoelomic route and invades the abdominal cavity extensively. The prognosis for patients with this tumor is poor, with 5-year survival of 15% [32]. There is a better prognosis when the malignant element is a squamous cell carcinoma and the tumor is confined to the ovary. In such cases the 5-year survival is 63% [32]. When the malignant element is other than squamous cell carcinoma, the prognosis is very poor. The treatment of mature cystic teratoma (dermoid cyst) with malignant transformation is surgical. The tumor does not respond to radiotherapy and at present there is no satisfactory chemotherapeutic combination active against it. Complete surgical excision of the tumor thus remains the best therapeutic modality at present.

Monodermal or Highly Specialized Teratomas

Struma Ovarii

Struma ovarii is a teratomatous tumor composed largely or entirely of thyroid tissue. It is regarded as a one-sided development of a teratoma. Struma ovarii is uncommon and comprises approximately 2% of ovarian teratomas. The age incidence is the same as in patients with mature cystic teratoma [55].

The symptomatology is the same as in cases of mature cystic teratoma, except for an occasional case where thyroid enlargement occurs and rare cases where there has been some evidence that the tumor may have been responsible for the development of thyrotoxicosis. The tumor varies in size from small to large and is unilateral. In 15% of cases it is associated with mature cystic teratoma in the contralateral ovary. The tumor is soft and its surface is smooth. On cross section it is glistening, light tan in color, and composed of normal mature thyroid tissue. This is confirmed on histologic examination [55] (Fig. 24). Occasionally the thyroid tissue may exhibit evidence of activity, or changes of nodular adenomatous goiter. Malignant transforma-

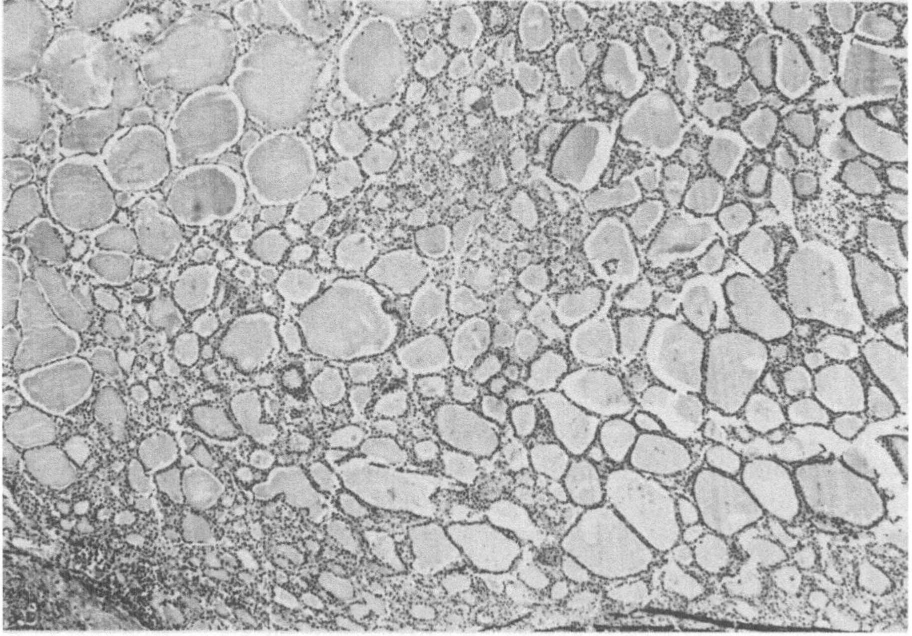

Fig. 24. Struma ovarii composed of normal thyroid tissue. HE, 60

tion with formation of papillary or follicular adenocarcinoma of the thyroid has been encountered on a few occasions. Occasionally struma ovarii spreads to the abdominal cavity, producing benign strumosis. Struma ovarii is treated by surgical excision and this is the treatment of choice in all cases except for those with thyroid carcinoma, where lymph node dissection, radioactive iodine (^{131}I), radiation therapy or chemotherapy may be used.

Carcinoid

Ovarian carcinoid tumors are classified as follows:

1. Primary
   a) Insular or islet carcinoid (carcinoid tumors of midgut derivation)
   b) Trabecular carcinoid (carcinoid tumors of foregut and hindgut derivation)
   c) Struma ovarii and carcinoid (strumal carcinoid) (carcinoid tumor combined with thyroid tissue)
   d) Mucinous (goblet, adenocarcinoid) carcinoid
2. Metastatic

Insular of islet carcinoid. Primary insular carcinoid tumors of the ovary are usually found in association with mature cystic teratoma, but may also be seen within a solid teratoma or a mucinous tumor [28]. They may also occur in a pure form, when they are considered to originate from argentaffin cells which may be present within the ovary, or as a one-sided development of teratoma. Primary islet cell carcinoid is uncommon, but it is the most common type of carcinoid tumor found in the ovary and more than 70 examples have been recorded [28, 32].

The age distribution is wide, but the majority of patients are perimenopausal or postmenopausal. The most common presentation is the presence of an ovarian mass, which may be accompanied by abdominal pain. One-third of cases have been associated with carcinoid syndrome. There is a correlation between the size of the tumor and the presence of the syndrome, and carcinoid syndrome is observed in patients with larger tumors [28, 32]. The presence of liver metastases is not necessary for the occurrence of the syndrome, as venous blood from the ovary enters systematic circulation and bypasses the liver, which is capable of detoxicating the serotonin produced by the neoplasm. Excision of the tumor is associated with remission of the symptoms and the disappearance of serotonin from the blood and 5-hydroxy-indole acetic acid (5-HIAA) from the urine.

Macroscopically carcinoid tumor forms a solid, yellow-gray homogeneous nodule within a mature cystic teratoma (dermoid cyst) or other type of tumor, or, when pure, forms a solid mass. It varies in size from microscopic to large. Primary carcinoids are nearly always unilateral, but may be associated with mature cystic teratoma in the contralateral ovary.

Microscopically the tumor is composed of collections of solid nests of polygonal epithelial cells with an ample amount of cytoplasm and round or oval centrally located nuclei and small acini composed of similar cells (Fig. 25). The cytoplasm is amphophilic or basophilic, and contains orange, brown, or red granules which exhibit the argentaffin or argyrophil reaction and when examined ultrastructurally contain

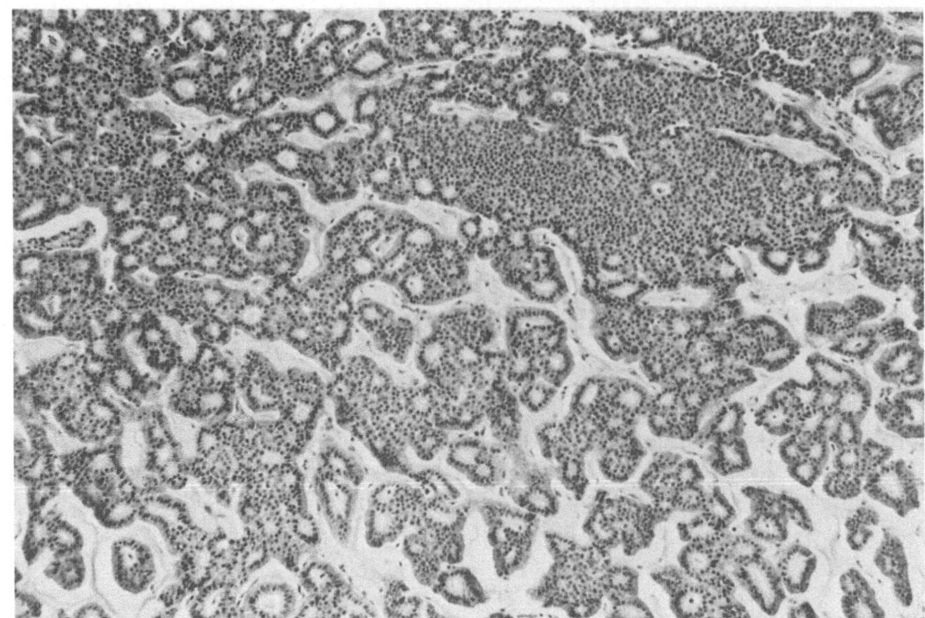

Fig. 25. Insular carcinoid composed of solid nests and small acini. HE, ×90

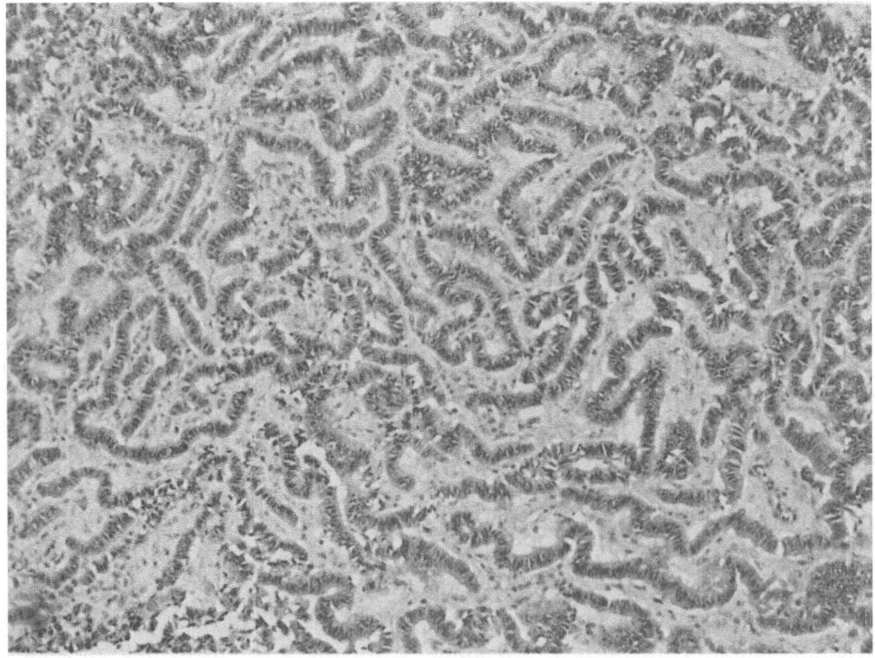

Fig. 26. Trabecular carcinoid composed of long cords or ribbons running in parallel and surrounded by connective tissue. HE, ×185

neurosecretory granules varying in size and shape [28, 32]. Very rarely primary insular carcinoids are associated with metastases, but these have been observed in only three cases [28, 32]. Estimation of serum serotonin and urinary 5-HIAA can be used to monitor disease activity in patients with insular carcinoid tumors.

Trabecular carcinoid. Primary trabecular carcinoid tumors of the ovary are usually found in association with mature cystic teratoma, but may sometimes occur in pure form. They are less common, than the insular type and only 20 cases have been recorded [29, 32]. The age distribution is similar to that ot the insular type, and the presenting symptoms are similar, except that the trabecular carcinoids in common with carcioid tumors of foregut or hindgut derivation are not associated with the carcinoid syndrome [29, 32]. Macroscopically they are similar to the insular carcinoid, forming a solid tumor mass which usually forms a part of mature cystic teratoma. The tumors are unilateral, but may sometimes coexist with mature cystic teratoma in the contralateral ovary.

Microscopically the tumor is composed of long wavy cords, ribbons or trabeculae running in parallel and surrounded by dense fibrous connective tissue stroma (Fig. 26). The cords are composed of one or two cell layers, and the cells have an ample amount of cytoplasm often containing orange to brown-red granules which stain positively with argyrophil stains. The nuclei are prominent, elongated, or ovoid. Mitoses are present, but are few in number. Ultrastructurally the cells contain neurosecretory granules, which are round or oval and uniform in size. Trabecular carcinoid of the ovary is not associated with metastases and therefore the prognosis is very favorable following the excision of the tumor. [29, 32]

Struma ovarii and carcinoid (strumal carcinoid). Struma ovarii and carcinoid is a tumor composed of thyroid tissue intimately admixed with carcinoid tumor, which in most cases shows the trabecular pattern. Struma ovarii and carcinoid is uncommon, but approximately 50 cases have been reported [26, 32]. The tumor has the same age incidence as the two types of ovarian carcinoid described above. It is not associated with the carcinoid syndrome.

Macroscopically this tumor shows similar features to insular and trabecular carcinoids. It may be a part of a mature cystic teratoma or may occur in a pure form. Microscopically it is composed of thyroid follicles which are usually small, merging with carcinoid tumor showing trabecular pattern [26, 32] (Fig. 27). Although some investigators have stated that the whole lesion represents a carcinoid tumor [12, 18, 24], it has been demonstrated by others that the thyroid follicles do contain thyroglobulin, confirming their thyroid nature [11, 53]. The tumor has only once been associated with metastases, and even in this case the patient was cured. In all other cases excision of the tumor resulted in a complete cure.

Mucinous (goblet, adenocarcinoid) carcinoid. Primary mucinous carcinoid is a newly described entity which is mainly observed in the vermiform appendix [14, 34, 54]; only rarely has it been observed in the ovary. On the other hand, it is considered that at least some cases described as primary Krukenberg tumors of the ovary have been examples of this entity.

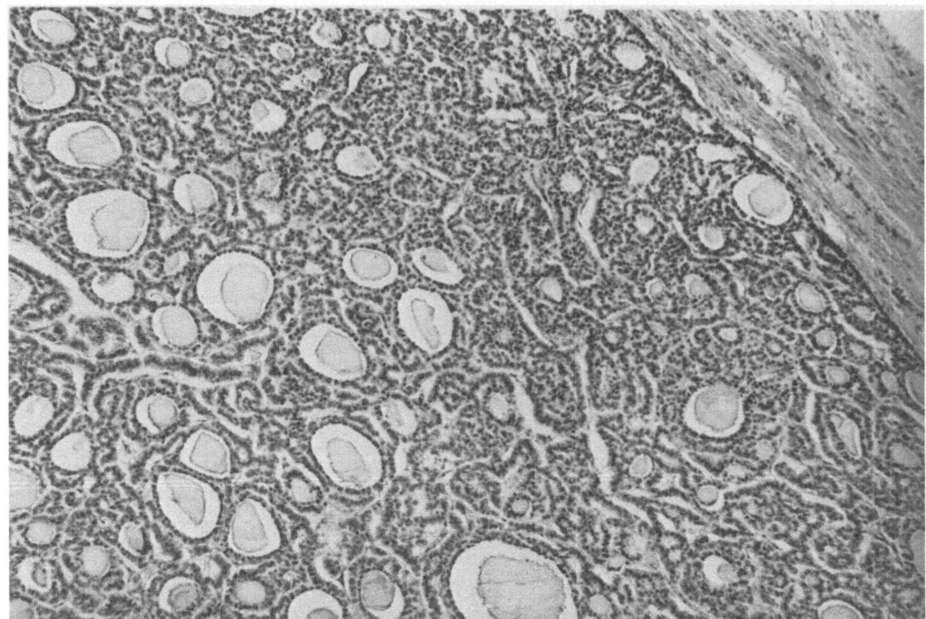

Fig. 27. Struma ovarii and carcinoid composed of thyroid follicles intimately admixed with cords of trabecular carcinoid. HE, ×150

In the ovary the tumor has been seen in younger patients than is the case with other types of primary ovarian carcinoid. It is usually seen in a pure form, but may be associated with teratomatous elements. The tumor is unilateral, but may be associated with metastatic lesions in the contralateral ovary.

Macroscopically the tumor is usually of considerable size and solid, but may contain cystic areas. Microscopically it is composed of numerous small glands lined by uniform cells distended with mucin and containing small round or oval nuclei (Figs. 28 and 29). The glands usually contain very small lumina. Some cells may be disrupted due to overdistention with the mucinous material. The glands are surrounded by stroma, which may vary from dense to loose and edematous. Some glands may be larger and some large cystic glands may also be present. Small pools of mucin are also seen. In some areas the tumor cells assume a signet-ring appearance, and this type of cell may predominate. In some areas the tumor cells form larger aggregates, show more atypical features, contain larger nuclei, and exhibit brisk mitotic activity. The mucinous carcinoid is more malignant than other carcinoid tumors. It tends to spread via the lymphatics and metastases may be present at the time of surgery. In such cases the treatment is surgical, followed by combination chemotherapy which includes 5-fluorouracil.

Argyrophil and sometimes argentaffin granules may be detected with the help of special stains. The number of granules is small and they are less evident than in the other types of carcinoid tumor. Ultrastructurally neurosecretory granules are observed in some of the cells. It is of interest that cells containing neurosecretory granules do not contain mucinous material and vice versa.

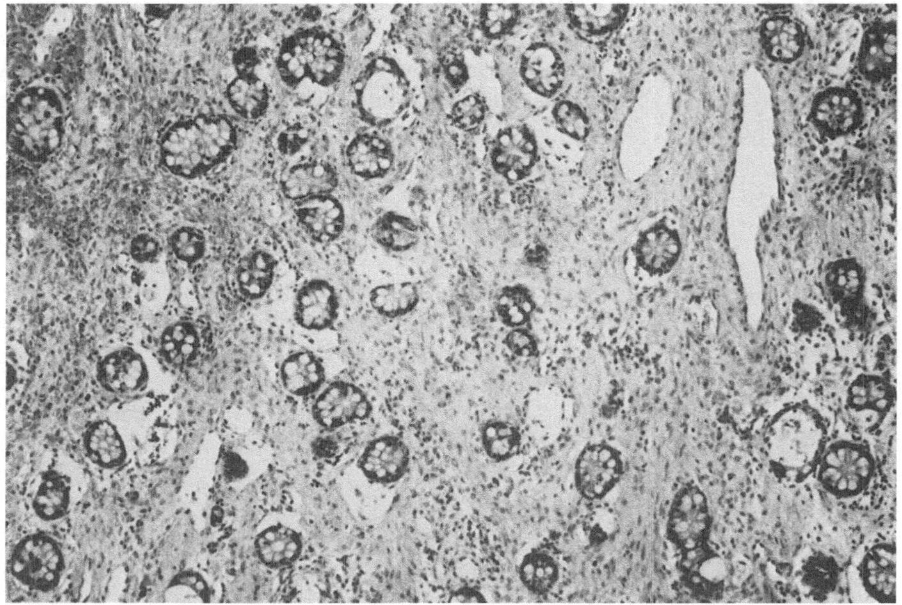

Fig. 28. Mucinous carcinoid composed of numerous small glands scattered within connective tissue. HE, ×90

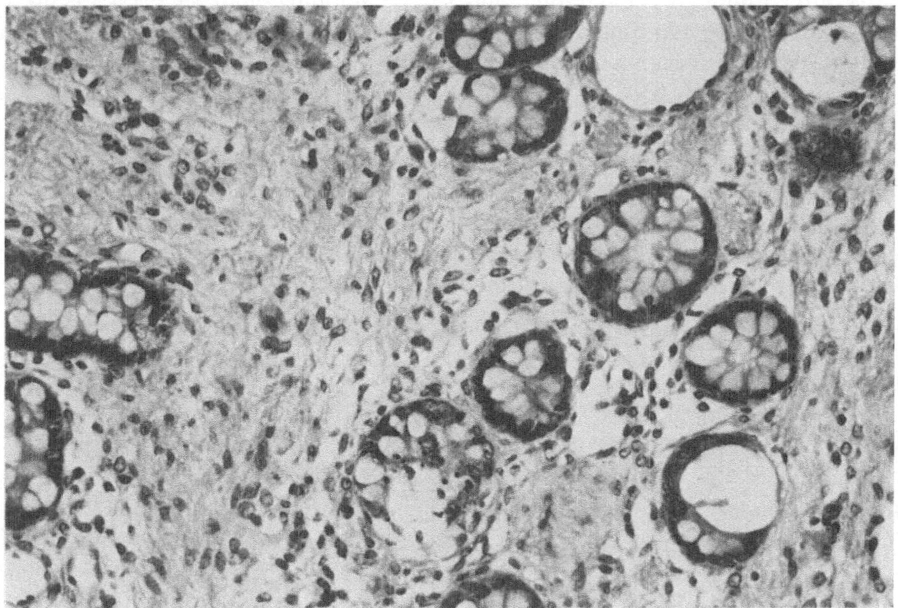

Fig. 29. Mucinous carcinoid. Higher magnification showing the tumor cells and presence of mucin. HE, ×360

Metastatic carcinoid. The ovary is also affected by metastases from carcinoid tumors, in most cases insular carcinoids of midgut origin, but occasionally also from carcinoids of foregut and hindgut origin and mucinous carcinoids. In these cases both ovaries are usually affected and the tumor deposits are scattered diffusely throughout the ovaries [27].

Other Types of Monodermal Teratoma

There are other types of monodermal teratoma occurring in the ovary and these have been described in larger texts [8, 32, 38]. It need only be mentioned in this context that approximately 10%–15% of mucinous tumors of the ovary which show intestinal differentiation are probably of teratomatous origin.

Mixed Germ Cell Tumors

Under the heading of mixed germ cell tumors are included all those composed of more than one germ cell element. Although tumors of this type have been considered uncommon, in recent years more extensive and judicious sampling of germ cell tumors has meant that many more germ cell neoplasms have been found to belong to this category [17, 38, 42]. It should be emphasized that germ cell neoplasms should always be extensively sampled, taking at least one section for each centimeter of the widest diameter of the tumor, as well as taking sections from any differing parts of the tumor. If possible the approximate amounts of all the elements present within the tumor should be quantitated and described in the report, thus giving an estimate of the exact composition of the tumor.

Tumors Composed of Germ Cells and Sex Cord Stroma Derivatives

Tumors composed of germ cells intimately admixed with sex cord stroma derivatives are uncommon. They are divided into two specific types: (a) gonadoblastoma, and (b) mixed germ cell-sex cord stroma tumor.

Gonadoblastoma

Gonadoblastoma occurs predominantly in young phenotypic females, and 80% of cases occur in this group. The remaining 20% of cases occur in phenotypic male pseudohermaphrodites. The majority of phenotypic females with gonadoblastoma (60%) show evidence of virilization. The great majority of patients with gonadoblastoma (96%) are chromatin-negative and have a Y chromosome. The most common karyotypes are 46XY, 46X/46XY and various other forms of mosaicism [31].

Gonadoblastoma has been reported in occasional subjects with Turner's syndrome or true hermaphroditism, and in females with normal 46XX karyotype. The

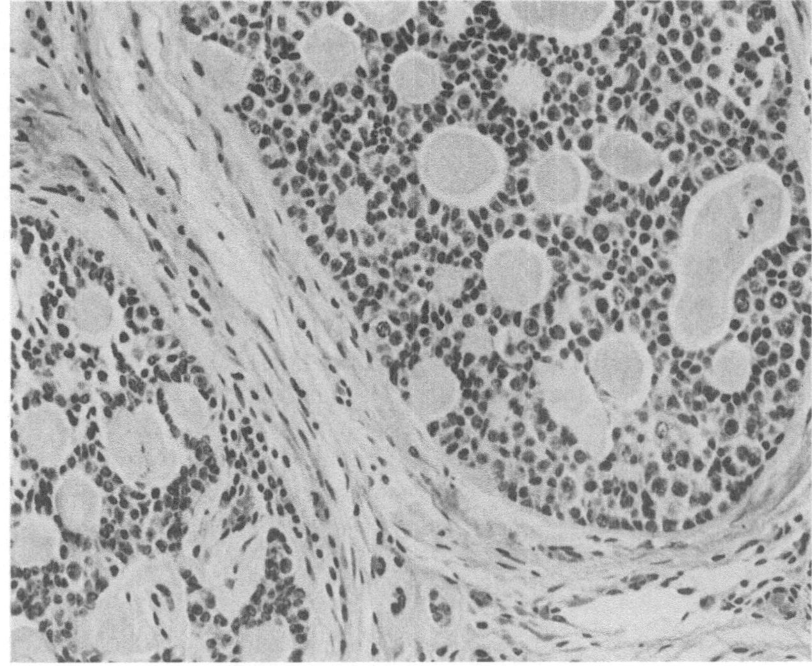

Fig. 30. Gonadoblastoma composed of tumor nests. Numerous hyaline Call-Exner-like bodies are in evidence. HE, ×150

gonad of origin is frequently indeterminate, but when discernible is a testis or a streak gonad. The contralateral gonad is either a testis, a streak, or a gonad of indeterminate nature [31].

Macroscopically gonadoblastomas form usually small or very small, solid, firm or hard, frequently partly calcified nodules. Microscopically gonadoblastoma presents a typical histologic pattern and is composed of collections of small cellular nests surrounded by connective tissue stroma (Fig. 30). The cellular nests contain a mixture of germ cells and sex cord derivatives resembling immature Sertoli and granulosa cells [30, 31]. These immature Sertoli and granulosa cells are arranged within the cell nests in three typical patterns:

1. They line the periphery of the nests in a coronal pattern
2. They surround individual or collections of germ cells
3. They surround small spaces containing amorphous hyaline eosinophilic and PAS-positive material resembling Call-Exner bodies.

Mitotic activity is seen in the germ cells but is not observed in the immature Sertoli and granulosa cells. The connective tissue stroma, which is usually dense, frequently contains collections of cells indistinguishable from Leydig cells, or luteinized cells of ovarian stromal origin. The amount of these cells is variable. Reinke crystalloids have not been demonstrated in these cells. The basic pattern of gonadoblastoma may be altered by hyalinization, calcification, and overgrowth by other neoplastic germ cell elements, usually dysgerminoma. All these processes are frequently seen in gonadoblastoma and may lead to distortion and obliteration of the gonadoblastoma nests. The resultant picture may be the presence of round, smooth, calcified concretions, or foci of hyalinization with calcific concretions surrounded by dysgerminoma. The histologic picture of gonadoblastoma has never been observed in metastatic lesions or outside the gonads. In at least 50% of cases gonadoblastoma is admixed with or overgrown by dysgerminoma, and in 10% of cases by other more malignant germ cell elements [31]. The prognosis in cases of gonadoblastoma associated with dysgerminoma is favorable, and metastases are rare. On the other hand, the prognosis is poor when gonadoblastoma is overgrown by more malignant germ cell elements [37].

As gonadoblastoma is frequently bilateral, careful investigation of the patient and excision of the contralateral gonad is mandatory. The contralateral gonad may harbour a minute gonadoblastoma, which may become overgrown by malignant neoplastic germ cell elements. A gonad containing gonadoblastoma is nonfunctional and as it contains a potentially malignant lesion it should be excised.

Mixed Germ Cell-Sex Card Stroma Tumor

Mixed germ cell-sex cord stroma tumor is a recently established entity which, like gonadoblastoma, is composed of germ cells intimately admixed with sex cord

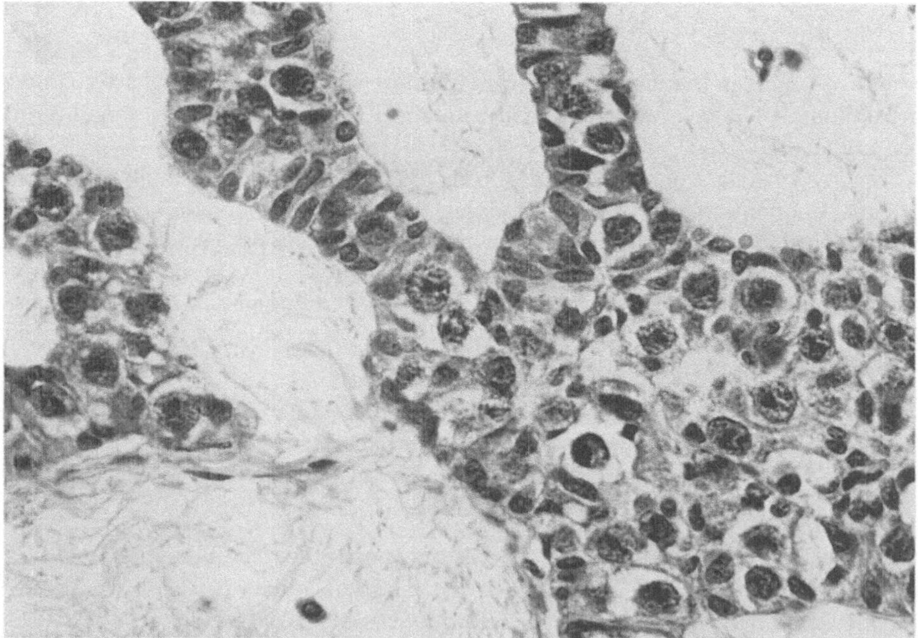

Fig. 31. Mixed germ cell-sex cord stroma tumor showing cord-like pattern. The cords or trabeculae expand forming large cellular aggregates. Note the large round germ cells and elongated sex cord derivatives. HE, ×600

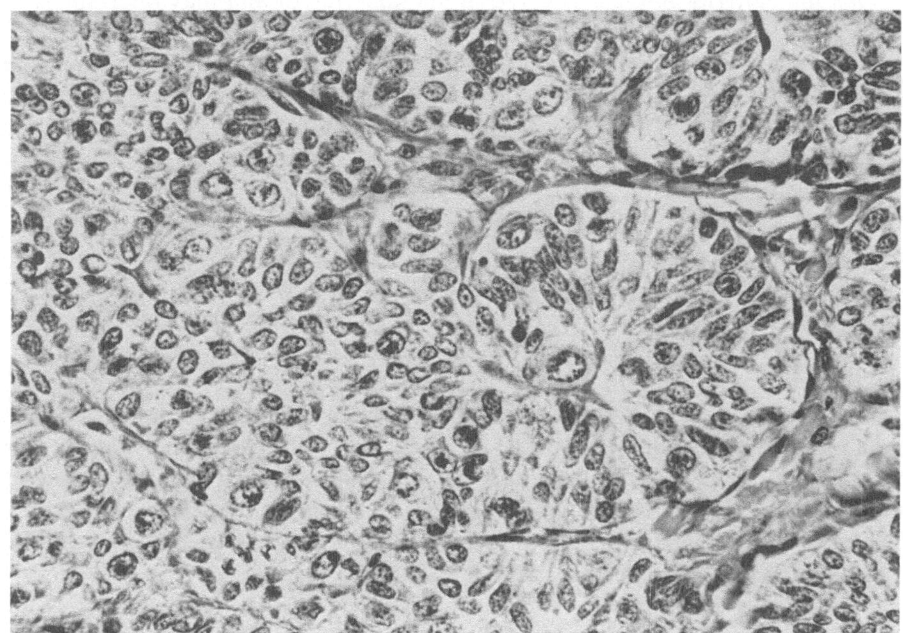

Fig. 32. Mixed germ cell-sex cord stroma tumor composed of tubular structures without a lumen and surrounded by fine connective tissue septa. Note the large germ cells and smaller sex cord derivatives. HE, ×460

stroma elements, but differs from it histologically, clinically, genetically, and endocrinologically [35, 36]. Mixed germ cell-sex cord stroma tumor is most frequently seen in normal ovaries of phenotypically and genetically normal female infants and children. It also occurs in ovaries of genetically normal young women, and in normally descended testes of phenotypically, anatomically, and genetically normal adult males, who are often elderly [38, 39].

Macroscopically the tumors are large, especially when compared with gonadoblastoma. They are round or oval, solid, firm, and gray-white. Microscopically the germ cell-sex cord stroma tumor is composed of germ cells intimately admixed with sex cord derivatives, which show greater resemblance to Sertoli cells than to granulosa cells (Figs. 31 and 32). The tumor may exhibit three different histologic patterns:

1. Composed of long, narrow, ramifying cords. or trabeculae, which in places expand forming large, round or oval cellular aggregates, or wide columns, which are surrounded by connective tissue stroma varying from loose and edematous to dense and hyalinized (Fig. 31)
2. Composed of solid, turbular structures devoid of a lumen and surrounded by fine connective tissue septa (Fig. 32)
3. Composed of large aggregates of germ cells and sex cord stroma derivatives devoid of any specific arrangement.

All the patterns may be observed in the same tumor and may intermingle with each other. The two components, the germ cells and the sex cord derivatives, are intimately admixed with each other, although in some areas sex cord elements may predominate, while in others there is a preponderance of germ cells. There is active proliferation, and mitotic activity is seen in the germ cells as well as in the sex cord derivatives. There are no regressive changes such as hyalinization and calcification, and no Call-Exner-like hyaline bodies. Cystic spaces lined by flattened epithelium or sex cord elements, and containing pale eosinophilic secretion, may be seen in some tumors and may occasionally be prominent [38, 39]. Presence or overgrowth by dysgerminoma is rare, and has been observed only when the tumor was encountered in patients in the third decade [39]. There were no metastases. The treatment of choice is excision of the tumor, or one-sided salpingo-oophorectomy. All the patients with this tumor, including those whose tumor was combined with dysgerminoma, are well and disease-free following this treatment, from a few months to 12 years. One patient, a girl of 8 years, who has been followed up for 9 years, is now menstruating normally. Two patients with this tumor had isosexual precocious puberty, which regressed following the excision of the tumor. The contralateral gonad was found to be normal in all cases [38, 39]. The prognosis is favourable following the excision of the affected adnexa.

References

1. Asadourian IA, Taylor HB (1969) Dysgerminoma. An analysis of 105 cases. Obstet Gynecol 33:370
2. Brody S (1961) Clinical aspects of dysgerminoma of the ovary. Acta Radiol (Stockh) 56: 209
3. Burkons DM, Hart WR (1978) Ovarian germinomas (dysgerminomas). Obstet Gynecol 51:221
4. Caruso PA, Marsh MR, Minkowitz S, Karten G (1971) An intense clinicopathologic study of 305 teratomas of the ovary. Cancer 27: 343
5. Chenot M (1911) Contribution a l'etude des epitheliomas primitifs de l'ovaire. Thesis, Paris
6. Dixon FJ, Moore RA (1952) Tumors of the male sex organs. Atlas of tumour pathology, Section VIII, Fasc. 31B and 32. Armed Forces Institute of Pathology, Washington, D. C.
7. Einhorn LH, Donohue J (1977) Cis-diamine dichloroplatinum, vinblastine, and bleomycin combination chemotherapy in disseminated testicular cancer. Ann Intern Med 87:293
8. Fox H, Langley FA (1976) Tumours of the ovary. Heinemann Medical Books, London
9. Gitlin D, Pericelli A (1970) Syntheses of serum albumin, pre-albumin, alphafetoprotein, alpha-1-antitrypsin and transferrin by the human yolk sac. Nature 228:995
10. Gitlin D, Pericelli A, Gitlin G (1972) Synthesis of alpha-fetoprotein by liver, yolk sac and gastro-intestinal tract of the human conceptus. Cancer Res 32:979
11. Greco MA, LiVolsi VA, Pertschuk LP, Bigelow B (1979) Strumal carcinoid of the ovary; an analysis of its components. Cancer 43:1380
12. Hart WR, Regezi JA (1978) Strumal carcinoid of the ovary. Ultrastructural observations and long term follow up study. Am J Clin Pathol 69:356
13. Itoh T, Shirai T, Naka A, Matsumato S (1974) Yolk sac tumour and alpha-fetoprotein. Clinicopathological study of four cases. Gann 65:215
14. Klein HZ (1974) Mucinous carcinoid tumour of the vermiform appendix. Cancer 33:770
15. Kurman RJ, Norris HJ (1976) Endodermal sinus tumour of the ovary. A clinical and pathologic analysis of 71 cases. Cancer 38:2404

16. Kurman RJ, Norris HJ (1976) Embryonal carcinoma of the ovary. A clinicopathologic entity distinct from endodermal sinus tumour resembling embryonal carcinoma of the adult testis. Cancer 38:2420
17. Kurman RJ, Norris HJ (1976) Malignant mixed germ cell tumours of the ovary. A clinical and pathologic analysis of 30 cases. Obstet Gynecol 48:57
18. Livnat EJ, Scommegna A, Recant W, Jao W (1977) Ultrastructural observations of the so-called strumal carcinoid of the ovary. Arch Pathol Lab Med 101:585
19. Meyer R (1931) The pathology of some special ovarian tumours and their relation to sex characteristics. Am J Obstet Gynecol 22:697
20. Novak ER, Woodruff JD (1967) Gynecologic and obstetric pathology, 6th edn. Saunders, Philadelphia
21. Pantoja E, Rodriguez-Ibanez I, Axtmayer RW, Noy MA, Pelegrina I (1975) Complications of dermoid tumours of the ovary. Obstet Gynecol 45:89
22. Peterson WT (1957) Malignant degeneration of benign cystic teratomas of the ovary: A collective review of the literature. Am J Obstet Gynecol 72:793
23. Peterson WF, Prevost EC, Edmunds FT, Huntley JM Jr, Morris FU (1955) Benign cystic teratomas of the ovary. A clinicostatistical study of 1007 cases with review of the literature. Am J Obstet Gynecol 70:368
24. Ranchod M, Kempson RL, Dorgeloh JR (1976) Strumal carcinoid of the ovary. Cancer 37:1913
25. Robboy SJ, Scully RE (1970) Ovarian teratoma with glial implants on the peritoneum. An analysis of 12 cases. Hum Pathol 1:643
26. Robboy SJ, Scully RE (1980) Strumal carcinoid of the ovary: An analysis of 50 cases of a distinctive tumour composed of thyroid tissue and carcinoid. Cancer 46:2119
27. Robboy SJ, Scully RE, Norris HJ (1974) Carcinoid metastatic to the ovary. A clinicopathologic analysis of 35 cases. Cancer 33:798
28. Robboy SJ, Norris HJ, Scully RE (1975) Insular carcinoid primary in the ovary-a clinicopathologic analysis of 48 cases. Cancer 36:404
29. Robboy SJ, Scully RE, Norris HJ (1977) Primary trabecular carcinoid of the ovary. Obstet Gynecol 49:202
30. Scully RE (1953) Gonadoblastoma. A gonadal tumour related to dysgerminoma (germinoma) and capable of sex hormone production. Cancer 6:455
31. Scully RE (1970) Gonadoblastoma. A review of 74 cases. 25:1340
32. Scully RE (1979) Tumours of the ovary and maldeveloped gonads. Atlas of tumour pathology, 2nd Series, Fascicle 16. Armed Forces Institute of Pathology, Washington D.C.
33. Serov SF, Scully RE, Sobin LH (1973) Histological typing of ovarian tumours. International histological classification of tumours, No. 9. WHO, Geneva
34. Subbuswamy SG, Gibbs NM, Ross CF, Morson BC (1974) Goblet cell carcinoid of the appendix. Cancer 34:338
35. Talerman A (1972) A mixed germ cell-sex cord stroma tumour in a normal female infant. Obstet Gynecol 40:473
36. Talerman A (1972) A distinctive gonadal neoplasm related to gonadoblastoma. Cancer 30:1219
37. Talerman A (1974) Gonadoblastoma associated with embryonal carcinoma. Obstet Gynecol 43:138
38. Talerman A (1977) Germ cell tumours of the ovary. Chapter 26. In: Blaustein, A (ed) Pathology of the female genital tract. Springer, Berlin Heidelberg New York
39. Talerman A (1980) Pathology of gonadal neoplasms composed of germ cells and sex cord stroma derivatives. Pathol Res Tract 170:24
40. Talerman, A. Unpublished observations
41. Talerman A, Haije WG (1974) Alpha-fetoprotein and germ cell tumours. A possible role of yolk sac tumour in production of alpha-fetoprotein. Cancer 34:1722
42. Talerman A, Huyzinga WT, Kuipers T (1973) Dysgerminoma, Clinicopathologic study of 22 cases. Obstet Gynecol 41:137
43. Talerman A, Haije WG, Baggerman L (1978) Serum alphafetoprotein (AFP) in diagnosis and management of endodermal sinus (yolk sac) tumour and mixed germ cell tumour of the ovary. Cancer 41:272

44. Teilum G (1944) Gonocytoma; Homologous ovarian and testicular tumours; 1; with discussion of "mesonephroma ovarii" (Schiller: Am J Cancer 1939). Acta Pathol Microbiol Scand 23:242
45. Teilum G (1950) "Mesonephroma ovarii", (Schiller) extraembryonic mesoblastoma of germ cell origin in ovary and testis. Acta Pathol Microbiol Scand 27:249
46. Teilum G (1959) Endodermal sinus tumours of the ovary and testis. Comparative morphogenesis of the so-called mesonephroma ovarii (Schiller) and extraembryonic (yolk sac-allantoic) structures of rat's placenta. Cancer 12:1092
47. Teilum G (1965) Classification of endodermal sinus tumour (mesoblastoma vitellinum) and so-called "embryonal carcinoma" of the ovary. Acta Pathol Microbiol Scand 64:407
48. Teilum G (1976) Special tumours of the ovary and testis. Comparative histology and identification, 2nd edn. Munksgaard, Copenhagen
49. Teilum G, Albrechtsen R, Norgaard-Pedersen B (1975) The histogenetic-embryomic basis for reappearance of alphafetoprotein in endodermal sinus tumours and teratomas. Acta Pathol Microbiol Scand [A] 83:80
50. Thurlbeck WM, Scully RE (1960) Solid teratoma of the ovary. Cancer 13:804
51. Tsuchida Y, Saito S, Ishida M, Ohmi K, Urano Y, Endo Y, Oda T (1973) Yolk sac tumour and alpha fetoprotein. A report of three cases. Cancer 32:317
52. Tsuchida Y, Kaneko M, Yokomori K et al. (1978) Alphafetoprotein, prealbumin, albumin, alpha-1-antitrypsin and transferrin as diagnostic and therapeutic markers for endodermal sinus tumours. J Pediatr Surg 13:25
53. Ueda G, Sato Y, Yamasaki M et al. (1978) Strumal carcinoid of the ovary. Histological, ultrastructural, and immunohistological studies with anti-human thyroglobulin. Gynecol Oncol 6:411
54. Warkel RL, Cooper PH, Helwig EB (1978) Adenocarcinoid, a mucin producing carcinoid tumor of the appendix. A study of 39 cases. Cancer 42:2781
55. Woodruff JD, Rauh JT, Markley RL (1966) Ovarian struma. Obstet Gynecol 27:194

Advances in Germ Cell Tumors of the Ovary

P. M. MOUNT and H. J. NORRIS [1]

Introduction

Malignant germ cell tumors are uncommon. In the past, their diagnostic criteria were not well established; reported series consisted of small heterogeneous mixtures of different tumors and therapeutic efforts met with little success. Until recently, germ cell tumors have been poorly understood.

Modern understanding of malignant germ cell tumors began with the pioneering comparative pathology studies of Teilum (reviewed by Teilum 1976). Further advances were made with the recognition that histologically pure tumors, unlike the combinations and mixtures reported earlier, have characteristic behaviors. Several new tumors have been recognized, requiring revision of older classifications. Embryonal carcinoma has been defined, and the category of gonadoblastoma has been revised. The WHO classification of ovarian neoplasms (Serov et al. 1973) established standard nomenclature and histologic criteria for pure tumors which have become generally accepted. This classification, applied in conjunction with more aggressive clinical staging procedures, has provided a uniform basis for understanding the behavior of malignant germ cell tumors and for predicting their response to therapy. The most important discovery has been the recognition that modern chemotherapy protocols produce a dramatic improvement in survival rates for patients with germ cell malignancies. Finally, the discovery of refined radioimmunoassays have led to the identification of alpha-fetoprotein (AFP) and human chorionic gonadotropin (HCG) as tumor markers in the diagnosis and management of germ cell tumors. Detected in the serum by use of highly specific and sensitive radioimmunoassays, these markers can reveal occult metastases and tumor recurrences before they become clinically evident (Kurman et al. 1979). Because certain marker patterns are frequently associated with specific tumor types, markers also may have diagnostic and prognostic value (Kurman et al. 1979).

1 Department of Gynecologic and Breast Pathology, Armed Forces Institute of Pathology, Washington, D.C. 20306, USA

The opinions and assertions contained herein are the private views of the author and are not to be construed as official or as reflecting the views of the Department of the Army or the Department of Defense

Based largely on experience with nearly 400 malignant germ cell tumors at the Armed Forces Institute of Pathology (AFIP) in Washington, DC, this review emphasizes new developments in the field. Pathologists must be taught that where a particular histologic type of tumor is described, this means a histologically proven *pure* tumor. It is no longer acceptable to bracket various types of mixed malignant germ cell tumors; to do so would only perpetuate the confusion of earlier years. Accurate classification of germ cell malignancies requires adequate sampling of the tumor. One block of tissue should be taken for every centimeter of maximum diameter.

Dysgerminoma

Dysgerminoma is rare in infants, but it is the commonest ovarian malignancy of children, adolescents, and pregnant women, and is the commonest associated with gonadoblastoma in dysgenetic gonads. The association with pregnancy is as high as 17% in some studies (Krepar et al. 1978). Only 4% of patients are over 40 years old (Asadourian and Taylor 1969). Dysgerminoma is the only malignant germ cell tumor that is regularly stage Ib. Eighty-six percent of stage I tumors are Ia (visibly confined to one ovary), and 14% are stage Ib (confined to both ovaries) (Asadourian and Taylor 1969). Although most of the stage Ib disease is macroscopically obvious at operation, nearly one-third of grossly normal contralateral ovaries contain micro-

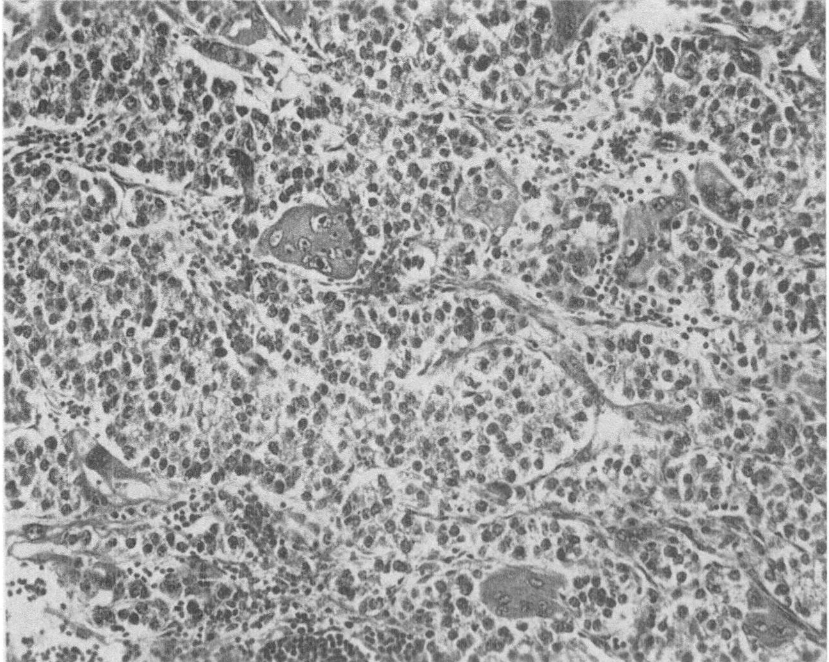

Fig. 1. Syncytiotrophoblastic giant cells in dysgerminoma. H&E, ×160

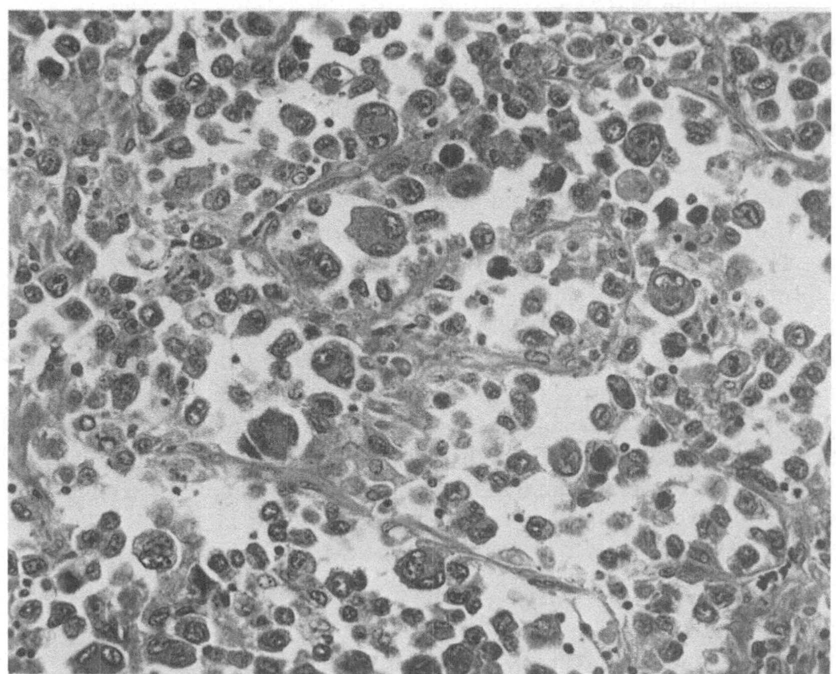

Fig. 2. Cytologic atypia and pleomorphism in anaplastic dysgerminoma. Mitotic activity is not evident in this field. H & E, ×250

scopic areas of dysgerminoma. This has important therapeutic implications. Obviously, biopsy of the contralateral ovary is indicated in dysgerminoma and in all malignant germ cell tumors that might contain dysgerminoma because of the existence of mixed tumors which contain occult areas of dysgerminoma overlooked at the time of frozen section.

Ordinarily, dysgerminoma has a distinctive microscopic appearance, identical with that of seminoma arising in the testis and the mediastinal, sacrococcygeal, and pineal regions. It is composed of cells that resemble primordial germ cells morphologically, histochemically, and ultrastructurally, but that tend to be smaller. About 20% of dysgerminomas contain foreign body type giant cells which, like the presence of a diffuse lymphocytic infiltrate, appear to correlate with a better prognosis (Asadourian and Taylor 1969).

Two distinctive subtypes of dysgerminoma have recently been recognized: a dysgerminoma with syncytiotrophoblastic giant cells (SGCS) and the anaplastic dysgerminoma. Approximately 3% of the dysgerminomas accessioned at the AFIP contain SGCS (Fig. 1), but a third of those have occurred in mixed germ cell tumors (Zaloudek et al. 1981). Production of HCG by SGCS has been documented by immunoperoxidase reactions. Serum elevation of HCG may cause this tumor to be clinically confused with ectopic pregnancy, embryonal carcinoma, or choriocarcinoma. The SGCS in dysgerminoma lack the two-cell population of admixed syncytiotrophoblast and cytotrophoblast found in choriocarcinoma. Thus, by growing convention, the SGCS are not sufficient by themselves for a diagnosis of choriocarcinoma. It is important to recognize dysgerminoma with SGCS as a subtype because as in choriocarcinoma serum HCG levels can be used to monitor the efficacy of therapy. Although few cases have been reported, all of the patients have had stage Ia tumors and none is known to have recurred over a follow-up period of from 1 to 19.5 years (Zaloudek et al. 1981). Thus, there is no evidence that the presence of SGCS alters the relatively good prognosis of an ordinary dysgerminoma.

The anaplastic dysgerminoma (Fig. 2) is analogous with anaplastic seminoma of the testis. It has the overall pattern of a dysgerminoma but with cellular pleomorphism, multinucleated cells, and increased numbers of mitotic figures. At present, few anaplastic dysgerminomas have been reported (Gillespie and Arnold 1978), and it is not yet possible to determine whether this is a distinctive subtype requiring more aggressive therapy. In one study Creasman et al. (1979) concluded that the prognosis is worse when anaplastic dysgerminoma is treated with surgery alone, but the value of resorting to chemotherapy rather than irradiation in stage I disease is not proven. The prognostic significance of testicular anaplastic seminoma is also unsettled. Some groups have reported a higher mortality rate, while others have identified no difference from ordinary seminoma (Mostofi 1980).

Endodermal Sinus Tumor

Endodermal sinus tumor is the second commonest ovarian malignant germ cell tumor after dysgerminoma in girls and young women (Norris and Jensen 1972). It represents about 1% of all ovarian malignancy. Originally confused with carcinoma of mesonephroid type (clear cell carcinoma), endodermal sinus tumors have been increasingly diagnosed, but collected series of pure tumors are still small.

The five interrelated growth patterns of endodermal sinus tumor have been described in detail by Teilum (1976). They include the reticular (microcystic), the endodermal sinus (festoon), the solid-cellular, the alveolar-glandular, and the polyvesicular vitelline patterns. There is no prognostic difference between the types and in approximately a third of cases the growth patterns are mixed (Kurman and Norris 1976 a). Schiller-Duval bodies, diagnostic of endodermal sinus tumor, are absent in one-fourth of tumors. Schiff PAS-positive hyaline droplets are always present, however (Kurman and Norris 1976 a). Immunochemical methods have established that some of these droplets contain AFP, but alpha-antitrypsin and other proteins are also present (Kurman and Norris 1976 a; Kurman et al. 1979).

Endodermal sinus tumors constitute a surgical and therapeutic emergency. The tumor growth rate is probably the fastest of any human malignancy, and some patients have had normal pelvic examinations a week before the removal of a large tumor. Prior to the advent of modern chemotherapy, the overall mortality was over 90% (Kurman and Norris 1976 a). Irradiation has no effect on this tumor. Aggressive chemotherapy with triple drug regimens such as vincristine, actinomycin D, and cyclophosphamide (VAC regimen), or similar protocols, is a major advance in medicine and is significantly changing the prognosis (Slayton et al. 1978). A survival rate greater than 50% over postoperative intervals of between 11 and 63 months (which includes some patients with stage III disease) has been achieved. Because stage Ib tumors are virtually nonexistent, the opposite ovary and uterus can be preserved in young patients with stage Ia neoplasms. Serial serum AFP determinations can be used to monitor the effectiveness of chemotherapy and to detect subclinical recurrences.

Immature Teratoma

Pure immature teratoma is the third most common malignant germ cell tumor of the ovary after dysgerminoma and endodermal sinus tumor (Norris and Jensen 1972). It represents nearly one-quarter of all ovarian germ cell tumors in children under 15 years old. The diagnosis of immature (malignant) teratoma is properly reserved for a pure teratoma that contains variable amounts of immature tissue derived from any of the three germ cell layers (Norris et al. 1976). In pure form, HCG is not produced. AFP is produced only in primitive areas of endodermal or hepatic differentiation. Generally, the presence of these markers within the tumor or the patient's serum is indicative of a mixed germ cell tumor (Kurman et al. 1979). In the past, much of the germ cell tumor literature, particularly in relation to testicular tumors, has not made a distinction between pure teratoma and neoplasms with combinations of malignant germ cell elements. Older reports also did not recognize that immaturity conveys metastatic potential. Immature teratoma should also be distinguished from those malignancies which arise in otherwise mature and benign teratomas. These tumors arise most frequently in postmenopausal women, and in up to three-quarters of cases consist of squamous cell carcinoma developing in the epidermal component (Scully 1979).

It has been established that immaturity in teratomas indicates a potential for recurrence and metastasis which is directly related to the degree of immaturity and the quantity of immature tissue present in the tumor. These two aspects of immaturity – degree and quantity – are combined in grading of an immature teratoma. Typically, a variety of immature tissues in different stages of maturity is present. The commonest element and easiest to grade is the neural tissue. Norris et al. (1976) proposed a simple quantitative method, amplifying that of Robboy and Scully (1970):

Grade 0: Wholly mature tissue
Grade 1: Abundant mature tissue but some immaturity, mainly glial, with loose, primitive mesenchyma. Mitoses are present, but neuroepithelium is absent or restricted to one low-power field (4 mm diameter) per slide
Grade 2: Greater immaturity, with neuroepithelium not exceeding three low-power fields per slide
Grade 3: Severe immaturity, with neuroepithelium found in four or more low-power fields per slide and frequently merging with sarcomatous stroma.

Modern triple agent chemotherapy is a notable advance and is curative in half of patients with advanced disease. Patients with stage I, grade 2 or grade 3 neoplasms require adjunctive chemotherapy. Chemotherapy is also probably indicated for any ruptured stage I tumor (Norris et al. 1976). Once metastasis has occurred, the grade of the metastasis is the major prognostic determination. Thorough sampling of metastases is, therefore, important for prognosis and therapy. Patients with stage II and III disease from grade 0 metastases all survive after surgery. They, therefore, need no treatment other than excision of the ovarian primary and debulking of the implants. It is not known to what extent mature deposits may continue to grow superficially. Grade 1 or 2 metastases imply 50% survival. No patient with grade 3 metastases has survived without modern chemotherapy. Irradiation has been abandoned as a therapeutic adjunct for immature teratomas.

Monodermal and Highly Specialized Teratomas

Struma ovarii, carcinoid tumors, and strumal carcinoids are the most common tumors in this category. The group also encompasses a variety of rare and unique neoplasms including highly malignant primitive neural tumors and sebaceous gland tumors. It is possible that some mucinous tumors, squamous neoplasms, and malignant mesenchymal tumors also have a teratomatous origin, but these are generally placed in other categories of ovarian neoplasms (Scully 1979).

Struma ovarii is a form of teratoma in which thyroid tissue represents more than half of the tumor. Clinical hyperthyroidism occurs in some patients, but the frequency of hyperfunction in ovarian struma is unknown. Although the malignancy rate in struma is stated to be 5%–10% (Yannopoulos et al. 1976), this figure is exaggerated. Many "malignant" strumas are now recognized as strumal carcinoids which are seldom malignant (Scully 1979). Thyroid tissue is not encapsulated in teratomas, giving a false impression of invasion. Peritoneal implants of benign thyroid tissue (strumosis) occur infrequently in struma and should not be confused with malignancy. Even papillary processes have no proven significance in ovarian thyroid tissue. Thus, the diagnosis of malignant struma ovarii should only be made when there is cytologic evidence of malignancy or documented metastases.

Carcinoid tumors of the ovary occur in pure form and admixed with other teratomatous elements. Carcinoids can be regarded as very low grade malignancies which have very limited potential for spread. Ninety percent remain confined to the ovary. In pure form ovarian carcinoid they must be distinguished from metastatic carcinoid. This distinction can be difficult, but primary ovarian carcinoids are unilateral and rarely have metastases (Scully 1979). Urinary 5-hydroxy-indoleacetic acid levels, when elevated, usually return to normal following excision of the ovary.

Both the insular (midgut) and trabecular (foregut and hindgut) forms of carcinoid occur in the ovary, depending on the type of tissue from which the carcinoid arises (Robboy et al. 1975, 1977). Argentaffin granules are identified in over 80% of the former and two-thirds of the latter type. Carcinoid syndrome develops only in the larger insular forms and is present in about one-third of cases. Because ovarian venous blood passes directly to the inferior vena cava, bypassing hepatic detoxification, presence of the carcinoid syndrome does not imply metastatic disease.

The strumal carcinoid includes tumors composed of thyroid tissue and carcinoid. These elements are usually admixed, but may be only contiguous. Mucinous elements are frequently present, suggesting that multidirectional differentiation of endodermal derivatives is occurring within the tumor (Scully 1979). Only one malignant example has been documented among more than 30 reported.

Despite being a newly described entity, the strumal carcinoid has been the subject of controversy. Several ultrastructural studies have challenged the view that the follicular component represents thyroid tissue (Livnat et al. 1977; Ranchod et al. 1976). All of the cells examined in these studies had ultrastructural characteristics of carcinoid cells. It is possible that the areas studied were ones in which the cells had biphasic characteristics, or perhaps carcinoid cells had invaded and replaced the normal follicular lining cells. Other investigators have identified calcium oxalate crystals typical of thyroid tissue, and immunofluorescent methods document the presence of thyroglobulin within the follicles (Greco et al. 1979; Ueda et al. 1978).

The identification of calcitonin in strumal carcinoids by immunoperoxidase methods has led to the suggestion that they represent medullary carcinomas of thyroid type (Greco et al. 1979). Although there is a histologic similarity, there is insufficient evidence to support this view. Strumal carcinoids do not behave clinically like thyroid medullary carcinomas, and calcitonin has been demonstrated in intestinal carcinoids where an association with parafollicular C cells is dubious (Scully 1979).

Embryonal Carcinoma

Morphologically analogous to embryonal carcinoma of the adult testis (Fig. 3), embryonal carcinoma of the ovary has only recently been characterized as a distinct clinicopathologic entity (Kurman and Norris 1976b). In the past, embryonal carcinoma was included with endodermal sinus tumor and both designations were used indiscriminately. The distinction between embryonal carcinoma and endodermal sinus tumor can be made on clinical, histologic, and immunochemical grounds. Microscopically, embryonal carcinoma is composed of solid sheets of large, primitive pleomorphic cells with amphophilic vacuolated cytoplasm and vesicular nuclei with one or more nucleoli. These cells may form gland-like spaces and clusters, but the reticular, polyvesicular vitelline, and festoon growth patterns of endodermal sinus tumor are not formed unless the tumor is a mixed germ cell neoplasm with an endodermal sinus tumor component. All embryonal carcinomas contain isolated clusters of syncytiotrophoblastic cells and mononuclear cells containing hyaline droplets. These different cell lines secrete HCG (Fig. 4) and AFP (Fig. 5) respectively, as demonstrable by immunoperoxidase methods in tissue sections. The tumor markers can also be demonstrated in serum by radioimmunoassay. Patients developing embryonal carcinoma are a few years younger on average than patients with endodermal sinus tumor. Because HCG is produced, precocious puberty is common in younger patients. It is less malignant than endodermal sinus tumor, and more patients are encountered with stage I neoplasms. The 5-year survival rate for patients with stage I disease prior to modern chemotherapy is 50% as compared with 7%–10% for those with endodermal sinus tumor.

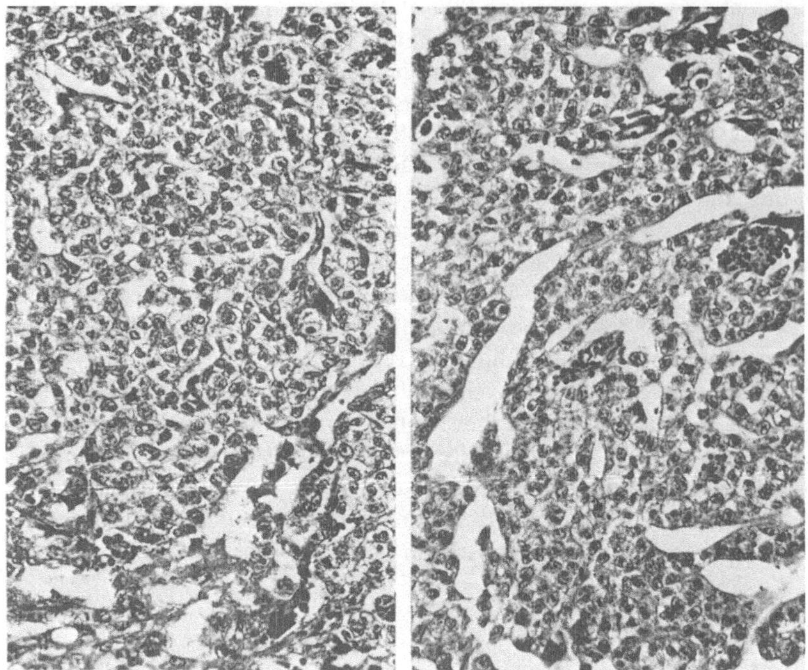

Fig. 3. Solid proliferation of primitive cells with gland-like clefts in embryonal carcinoma of ovary (*right*) and testis (*left*). H&E, ×160

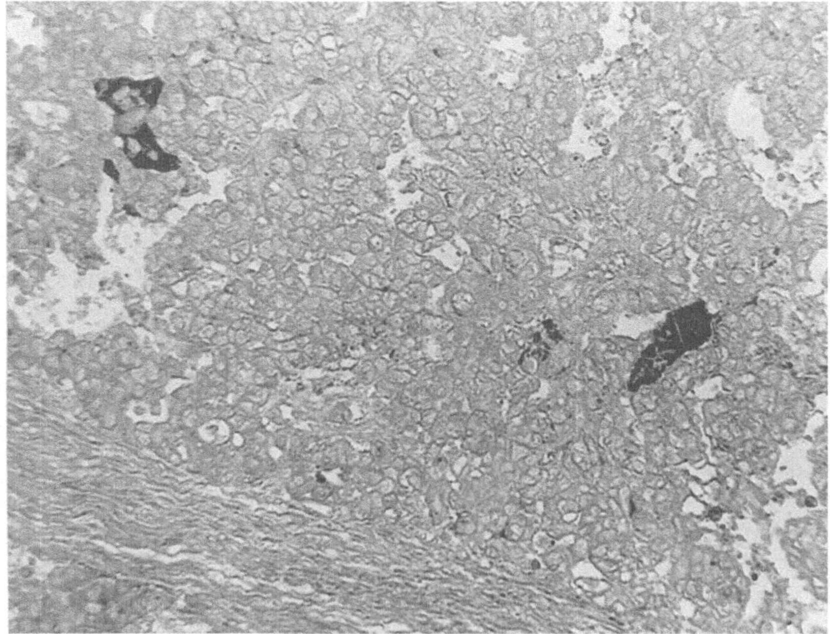

Fig. 4. Embryonal carcinoma. Positive immunoperoxidase reaction for HCG in syncytiotrophoblastic giant cells. Kurman and Norris 1976b, ×42

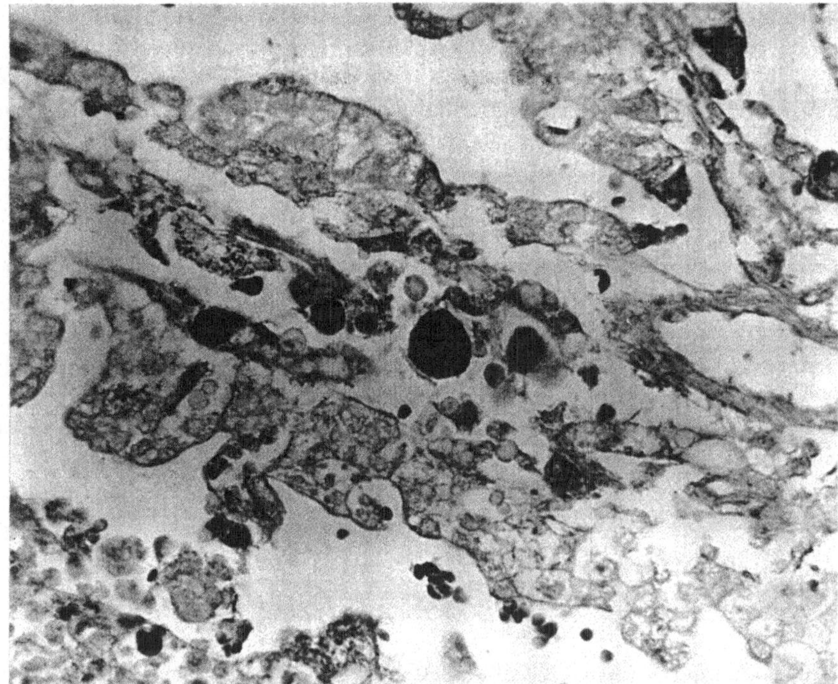

Fig. 5. Embryonal carcinoma. Positive immunoperoxidase reaction for AFP. Kurman and Norris 1976b, ×200

Choriocarcinoma

Primary ovarian choriocarcinoma is extremely rare and is most commonly a component of a mixed germ cell tumor (Fox and Langley 1976). When pure, it is more likely to be gestational than derived from germ cells. If it is gestational, a primary uterine or tubal malignancy is more likely than a primary choriocarcinoma arising in an ovarian pregnancy. To have been unequivocally derived from germ cells, the tumor should have arisen in a prepubertal child. In older reports, nongestational choriocarcinoma of the ovary has not been as amenable to methotrexate-based therapy as gestational choriocarcinomas of the uterus. It is probable, however, that some cases either represented misdiagnosed embryonal carcinoma or were poorly sampled combinations and mixtures of malignant germ cell tumors. Modern therapy is based on surgical excision and combination chemotherapy including methotrexate (Gerbie et al. 1975).

Mixed Germ Cell Tumors

Mixed germ cell tumors contain a combination of two or more malignant components. Approximately 8% of malignant germ cell tumors accessioned at the AFIP are of the mixed type (Kurman and Norris 1976c). Because of inadequate sampling in many instances, this figure probably underestimates slightly the frequency of mixed forms. In the testis, mixtures comprise 32%–40% of all germ cell tumors.

The most common component is dysgerminoma, found in 80% of mixed germ cell tumors, followed by endodermal sinus tumor in 70%, immature teratoma in 53%, choriocarcinoma in 20%, and embryonal carcinoma in 13% (Kurman and Norris 1976c). In two-thirds of tumors, only two malignant components are present. Mixtures of dysgerminoma and endodermal sinus tumor are the most common, representing a third of the combination tumors.

The most important factors in predicting the prognosis in stage I disease are the size and composition of the neoplasm (Kurman and Norris 1976c). If more than one-third of a stage I tumor is composed of endodermal sinus tumor, choriocarcinoma or grade 3 teratoma, the prognosis is poor, whereas if it contains less than one-third of these components or contains combinations of dysgerminoma, embryonal carcinoma or grade 1 or 2 teratoma, the outlook is more favourable. Patients with tumors less than 10 cm in diameter are likely to survive, regardless of the composition of the tumor. Modern treatment depends upon surgical excision, proper sampling, and a choice of combinations of chemotherapeutic agents based upon histologic evaluation of all elements present.

Mixed Germ Cell and Sex Cord Stromal Tumors

This category includes tumors composed of mixtures of germ cells and neoplastic gonadal stromal cells. The majority of these tumors are gonadoblastomas. Although the gonadoblastoma is not new, it is becoming better understood. What is new is the small number of tumors with clinical and pathologic features distinct from gonadoblastoma recently described as mixed germ cell-sex cord stroma tumors (Talerman tumor).

Gonadoblastoma arises almost exclusively in dysgenetic gonads (Scully 1970). Over 80% of patients are phenotypic females who are frequently virilized. Although a Y chromosome has been demonstrated in over 90% of patients, gonadoblastoma has been reported in patients with a 46XX karyotype, some of whom have been fertile (Garvin et al. 1976). This latter group may represent patients with gonadal mosaicism.

The most common tumor to arise in dysgenetic gonads, approximately 50% of gonadoblastomas are overgrown by dysgerminoma and an additional 10% are associated with endodermal sinus tumor, embryonal carcinoma, or choriocarcinoma (Scully 1979). While the prognosis for dysgerminoma in gonadoblastoma is favorable, none of the patients with one of the more malignant forms of germ cell tumor has survived more than 18 months. Presumably modern chemotherapy, selected on the basis of adequate histologic examination, will improve this prognosis. Because of the high incidence of malignancy, phenotypic females with a Y chromosome should have a bilateral gonadectomy (Scully 1979).

Mixed germ cell–sex cord stroma tumors of a type other than gonadoblastoma were described originally by Talerman (1972a, b). Although composed of a mixture of germ cells and stromal elements (Fig. 6), tumors in this category are histologically

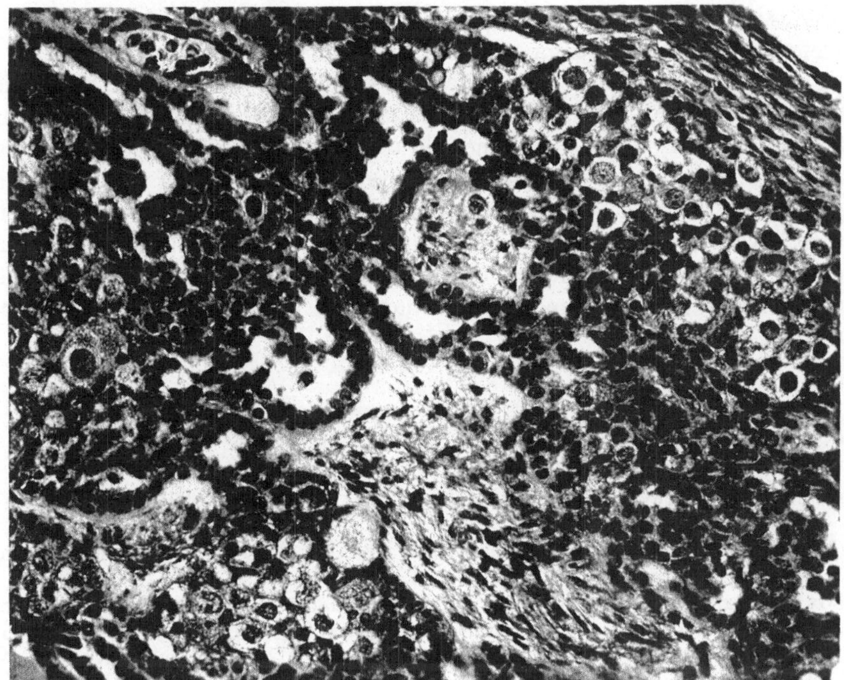

Fig. 6. Primitive germ cells and cords of stromal cells in mixed germ cell-sex cord stroma tumor. H&E, ×250

and clinically distinct from gonadoblastoma. All patients have had a normal 46XX karyotype and none have been virilized. Isosexual precocious puberty occurred in one 8-year-old girl (Talerman and van der Harten 1977), probably from abnormal endocrine activity of the stromal component. The tumors are unilateral and large. The germ cells are easy to overlook, as they appear intermingled with cells differentiating to granulosa and Sertoli cells. The gonadal stromal component may have trabecular, solid, or tubular patterns. A cord-like arrangement was present in one. Mitotic activity occurs in both the germ cell and stromal components. Biopsy of the contralateral gonad has revealed a normal ovary in these patients. Association with malignant germ cell neoplasms, common in gonadoblastoma, has not been reported in any of the forms of Talerman tumors, except for dysgerminoma in one case.

Summary

In recent years, important advances have been in the understanding of malignant germ cell tumors. Several new tumors have been described and older forms have been better delineated. Gradually it has become recognized that histologically pure types have a characteristic behavior. Because germ cell tumors may be mixed, all lesions must be thoroughly sampled and examined histologically. Only with a complete knowledge of the composition of a particular neoplasm can the proper therapy be selected on a rational basis. Adequate evaluation must include histologic evaluation of peritoneal implants and metastases, particularly in the case of immature teratoma. Biopsy of the grossly normal contralateral ovary is probably indicated in all cases and provides the only effective means of ruling out a bilateral dysgerminoma (stage Ib). Aggressive modern chemotherapy following debulking of the tumor has yielded dramatic improvals in survival rates in highly malignant neoplasms. The identification of the tumor markers HCG and AFP has opened new vistas in diagnosis, detection of occult metastases, and monitoring the response to therapy.

References

Asadourian LA, Taylor HB (1969) Dysgerminoma. An analysis of 105 cases. Obstet Gynecol 33:370–379

Creasman WT, Fetter BF, Hammond CB, Parker RT (1979) Germ cell malignancies of the ovary. Obstet Gynecol 53:226–230

Fox H, Langley FA (1976) Tumours of the ovary. Year Book Medical Publishers, Chicago

Garvin AJ, Pratt-Thomas HR, Spector M, Spicer SS, Williamson HO (1976) Gonadoblastoma: Histologic, untrastructural and histochemical observations in five cases. Am J Obstet Gynecol 125:459–471

Gerbie MV, Brewer JI, Tamimi H (1975) Primary choriocarcinoma of the ovary. Obstet Gynecol 46:720–723

Gillespie JJ, Arnold LK (1978) Anaplastic dysgerminoma. Cancer 42:1886–1889

Greco MA, LiVolsi VA, Pertschuk DO, Bigelow B (1979) Strumal carcinoid of the ovary. An analysis of its components. Cancer 43:1380–1388

Krepart G, Smith JP, Rutledge F,Delclos L (1978) The treatment for dysgerminoma of the ovary. Cancer 41:986–990

Kurman RJ, Norris HJ (1976a) Endodermal sinus tumor of the ovary. A clinical and pathologic analysis of 71 cases. Cancer 38:2404–2419

Kurman RJ, Norris HJ (1976b) Embryonal carcinoma of the ovary. A clinicopathologic entity distinct from endodermal sinus tumor resembling embryonal carcinoma of the adult testis. Cancer 38:2420–2433

Kurman RJ, Norris HJ (1976c) Malignant mixed germ cell tumors of the ovary. A clinical and pathologic analysis of 30 cases. Obstet. Gynecol 48:579–589

Kurman RJ, Scardino PT, McIntire KR, Waldman TA, Janadpour N, Norris HJ (1979) Malignant germ cell tumors of the ovary and testis. An immunohistologic study of 69 cases. Ann Clin Lab Sci 9:462–466

Livnat EJ, Scommegna A, Recant W, Jao W (1977) Ultrastructural observations of the so-called strumal carcinoid of the ovary. Arch Pathol Lab Med 101:585–589

Mostofi FK (1980) Pathology of germ cell tumors of the testis. A progress report. Cancer 45:1735–1754

Norris HJ, Jensen RD (1972) Relative frequency of ovarian neoplasms in children and adolescents. Cancer 30:713–719

Norris HJ, Zirkin HJ, Benson WL (1976) Immature (malignant) teratoma of the ovary. A clinical and pathologic study of 58 cases. Cancer 37:2359–2372

Ranchod M, Kempson RL, Dorgeloh JR (1976) Strumal carcinoid of the ovary. Cancer 37:1913–1922

Robboy SJ, Scully RE (1970) Ovarian teratoma with glial implants on the peritoneum. An analysis of 12 cases.Hum Pathol 1:643–653

Robboy SJ, Norris HJ, Scully RE (1975) Insular carcinoid primary in the ovary. A clinicopathologic analysis of 48 cases. Cancer 36:404–418

Robboy SJ, Scully RE, Norris HJ (1977) Primary trabecular carcinoid of the ovary. Obstet Gynecol 49:202–207
Scully RE (1970) Gonadoblastoma. A review of 74 cases. Cancer 25:1340–1356
Scully RE (1979) Tumors of the ovary and maldeveloped gonads. Atlas of Tumor Pathology, 2nd Ser, Fasc 16. Armed Forces Institute of Pathology, Washington
Serov SF, Scully RE, Sobin LH (1973) International histological classification of tumors, No. 9. Histological typing of ovarian tumours, WHO, Geneva
Slayton RE, Hreshchyshyn MM, Silverberg SG, Shingleton HM, Park RC, DiSaia PJ, Blessing JA (1978) Treatment of malignant ovarian germ cell tomors. Cancer 42:390–398
Talerman A (1972a) A distinctive gonadal neoplasm related to gonadoblastoma. Cancer 30:1219–1224
Talerman A (1972b) A mixed germ cell-sex cord stroma tumor of the ovary in a normal female infant. Obstet Gynecol 40:473–478
Talerman A, van der Harten JJ (1977) A mixed germ cell-sex cord stroma tumor of the ovary associated with isosexual precocious puberty in a normal girl. Cancer 40:889–894
Teilum G (1976) Special tumors of ovary and testis. Comparative pathology and histological identification, 2nd edn. Lippincott, Philadelphia
Ueda G, Sato Y, Yamasaki M, Inoue M, Hiramatsu K, Kurachi K, Amino N, Miyai K (1978) Strumal carcinoid of the ovary. Histological, untrastructural, and immunohistological studies with anti-human thyroglobulin. Gynecol Oncol 6:411–419
Yannopuolos D, Yannopoulos K, Ossowski R (1976) Malignant struma ovarii. In: Sommers Sc (ed) Pathology annual. Appleton-Century Croft, New York, pp 403–413
Zaloudek CJ, Tavassoli FA, Norris HJ (1981) Dysgerminoma with syncytiotrophoblastic giant cells: A histologically distinctive subtype of dysgerminoma. Am J Surg Path 5: 361–367

Follikuläre (endokrin aktive) Stromatumoren

J. H. Holzner[1]

Die Klassifikation der Ovarialtumoren basiert hauptsächlich auf histogenetischen Prinzipien. Da aber die Entwicklungsgeschichte der Keimdrüsen noch keineswegs restlos geklärt ist, schließt eine Klassifizierungsmethode auf dieser Basis von vorneherein mögliche Kontroversen ein. Diese sind jedoch weniger von praktisch-klinischer als von akademisch-wissenschaftlicher Bedeutung.

Zum Verständnis der sog. „Stromatumoren" der Gonaden sind einige Grundkenntnisse der Embryologie notwendig. Die Entwicklung der Keimdrüsenanlage erfolgt schon frühzeitig an der Vorderseite des Wolff-Körpers an der Hinterwand der Zölomhöhle. Durch Verdickung des Zölomepithels entsteht hier zunächst eine Zellaggregation, die sich bald in eine submesotheliale Zellmasse und in das diese oberflächlich überkleidende Zölomepithel differenziert. Die geschlechtliche Differenzierung der Gonaden erfolgt unter dem Einfluß genetischer Faktoren und eines lokalen Polypeptidenzyms. Bei der Entwicklung zur männlichen Keimdrüse bilden sich sehr früh sog. Keimstränge, die primitiven Samenkanälchen entsprechen. Bei weiblicher Differenzierung bleibt zunächst der Status quo erhalten. Erst später ändert auch hier ein Teil der zunächst undifferenzierten Zellen der submesothelialen Zellmasse seinen Charakter und bildet primitive Zellballen und -stränge. In der Zwischenzeit sind die Keimzellen in die Keimdrüsenanlage gewandert und nehmen wahrscheinlich auch aktiven Einfluß auf die weitere Differenzierung des Gonadenmesenchyms.

Über die Entwicklung und Differenzierung des Gonadenstroma bestehen verschiedene Anschauungen. Gillmann, Fischer, Meyer, Politzer, von Wagenen u. Simpson nehmen an, daß das indifferente Gonadenstroma direkt aus dem Zölomepithel (sog. Keimepithel) entsteht, während Pinkerton der Ansicht ist, daß es sich aus einem primitiven subzölomischen Mesenchym entwickelt.

Auch bezüglich der weiteren Differenzierung des zunächst indifferenten Gonadenstroma in einen epithelartigen Anteil (Granulosazellen und Sertoli-Stütz-zellen) und in einen mesenchymalen (Thekazellen und Leydig-Zwischenzellen) sind die Meinungen geteilt. Novak et al. (1971) sowie Busby u. Anderson (1957) nehmen eine Entstehung dieser beiden Gewebsanteile aus einem einheitlichen Muttergewebe an. Morris u. Scully (1958) sind der Auffassung, daß sich Thekazellen, undifferenziert bleibende Stromazellen und Leydig-Zwischenzellen aus der subzölomischen Zellmasse entwickeln, während Granulosazellen und Sertoli-Stützzellen Abkömmlinge des oberflächlichen Zölomepithels sind.

---

1 Institut für Pathologische Anatomie der Universität Wien, A-1090 Wien

Die verschiedenen Auffassungen haben auch zu unterschiedlichen Benennungen der aus diesen Geweben entstehenden Neoplasmen geführt. Die Vertreter der erstgenannten Anschauung sprechen von „gonadalen Stromatumoren“ oder „Keimdrüsenmesenchymomen“, während Scully die Bezeichnung „Sex cord – mesenchyme tumors“ vorschlägt. Die WHO hat aus beiden Nomenklaturvorschlägen einen Kompromiß gezogen und die Bezeichnung „Sex cord – stromal tumors“ (Keimstrang-Keimdrüsenstroma-Tumoren) eingeführt. Damit soll dem Umstand Rechnung getragen werden, daß sich diese Tumoren einerseits aus den primitiven Keimsträngen und Keimballen, andererseits auch aus dem speziellen Keimdrüsenstroma entwickeln können.

In der weiblich determinierten Keimdrüse sind die Matrix dieser Neoplasmen die Granulosazellen, Thekazellen und deren luteinisierte Varianten, in der männlich determinierten Gonade sind es die Sertoli-Stützzellen und die Leydig-Zwischenzellen. Ferner gibt es Tumoren, die sich aus nicht in eine bestimmte geschlechtliche Richtung differenzierten, sondern indifferenten Keimstrangelementen und indifferenten Stromazellen mit der Fähigkeit kollagene Fasern zu produzieren entwickeln.

In den Keimstrang-Stroma-Tumoren können alle genannten Zelltypen repräsentiert sein, in unterschiedlichem Differenzierungsgrad und in verschiedenen Kombinationen vorkommen. Es kann unterschieden werden zwischen:

a) *Reinen Keimstrangtumoren* mit einem mehr oder weniger epithelartigen Charakter (Granulosazelltumor, Sertoli-Zell-Tumor, undifferenzierter Keimstrangtumor);
b) *reine mesenchymale Tumoren* (Leydig-Zell-Tumor, Thekazelltumor, undifferenzierter Stromatumor);
c) *gemischte Tumoren* aus Keimstrangelementen und mesenchymalen Zellen;
d) *Mischformen* aus männlich und weiblich differenzierten Keimstrang- und Stromazellen.

Aus praktischen Gründen werden diese Tumoren, die etwa 6–8% aller Ovarialtumoren ausmachen, in vier Gruppen gegliedert:

I. Granulosa-Stromazell-Tumoren
II. Sertoli-Leydig-Zell-Tumoren (Androblastome)
III. Gynandroblastome
IV. Unklassifizierbare Keimstrang-Keimdrüsenstroma-Tumoren

Granulosa-Stromazell-Tumoren

Wesentliche zelluläre Komponenten dieser Tumorgruppe, für die auch eine Reihe anderer Namen verwendet werden und wurden (z. B. Granulosa-Thekazell-Tumoren, feminisierende Mesenchymome, Gynoblastome, Kahlden-Tumor u. a.), sind Granulosazellen, Thekazellen sowohl der Theca externa wie interna und kollagenbildende Stromazellen (Fibroblasten). Dementsprechend kann diese Tumorgruppe in zwei Untergruppen unterteilt werden:

a) Granulosazelltumoren und
b) Thekoma-Fibrom-Gruppe (Thekom, Fibrom, unklassifizierbare Varianten dieser Gruppe).

Granulosazelltumor

Wesentlicher und repräsentativer Zellanteil dieser Neoplasmen sind Zellelemente, die Granulosazellen entsprechen. Daneben können jedoch in unterschiedlicher, aber nicht repräsentativer Menge auch Thekazellen und faserbildende Stromazellen enthalten sein.

Granulosazelltumoren sind unter den Ovarialtumoren mit weniger als 2%, unter den malignen mit weniger als 10% vertreten (Scully 1968). Sie kommen in allen Altersgruppen vor, jedoch nur selten vor der Pubertät.

Makroskopisch können sie solide oder zystisch, oft auch multizystisch sein und haben meist eine mehr oder weniger deutlich gelbe Farbe. In den Zysten findet sich seröser Inhalt oder Blut. Bei Ruptur von Zysten kann ein Hämatoperitoneum entstehen.

Histologisch können verschiedene Typen, jedoch ohne prognostische Signifikanz, unterschieden werden:

a) Ein *mikrofollikulärer Typ* mit zahlreichen, von Granulosazellen radiär umgebenen Call-Exner-Körperchen;
b) ein *makrofollikulärer Typ,* der größere Zysten bildet und einem Graaf-Follikel ähnlich sieht;
c) ein *trabekulärer Typ* mit soliden Zellbalken;
d) ein *insulärer Typ* mit karzinoidähnlichen Zellbändern und -inseln, umgeben von Stroma- und Thekazellen;
e) ein *„watered-silk“-Typ,* bei dem ein Mosaik von in Reihen angeordneten Granulosazellen an gewässerte Seide erinnert;
g) ein diffuser (sarkomatoider, parenchymatöser) Typ mit dichtliegenden ungeordneten Granulosazellen, zwischen denen nur andeutungsweise manchmal Call-Exner-Körperchen erkennbar sind.

Die Tumorzellen enthalten meist wenig Zytoplasma, so daß die Kerne dicht beisammen liegen. Nur bei luteinisierten Formen ist das Zytoplasma reichlich entwikkelt, eosinophil oder vakuolisiert und deutlich begrenzt. Die typischen, meist runden oder ovalen Kerne besitzen keine auffälligen Nukleolen, zeigen jedoch eine charakteristische Längsfurchung, durch welche sie kaffeebohnenartiges Aussehen erhalten. Manchmal können sie eine stärkere Polymorphie und vermehrt Mitosen zeigen.

Der Stromaanteil ist außerordentlich variabel. Bei zellreichem Stroma ist eine Differenzierung zwischen Granulosazellen und Stromazellen durch Darstellung der Retikulinfaser meist leicht möglich.

Dickersin u. Scully (zitiert nach Scully 1979) haben bei jugendlichen Patientinnen eine Sonderform (*„juveniler Granulosazelltumor“*) beschrieben, die in der

Hauptsache aus großen unreifen Granulosazellen und Thekazellen aufgebaut ist, in denen reichlich Lipide nachweisbar sind.

Manchmal sind Übergänge zwischen Granulosazellen und Thekazellen zu sehen, was als möglicher Hinweis auf eine Entstehung aus einer gemeinsamen Mutterzelle sein könnte (s. S. 96).

Differentialdiagnostisch sind solide undifferenzierte Karzinome (diffuser Typ), kleinalveoläre Adenokarzinome (tubulärer Typ) und Karzinoide (insulärer Typ), ferner auch undifferenzierte Androblastome (s. S. 101) abzugrenzen.

Besondere klinische Bedeutung haben die endokrinen Wirkungen der Granulosazelltumoren infolge ihrer Produktion von Östrogenen. Die Mehrzahl der präpubertalen Granulosazelltumoren führen zur Pubertas praecox. In der reproduktiven Phase stehen Zyklusstörungen (Amenorrhöen und Metrorrhagien), aber auch Endometriumhyperplasien oder endometriale Karzinome im Vordergrund. Nach der Menopause manifestiert sich die endokrine Aktivität des Tumors vor allem im Auftreten von Metorrhagien, als deren morphologisches Substrat eine Hyperplasie oder ein Karzinom des Endometriums vorliegt. Auch andere Effekte des Hyperöstrogenismus (z. B. Ausreifung des Vaginalepithels) sind diagnostisch verwertbar.

Granulosazelltumoren sind maligne Tumoren, jedoch mit einer relativ langen Überlebenserwartung. Kottmeier (1953) berichtet über 88%, Norris u. Taylor (1968) über 93% 10-Jahres-Überlebensquoten. Bei einem Teil der Patienten traten jedoch auch nach 10 Jahren Rezidive auf, so daß diese Zahlen über die tatsächliche Dignität wenig aussagen. Wenn auch der histologische Typ wenig prognostische Signifikanz hat, so scheinen diffuse sarkomatoide Typen i. allg. eine kürzere Lebenserwartung aufzuweisen als differenzierte follikuläre und trabekuläre Formen. Die Rezidive sind meist auf Abdomen und Becken beschränkt, hämatogene Fernmetastasen werden selten beobachtet (Lunge, Leber, Knochen, Gehirn).

Thekom

Die etwa 1% aller Ovarialtumoren ausmachenden Thekome (auch: Thekazelltumoren, Fibroma thecocellulare xanthomatodes, Löffler-Priesel-Tumor) werden meist im höheren Lebensalter und nur sehr selten vor der Pubertät beobachtet.

Makroskopisch sind Thekome derbe, faserige, weißlich-gelbliche bis orangefarbene Bildungen, die manchmal auch multinodulär und bilateral auftreten können.

Histologisch sind die typischen Thekome aus ovalen oder spindeligen Zellen mit runden Kernen und blassem vakuolisiertem, lipidhaltigem Zytoplasma aufgebaut. Dazwischen finden sich kollagenbildende Bindegewebszellen und oft girlandenförmige hyaline Bänder. Luteinisierte Thekome mit Haufen von Zellen, die sowohl Thekalutein- wie Stromaluteinzellen imitieren, sind oft schwierig von Leydig-Zell-Tumoren abzugrenzen, besonders vom stromalen Typ dieser Neoplasmen. Ferner sind Übergangsformen zwischen Thekomen und Fibromen möglich.

Die endokrinologische Wirkung der Thekome entspricht jener der Granulosazelltumoren. Wegen der Seltenheit dieser Neoplasmen vor der Pubertät verursachen sie nur sehr selten eine Pubertas praecox. Aszites oder Meigs-Syndrom wird nur ausnahmsweise beobachtet.

Das Thekom ist ein gutartiger Tumor. Die seltenen malignen Thekome, über die in der Literatur berichtet wird, sind nach der Auffassung von Scully (1968) eher als diffuse Granulosazelltumoren oder Fibrosarkome einzustufen.

Die Differentialdiagnose von Fibromen, Stromahyperplasie der Ovars, Hyperthekose und stromalem Leydig-Zell-Tumor kann manchmal große Schwierigkeiten bereiten.

Fibrom

Etwa 4% der Ovarialtumoren sind Fibrome, die alle Altersgruppen, besonders aber die mittleren Lebensalter betreffen.

Das Fibrom des Ovars nimmt unter den kollagenbildenden Tumoren eine Sonderstellung ein, so daß die Annahme der Abkunft dieses Tumors von den gonadalen Stromazellen zu Recht besteht. Zwischen Fibrom und Thekom bestehen fließende Übergänge, so daß die Zuordnung eines Tumors der Grenzzone oft willkürlich erfolgt.

Zum Unterschied vom typischen Thekom ist das Fibrom gewöhnlich weißlich, fest-faserig und oft ödematös oder zystisch. Verkalkungen und Bilateralität sind möglich.

Histologisch erweist sich das Ovarialfibrom als zellreicher Tumor mit spindeligen Zellen, die Fibroblasten entsprechen, und reichlich kollagenen Fasern. Manchmal zeigen die Zellbündel feuerradartige Muster, manchmal ist das Interstitium stark ödematös aufgelockert.

Differentialdiagnostisch sind vor allem Thekome (Übergangsformen) abzugrenzen, was nicht immer möglich ist, ferner nichtneoplastische Ovarialveränderungen wie das massive Ovarialödem (ödematöses Fibrom), die Stromahyperplasie und die Hyperthekose.

Klinisch verhält sich das Fibrom gutartig, ist aber häufig mit Aszites (besonders größere Tumoren), seltener mit Aszites und Hydrothorax (Meigs-Syndrom) vergesellschaftet. Maligne Fibrosarkome werden wie andere maligne mesenchymale Tumoren (Leiomyosarkome, Rhabdomyosarkome, Chondrosarkome und osteogene Sarkome) den unspezifischen Ovarialtumoren zugeordnet.

Unklassifizierbare Tumoren der Thekom-Fibrom-Gruppe

Dazu gehören vor allem Übergangsformen zwischen Thekomen und Fibromen, die aus intermediären Zelltypen, Fibroblasten und lipidhaltigen Thekomzellen aufgebaut sind und selten auch Östrogenaktivität aufweisen können. Zu dieser Gruppe wird auch der seltene *„sklerosierende Stromatumor des Ovars"*(Chalvardjian u. Scully 1973) gerechnet, der oft eine charakteristische Pseudolobulation zeigt und in seinem Lipidgehalt zwischen dem Thekom und dem Fibrom steht. Der Name beruht auf sklerosierenden Veränderungen innerhalb und außerhalb der Pseudolobuli.

Sertoli-Leydig-Zell-Tumoren (Androblastome)

Sertoli-Leydig-Zell-Tumoren sind mit weniger als 0,2% der Ovarialtumoren seltener als die feminisierenden Keimstrang-Stroma-Tumoren. Sie kommen vorwiegend bei jüngeren Patienten, meist zwischen dem 20. und 40. Lebensjahr, vor.

Makroskopisch sind sie solide oder zystische, meist gelbliche Bildungen, die – besonders die maligneren Formen – oft Blutungen und Nekrosen aufweisen.

Histologisch können verschiedene Formen aufgrund ihres Differenzierungsgrades unterschieden werden:

a) *Differenzierte Formen,* die entweder aus Sertoli-Zellen (*Sertoli-Zell-Tumor, tubuläres Androblastom, Picksches tubuläres Adenom*), aus lipidspeichernden Sertoli-Zellen (*Sertoli-Zell-Tumor mit Lipidspeicherung, Folliculome lipidique Lecene*), aus Sertoli- und Leydig-Zellen (*Sertoli-Leydig-Zell-Tumor*), aus Leydig-Zwischenzellen (*Leydig-Zell-Tumor, Hiluszelltumor*) oder aus Leydig-Zellen, eingelagert in thekomatös-fibromatöses Gewebe (*stromaler Leydig-Zell-Tumor*), aufgebaut sind. Während die Sertoli-Zellen mehr oder weniger differenzierte tubuläre Strukturen bilden, sind die lipidhaltigen Leydig-Zellen vor allem durch die Reinke-Kristalloide erkennbar.

b) *Intermediäre und undifferenzierte Androblastome* zeigen eine große Variabilität ihres histologischen Aufbaus. Sertoli-Zellen sind nur teilweise in Form tubulärer Strukturen nachweisbar, daneben bilden sie solide Nester und Trabekel und – bei undifferenzierten Typen – zellreiche Areale, die nur schwer von sarkomatoiden Typen eines Granulosazelltumors unterscheidbar sind. Dazwischen eingestreut liegen mehr oder weniger reife Leydig-Zwischenzellen mit reichlichem Zytoplasma, das Lipidvakuolen oder Lipochromgranula enthält. Reinke-Kristalloide sind meist nur selten nachweisbar. Neben undifferenzierten Sertoli-Leydig-Zell-Tumoren gibt es auch reine undifferenzierte Sertoli-Zell-Tumoren und Sertoli-Leydig-Zell-Tumoren mit heterologen Gewebseinlagerungen endodermalen oder mesodermalen Ursprungs (Muskelgewebe, Knorpel, Knochen, muzinöse Zysten u. a.).

In Abhängigkeit vom Anteil der im Tumor vorhandenen Leydig-Zwischenzellen haben die Androblastome in 70 bis 85% der Fälle einen virilisierenden Effekt, reine Sertoli-Zell-Tumoren selten auch einen Östrogeneffekt.

Ähnlich wie die Granulosa-Stromazell-Tumoren sind Rezidive relativ häufig – besonders bei den undifferenzierten Formen –, Metastasen jedoch selten. Die Fünfjahresüberlebenschance wird mit 70–90% (Scully 1968) angegeben.

Differentialdiagnostisch können Abgrenzungsschwierigkeiten gegen Granulosa-Stromazell-Tumoren (besonders sarkomatoide Typen), Klarzellenkarzinome, endometroide Karzinome, muzinöse epitheliale Tumoren und Karzinome entstehen.

Gynandroblastom

Beim echten Gynandroblastom sind feminisierende (Granulosa- und Thekazellen) und maskulinisierende (Sertoli- und Leydig-Zellen) Tumoranteile in gleicher Weise repräsentativ enthalten. Da sowohl Granulosa-Stromazell-Tumoren Sertoli- und Leydig-Zellen enthalten können, wie umgekehrt in Androblastomen weiblich differenzierte Tumoranteile vorkommen können, sind echte Gynandroblastome wahrscheinlich sehr selten, und ihre Berechtigung als eigene Tumorgruppe wird von manchen Autoren angezweifelt (Scully 1968). Die Tatsache, daß in einem Tumor sowohl weiblich determinierte wie männlich differenzierte Gonadengewebsanteile enthalten sein können, ist eine Unterstützung der Annahme, daß sich beide Gewebskomponenten aus dem gleichen Muttergewebe entwickeln.

Unklassifizierbare Keimstrang-Keimdrüsenstroma-Tumoren

Ungefähr 10% aller Tumoren der Keimstrang-Stroma-Gruppe zeigen keine eindeutige Differenzierung in männlicher oder weiblicher Richtung und bauen sich aus undifferenzierten Keimstrang- und Keimdrüsenstromaelementen auf. Wegen ihres undifferenzierten Charakters ist ihre potentielle Malignität etwas höher als bei den geschlechtlich differenzierten Tumortypen. Endokrinologisch können sie inaktiv sein oder androgene oder östrogene Wirkungen entfalten. Alle Lipidzelltumoren, deren Zellen nicht eindeutig als Luteinzellen oder Leydig-Zellen identifizierbar sind, sind dieser Tumorgruppe zuzurechnen.

Ein in der WHO-Klassifikation dieser Gruppe zugeordneter Tumor wurde erstmals 1970 von Scully als *„Keimstrangtumor mit anulären Tubuli"* beschrieben.

Er besteht aus ringförmig angeordneten Tubuli, die im Zentrum aus solidem Zytoplasma bestehen, während die peripher liegenden Kerne an der Innenseite des „Ringes" hyaline Körper umgeben und sich an der Außenseite gleichartig verhaltendes Basalmembranmaterial findet, das manchmal mit den hyalinen Körpern in direkter Verbindung steht. Die Zellen gehen manchmal in wenig differenzierte tubuläre und solide Zellareale über, die Sertoli-Zellen gleichen. Das Stroma ist oft hyalinisiert, in den Zellnestern können Verkalkungen auftreten, die Epithelzellen enthalten reichlich Lipide. Elektronenmikroskopische Untersuchungen der hyalinen Körper (Waisman et al. 1975) sprechen für deren Aufbau aus Basalmembranmaterial und unterscheidet sie damit von Call-Exner-Körperchen.

Etwa 50% dieser Tumoren sind primär multipel und dann häufig mit einem Peutz-Jeghers-Syndrom kombiniert. Bei den größeren solitären und meist nicht verkalkenden Formen fehlt diese Kombination.

Literatur

Busby T, Anderson GW (1959) Feminizing mesenchymomas of the ovary. Am J Obstet Gynecol 68:1391–1420

Chalvardjian A, Scully RE (1973) Sclerosing stromal tumors of the ovary. Cancer 31:664–670

Fischel A (1930) Über die Entwicklung der Keimdrüsen des Menschen. Z gesamte Anat 92:34–72

Gillman J (1948) The development of the gonads in man, with a consideration of the role of fetal endocrines and the histogenesis of ovarian tumors. Carnegie Inst Washington Publ 210 [Contrib Embryol] 32:81–132

Kottmeier HL (1953) Carcinoma of the female genitalia. The Abraham Flexner Lectures. Ser 11.Williams & Wilkins, Baltimore

Meyer R (1930) Handbuch der speziellen pathologischen Anatomie und Histologie. Springer, Berlin

Meyer R (1931) Pathology of some special ovarian tumors and their relation to sex characteristics. Am J Obstet Gynecol 22:697–713
Morris JM, Scully RE (1958) Endocrine pathology of the ovary. Mosby, St. Louis
Norris HG, Taylor HB (1968) Prognosis of granulosa-theca tumors of the ovary. Cancer 21:255–263
Novak ER, et al. (1971) Feminizing gonadal stromal tumors. Analysis of the granulosa-theca cell tumors of the ovarian tumor registry. Obstet Gynecol 38:701–713
Pinkerton JHM (1961) Development of the human ovary – a study using histochemical technics. Obstet Gynecol 18:152–181
Scully RE (1968) Sex cord-mesenchyme tumours. In: UICC Monographs ovarian cancer Vol 11. Springer, Berlin Heidelberg New York
Scully RE (1970) Sex cord tumor with annular tubules. A distinctive ovarian tumor of the Peutz-Jeghers syndrome. Cancer 25:1107–1121
Scully RE (1979) Tumors of the ovary and maldeveloped gonads. In: Atlas of Tumor Pathology, 2nd Ser, Fasc 16. AFIP, Washington
Serov SF, Scully RE, Sobin LH (1973) Histological typing of ovarian tumors. Internat. Histol. Classification of Tumors, 9. WHO, Geneva
Teilum G (1950) Classification of testicular and ovarian androblastoma and Sertoli cell tumor. Cancer 11:769
Teilum G (1971) Special tumors of ovary and testis. Munksgaard, Kopenhagen
Wagenen G Van, Simpson ME (1965) Embryology of the ovary and testis, Homo Sapiens and Macaca Mulatta. Yale University Press, New Haven
Waisman J (1975) The ultrastructure of a feminizing granulosa theca tumor. Am J Obstet Gynecol 123:147–150

Diskussion: Ovarialbefunde bei gesteigerter Androgenproduktion während der Gravidität

H. Pickartz: Es wird über die morphologischen Ovarbefunde bei 2 graviden Frauen berichtet, welche wegen Zeichen der Androgenisierung endokrinologisch untersucht wurden. Nach Messung stark erhöhter Testosteronwerte im peripheren Blut ergab die selektive Katheterisierung von Nebennieren- und Ovarialvenen in beiden Fällen unilateral in einer Ovarialvene eine tumorverdächtige Androgenerhöhung.

Nach der Operation sank bei beiden Patientinnen binnen einer Woche der Testosteronspiegel im peripheren Blut auf Normalwerte ab.

Die morphologische Untersuchung der ektomierten Ovarien ergab in einem Fall (14. Schwangerschaftswoche; 5,7 ng Testosteron/ml Serum) einen 10 mm großen Sertoli-Leydig-Zell-Tumor mit mäßiger Differenzierung in der ovariellen Medulla. Der zugehörige ovarielle Kortex zeigte Veränderungen im Sinne polyzystischer Ovarien, welche wir teilweise als Folge der erhöhten Androgenwerte betrachten.

Das Ovar der zweiten Patientin (19. Schwangerschaftswoche; 5,1 ng Testosteron/ml Serum) zeigte eine starke Hyperreactio luteinalis, welche mit einer erhöhten Androgenproduktion verbunden sein kann.

In der Literatur finden sich Mitteilungen über erhöhte Androgenwerte während der Gravidität. Die höchsten gemessenen Testosteronwerte im Serum betragen danach zu einem vergleichbaren Schwangerschaftstermin bis zu 4,5 ng Testosteron/ml Serum. Die Befunde unterstreichen die Problematik einer endokrinologischen Tumordiagnostik bei Verdacht auf einen androgenproduzierenden Tumor. Tumorverdächtige Testosteron-Werte bei nichtgraviden Frauen (> 1,5 ng Testosteron/ml Serum) sind während der Gravidität nur eingeschränkt aussagekräftig.

Sertoli-Leydig Cell Tumors of the Ovary

C. Y. GENTON [1]

Introduction

The Sertoli-Leydig cell tumors of the ovary, also called androblastomas, belong to the group of the sex cord stromal tumors. Although apparently pure Sertoli or Leydig cell tumors do occur, most of the androblastomas are composed of both Sertoli and Leydig cells and exhibit, at least focally, histologic features reminiscent of various developmental stages of the testis.

These tumors may have no recognizable endocrine activity, or rarely be associated with estrogenic clinical manifestations, but the majority prove to be androgenic and cause virilization. As in other gonadal stromal tumors, the microscopic features of the tumor tissue allow neither prediction of the endocrine activity nor evaluation of the degree of malignancy.

In the WHO classification (Serov and Scully 1973) these tumors are divided into three groups according to the degree of differentiation, a fourth group comprising the androblastomas that contain heterologous elements such as mucinous cysts, argentaffin cells, carcinoid, rhabdomyoblast or cartilage.

Incidence

Sertoli-Leydig cell tumors are rare and constitute well under 1% of all ovarian neoplasms. The vast majority occur in the reproductive age-group, with a peak incidence in the third decade. The youngest reported patient was 2½ years of age (Novak and Long 1965). At the other extreme is a 72-year-old woman (Genton 1978). Probably because of sterility due to excessive androgens, or because of age, or marital status, more than half of the reported patients were nulliparous at time of diagnosis. The tumor has rarely been found during pregnancy (Pedowitz and O'Brien 1960; Galle et al. 1978).

1 Pathologisches Institut der Universität (Prof. Chr. Hedinger und Prof. J. R. Rüttner) und Universitäts-Frauenklinik (Prof. W. E. Schreiner), CH-Zürich

Gross Pathology

The smallest androblastomas have microscopic dimensions and are characteristically located in the hilar region. The larger tumors may replace the ovary and form bulky masses filling the pelvis. The opposite ovary is involved in 4%–5% of patients.

The surface of the tumor is usually smooth and glistening, without adhesions to surrounding structures. Local invasion and peritoneal metastases are quite unusual; visceral metastases are exceedingly rare. The cut surface is most often grey to golden yellow, the tumor tissue being lobulated by fibrous septa. The neoplasm is generally solid and soft in consistency. Rarely cystic spaces as well as areas of hemorrhage or necrosis may be present.

Histology

The microscopic appearance of Sertoli-Leydig cell tumors depends on the grade of differentiation and may be quite variable within the same tumor. About one-fourth of the neoplasms are well differentiated, one-half are of intermediate type, and the rest are undifferentiated or so-called sarcomatoid.

The tubular adenoma first described by Pick (1905) is composed essentially of tubular structures lined by well-differentiated Sertoli cells. Some Leydig cells may be present between the tubules. In such well-differentiated tumors the Sertoli cells are cylindrical or cuboidal; their nuclei are oval with evenly distributed chromatin. The cytoplasm is generally pale eosinophilic but may contain numerous lipid vacuoles (Fig. 1).

In the intermediate type of androblastomas the Sertoli cells form solid nests, anastomosing cords, and pseudotubules (Fig. 2). Small cystic spaces reminiscent of the Call-Exner bodies in granulosa cell tumors may be present in the solid islands (Fig. 3). The moderately differentiated Sertoli cells often exhibit dark nuclei that may be somewhat pleomorphic. Mitoses are uncommon.

In the undifferentiated androblastomas the Sertoli cells are mostly spindle shaped and resemble neoplastic granulosa cells (Fig. 4). They are arranged in broad interlacing strands conferring a sarcomatous appearance on the tumor tissue. Their nuclei are oval, the chromatin is often bulky and irregularly distributed, and the nucleoli are prominent. Such neoplasms, in particular when associated with estrogenic clinical manifestations, may be misinterpreted as sarcomatoid granulosa cell tumors (Morris and Scully 1958; Kempson 1968; Genton 1981).

The neoplastic Leydig cells are histologically and biochemically identical with the ovarian hilus cells first described by Berger (1923) (Cervos-Navarro et al. 1964; Jones et al. 1967). The cytoplasm of these cells is mostly eosinophilic with occasional lipochrome granules, but may appear clear because of the presence of lipids in large amounts. Therefore the Leydig cells may be very difficult to distinguish from luteinized stromal cells as seen in ovaries with hyperthecosis. The nuclei of the Leydig cells are round and exhibit a prominent eccentric nucleolus. Conclusive evidence for the identification of Leydig cells as such can be furnished only by the presence of the crystals described by Reinke (1896). A careful search for them is therefore war-

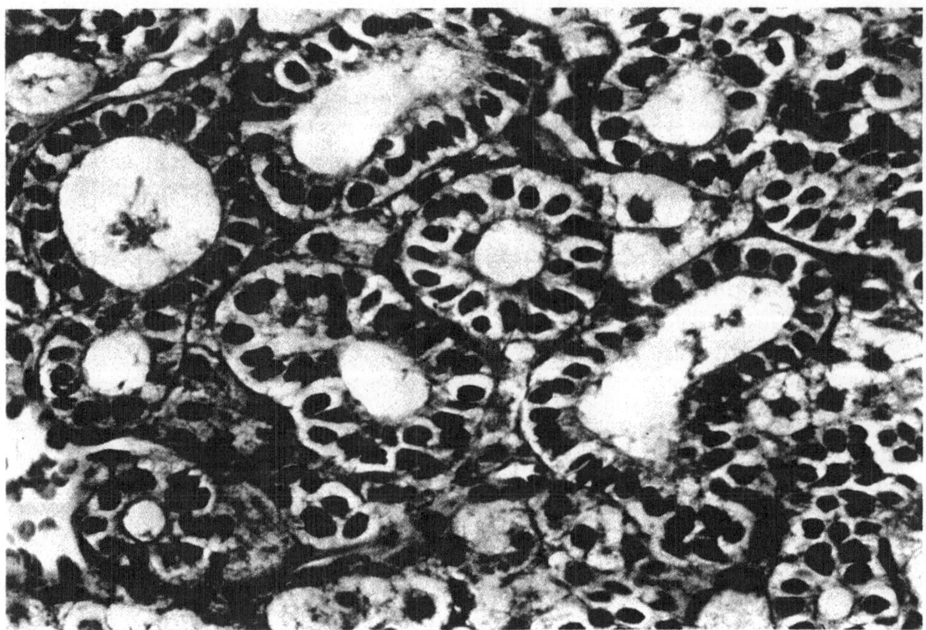

Fig. 1. Well-differentiated Sertoli-Leydig cell tumor. The Sertoli cells form obvious tubular structures and have a faintly eosinophilic cytoplasm and regular nuclei. Between the tubules a few lipid-laden Leydig cells. H & E, ×400

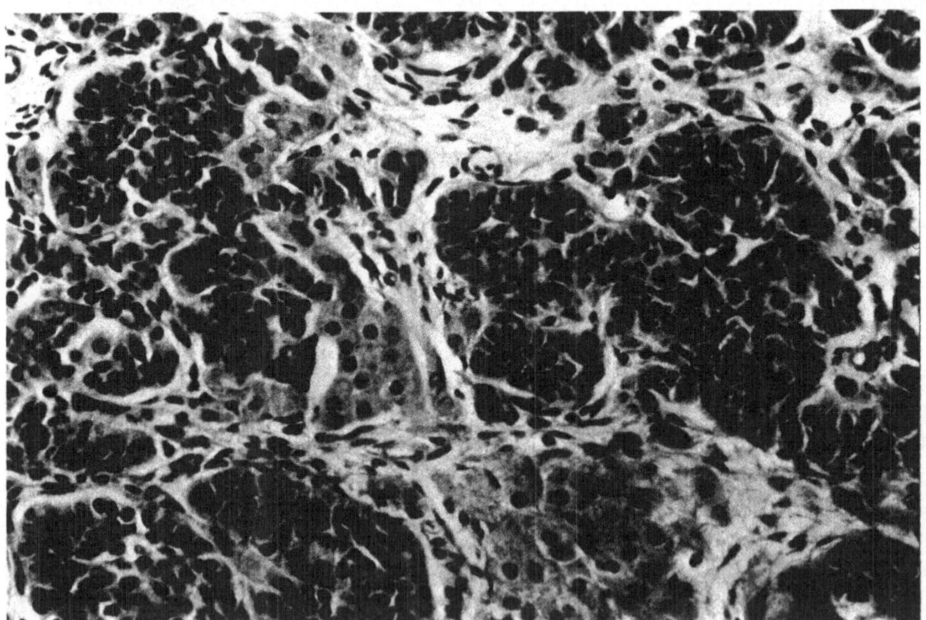

Fig. 2. Androblastoma of intermediate type. The Sertoli cells are arranged in solid cords and islands between which lie groups of typical Leydig cells. H & E, ×250

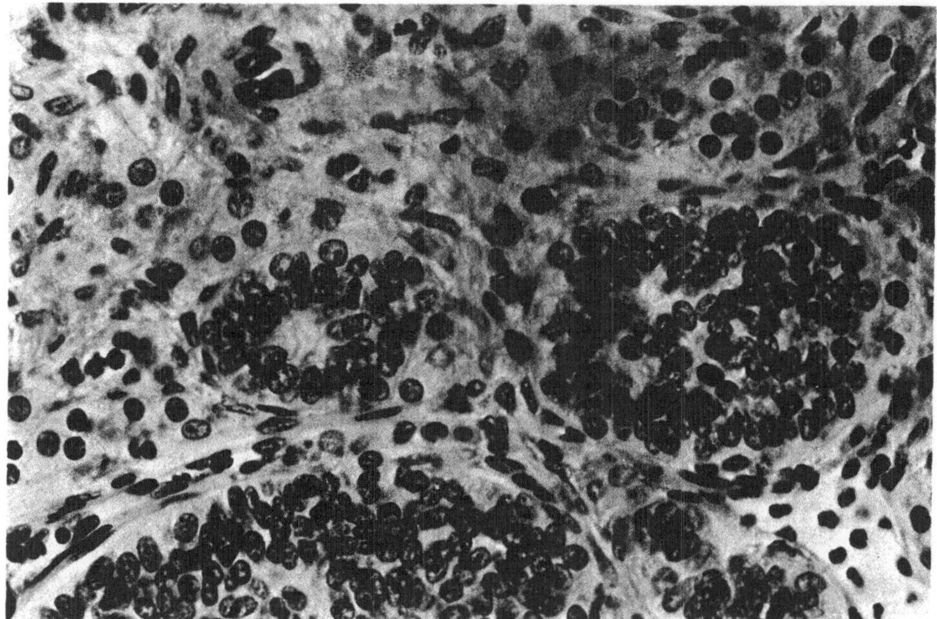

Fig. 3. Androblastoma of intermediate type. Some solid islands of Sertoli cells display cribriform structures reminiscent of Call-Exner bodies seen in granulosa cell tumors. H&E, ×400

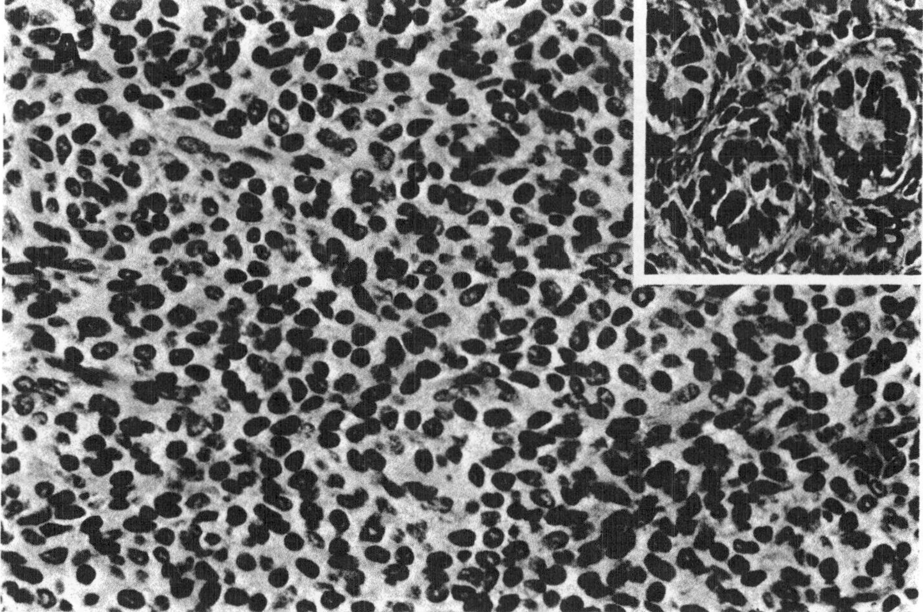

Fig. 4. A Undifferentiated or sarcomatoid type of androblastoma. Solid pattern without tubular formation. The Sertoli cells are spindle-shaped and exhibit somewhat pleomorphic nuclei. H&E, × 400. *B* In a few areas distinct tubules are present. (Same tumor as in Fig. 4 A.) H&E, ×320

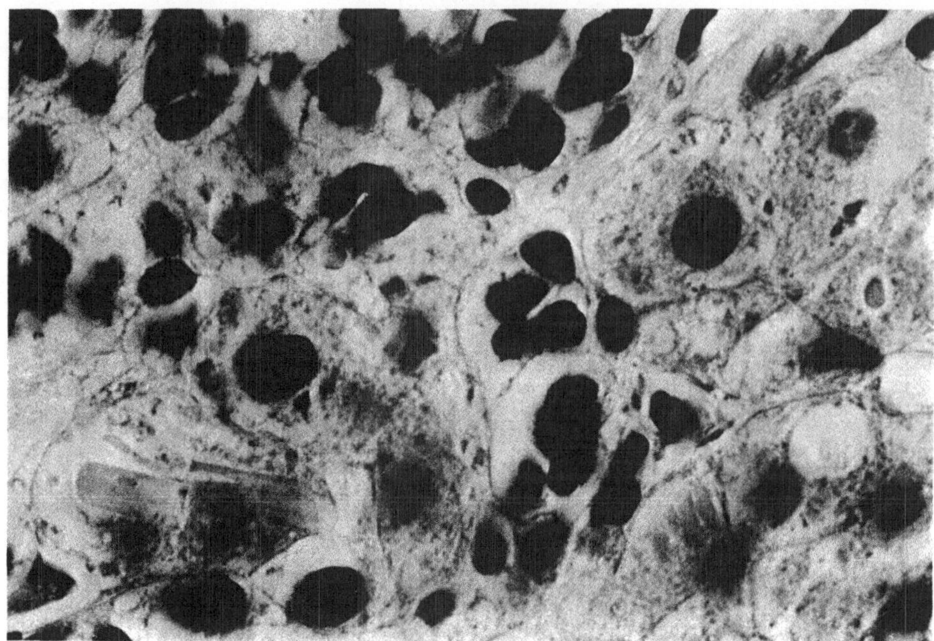

Fig. 5. Typical Leydig cells with their round nucleus displaying an eccentric nucleolus. A few crystals of Reinke are present. H & E, × 1000

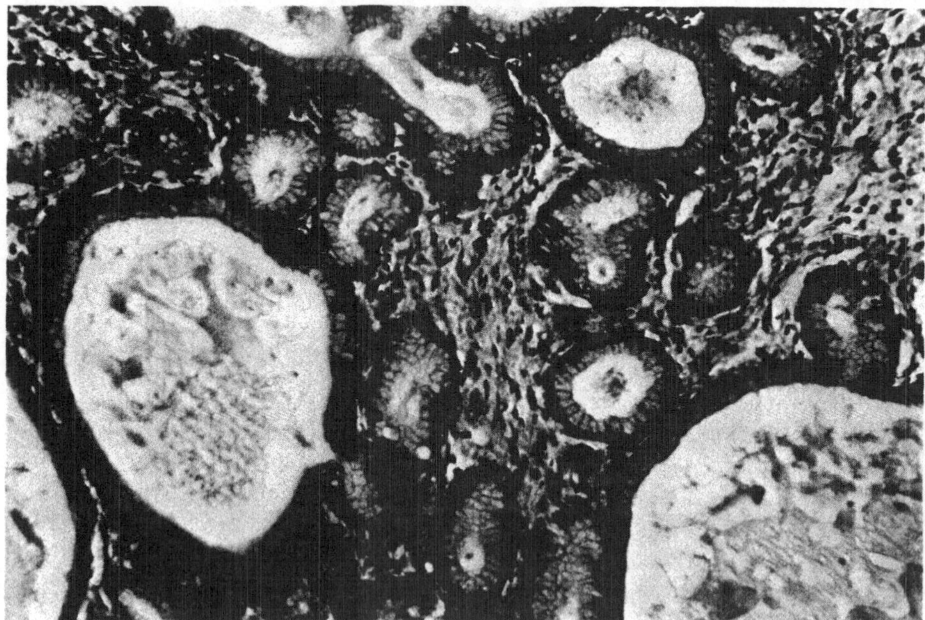

Fig. 6. Multiple mucinous cysts of variable size in an androblastoma of intermediate differentiation. H & E, × 100

ranted. These eosinophilic rod-shaped structures with rounded extremities (Fig. 5) can readily be identified in testicular Leydig cells, as well as occasionally in ovarian hilus cells.

In addition to Sertoli and Leydig cells unusual types of tissue may be found in the tumor (Scully 1977). Most frequent among these are numerous cysts of variable size and lined by mucus-producing cells (Fig. 6). The presence of mature cartilage, rhabdomyoblasts, or carcinoid areas is very rare.

The stroma of androblastomas consists mostly of spindle-shaped, fibroblast-like cells separated by collagen fibers, and may exhibit extensive hyalinization.

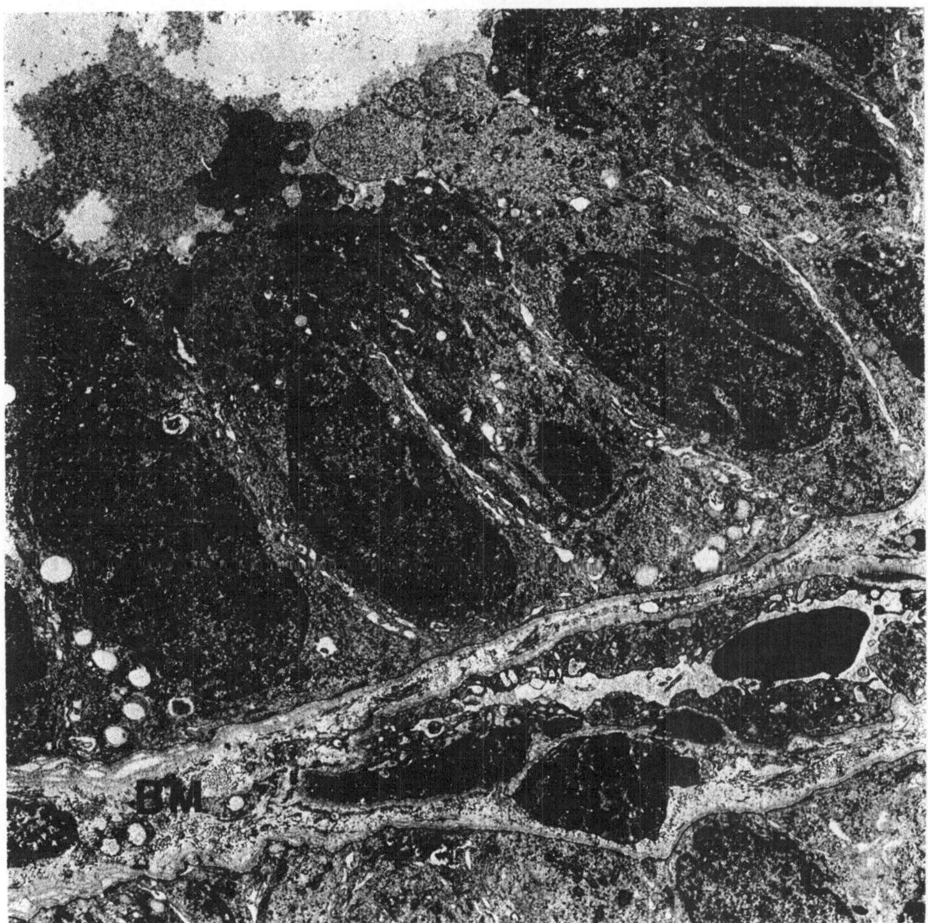

Fig. 7. Well-differentiated tubules surrounded by a multilayered basement membrane (*BM*). The Sertoli cells are cylindrical with indented nuclei. Numerous desmosomes are present in the apical portions of the cells. Slender cytoplasmic projections intermingle in widened intercellular spaces. ×4200

Ultrastructure

Sertoli Cells

The ultrastructural features of the Sertoli cells depend on the degree of differentiation, but the epithelial character of these cells has been noted in all cases investigated (Kempson 1968; Jenson and Fechner 1969; Murad et al. 1973; Kalderon and Tucci 1973; Roth et al. 1974; Ramzy and Bos 1976; Ueda et al. 1976).

The well-defined tubules are lined by a single layer of columnar cells and surrounded by a multilayered basement membrane (Fig. 7). The lumen contains pinched-off cytoplasmic fragments and cellular detritus. The nuclei are mostly oval but may be severely indented. Their solitary nucleoli are irregular and heteroge-

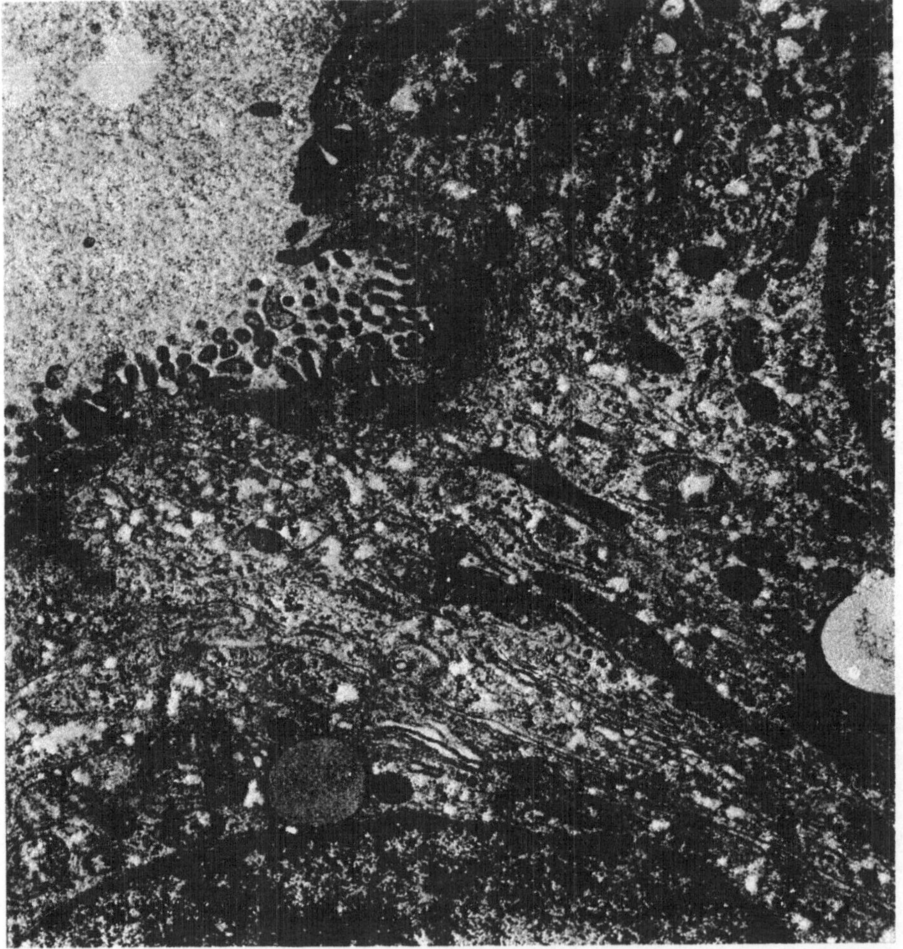

Fig. 8. Apical portion of Sertoli cells in a well-differentiated tubule. At their luminal border the cells exhibit numerous microvilli with a filamentous core as well as some cilia. In the cytoplasm partly pleomorphic mitochondria, endoplasmic reticulum, lipid droplets, and bundles of microfilaments. ×13 300

neous. The cell membranes are well defined and run mostly parallel to one another. However, small widenings of the intercellular spaces containing villous-like cytoplasmic projections are commonly found. At their luminal border the cells often present numerous microvilli and some micropinocytic vesicles, and rarely cilia (Kalderon and Tucci 1973; Ramzy and Bos 1976; Genton 1980b). Well-developed desmosomes are present, especially in the apical portions of the cells, which exhibit some degree of polarity, the numerous organelles often being mainly in supranuclear location (Fig. 8). The endoplasmic reticulum is sparse, mainly granular in type, and occasionally arranged in whorls (Fig. 9) (Jenson and Fechner 1969; Fiz et al. 1971; Roth et al. 1974). Free ribosomes are numerous. Golgi complexes are seldom found and mostly poorly developed. Mitochondria are present in moderate numbers, some of them displaying bizarre contours. Their plate-like cristae are

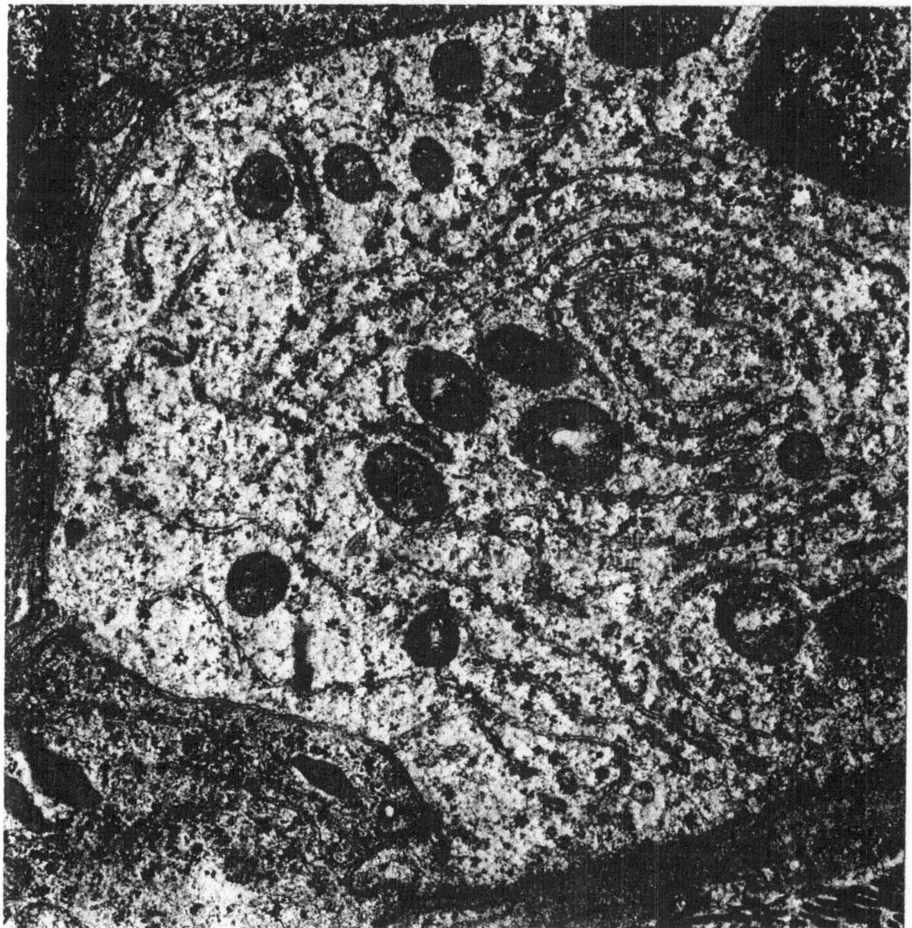

Fig. 9. Basal portion of a Sertoli cell resting on a multilayered basement membrane surrounded by collagen fibers. The cytoplasm contains numerous membranes of partly agranular endoplasmic reticulum occasionally in close association with mitochondria or arranged in whorls. ×18 800

sparse and irregularly orientated. Lipid droplets, lysosomes, bundles of microfibrils, and microtubules are occasionally found.

In the less differentiated areas the Sertoli cells are arranged in pseudotubules and solid nests surrounded by a multilayered basement membrane (Fig. 10). The tumor cells are irregular in shape and display no polarity, the sparse organelles being randomly distributed throughout the cytoplasm. Widenings of the intercellular spaces are large and more numerous. The nuclei are often deeply indented; junctional complexes are sparse and poorly developed.

At some locations the Sertoli cells form structures very similar to the Call-Exner bodies found in granulosa cell tumors (Fig. 11). Charcot-Böttcher crystals as observed in normal mature testicular Sertoli cells have never been found in andro-

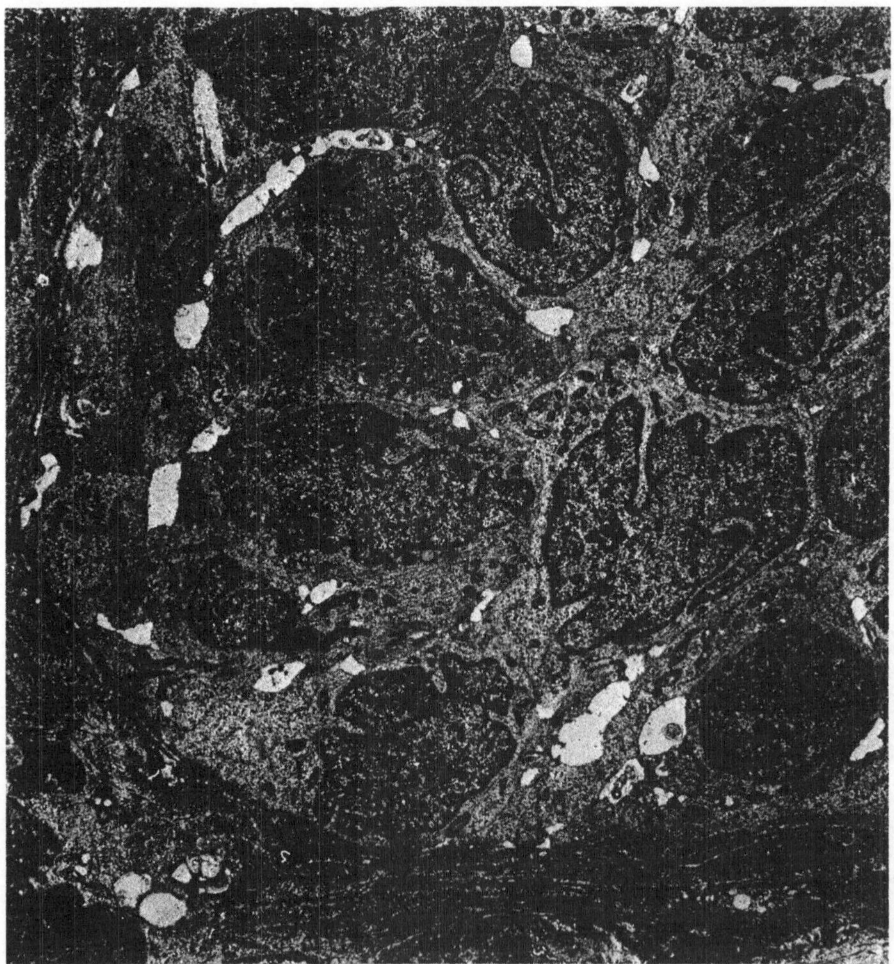

Fig. 10. Pseudotubule surrounded by a multilayered basement membrane and collagen fibers. The nuclei of the Sertoli cells are severely indented, the organelles are randomly distributed throughout the cytoplasm, and desmosomes are sparse. ×4200

blastomas. The virus-like particles described by Murad et al. (1973) probably represent non specific cytoplasmic bodies, the significance of which are unknown.

Leydig Cells

The Leydig cells lie isolated or in small groups surrounded by some collagen fibers. Their nuclei are round, the heterochromatin being characteristically concentrated along the nuclear membrane. The nucleolus is large and eccentric (Fig. 12). The cytoplasm contains the typical organelles which are associated with steroid synthesis: a strongly developed tubular and vesicular agranular endoplasmic reticulum

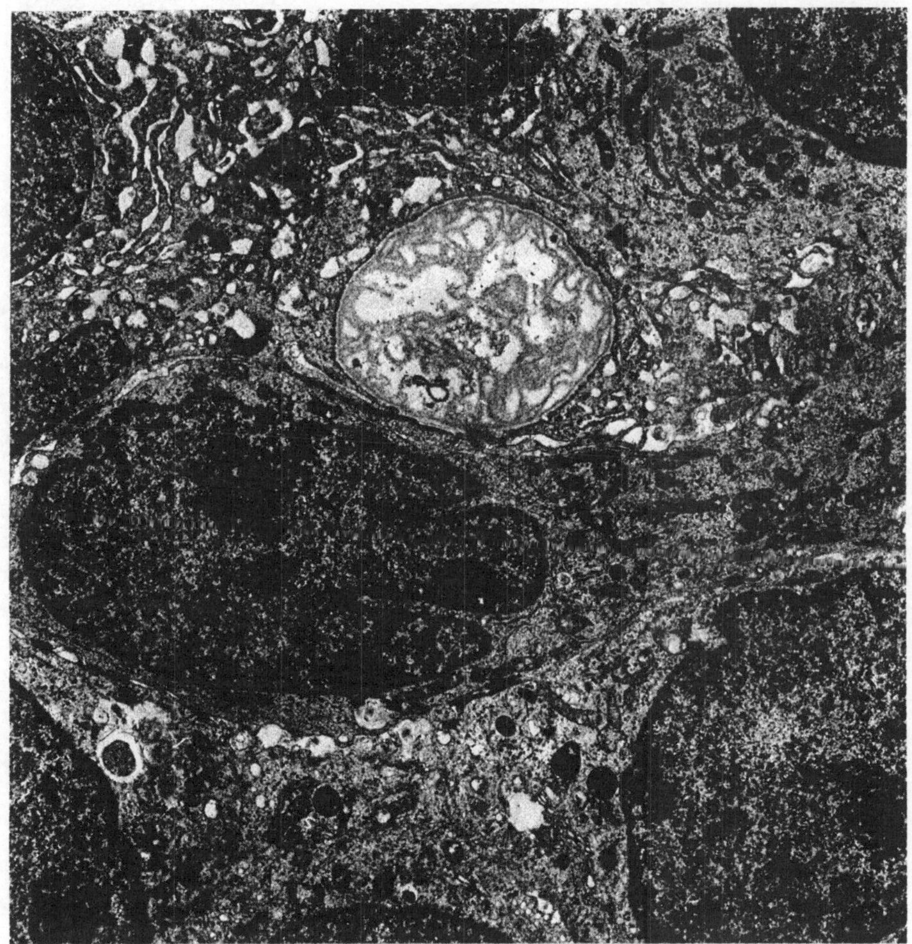

Fig. 11. Small cystic space surrounded by Sertoli cells, quite reminiscent of a Call-Exner body as seen in granulosa cell tumors (Genton 1980a). It contains basement-membrane-like material and cellular detritus. ×6400

and numerous mitochondria with tubular cristae (Fig. 13). Similar features have also been observed in normal and neoplastic testicular Leydig cells (Fawcett and Burgos 1960; Cervos-Navarro et al. 1964; De Kretser 1967) and in ovarian hilus cells (Motta 1972), as well as in neoplastic hilus cells, luteinized neoplastic granulosa cells, and so-called lipid cell tumors (Green and Maqueo 1966; Koss et al. 1969; Ishida et al. 1977; Genton 1980a). The granular endoplasmic reticulum is sparse and often arranged in parallel stacks. Some lysosomes, pigment granules, lipid droplets, and numerous free ribosomes, are commonly found. The cell membrane is indistinct and occasionally exhibits small cytoplasmic projections in the widened intercellular spaces, as well as a few micropinocytic vesicles.

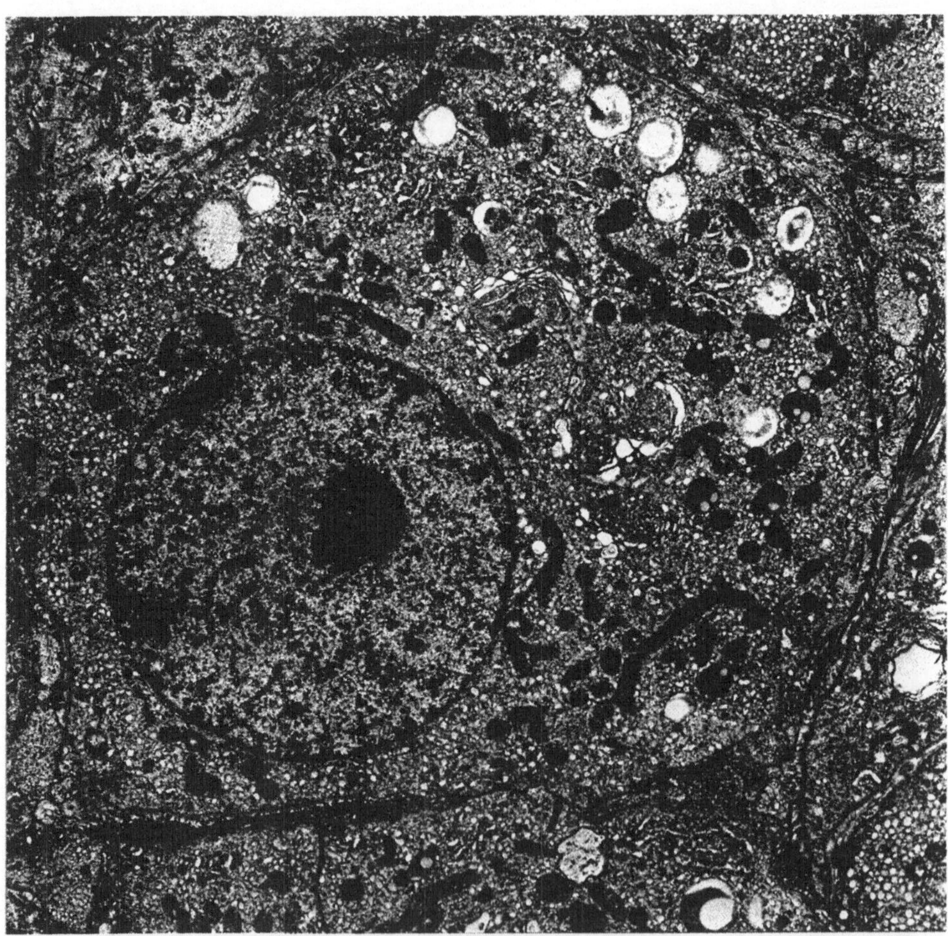

Fig. 12. Typical Leydig cell with its round nucleus, the chromatin being concentrated at the periphery. The nucleolus is solitary and in eccentric location. In the cytoplasm strongly developed agranular endoplasmic reticulum, pleomorphic mitochondria, and pigment granules. ×6400

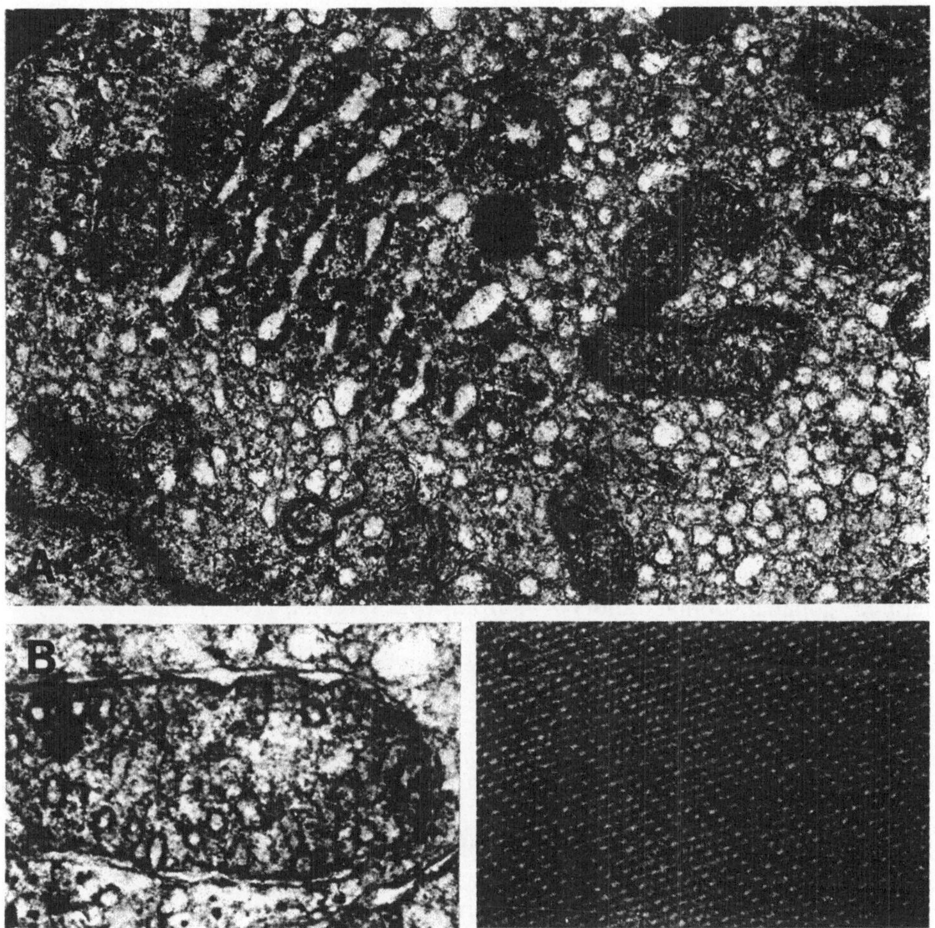

Fig. 13A–C. Details of Leydig cells. *A* Higher magnification of the cytoplasm exhibiting a markedly developed vesicular and tubular endoplasmic reticulum and mitochondria with tubular cristae. Some parallel strands of granular endoplasmic reticulum are also present, as well as free ribosomes. ×26 100. *B* High magnification of a mitochondrion with its characteristic tubular cristae. ×59 800. *C* High magnification of a Reinke crystal showing its typically lattice-like crystalline structure. ×52 900

Ultrastructurally the crystals of Reinke, consisting of proteins (Janko and Sandberg 1970), have a typical lattice-like structure (Fig. 13c) which has been exhaustively analyzed in particular by Merkow et al. (1971). In the tumor that they investigated Berendsen et al. (1969) observed filaments with a periodicity of 150 Å and postulated that these structures possibly constitute precursors of the crystals.

Some Leydig cells seem to be degenerating. Their nuclei are shrunken, the cytoplasm is packed with lipid droplets of varying size and electron density, and the mitochondria are swollen and hardly recognizable.

Histogenesis

There is still doubt about the pathogenesis and histogenesis of androblastomas. Such tumors have occasionally been reported to occur in the same family (Accardo and Condorelli 1966; Goldstein and Lamb 1970), and can be induced experimentally in animal ovaries (Warner et al. 1960).

Since a small number of androblastomas contain such tissues as cartilage or argentaffin cells, a teratomatous origin has been proposed (Hartz 1945). Vestigial remnants of the testis possibly present in the ovarian hilus may give rise to neoplasia (Meyer 1931; Teilum 1958). However, the tumor cells were shown to be chromosomally female (Rüttner 1957; Teilum 1971). The few available studies of ultrastructure have led to contradictory interpretations. Some authors observed similarities between the neoplastic cells of androblastomas and the immature testicular Sertoli cells (Roth et al. 1974; Ramzy and Bos 1976). Several investigators came to the conclusion that the neoplastic Sertoli cells probably derive from specific ovarian stroma cells (Kempson 1968; Jenson and Fechner 1969; Fiz et al. 1971; Murad et al. 1973). Thus the opinion has been expressed that such ovarian Sertoli-Leydig cell tumors displaying obvious morphologic similarities to testicular structures should be termed "gonadal stromal tumors of android type" (Genton 1980b).

Clinical Manifestations

The classic symptoms caused by the Sertoli-Leydig cell tumors are amenorrhea and sterility followed by defeminization and virilization. There exists no strict correlation between histology and androgenicity of the androblastomas but moderately or poorly differentiated tumors seem to be more likely to produce endocrine effects (Morris and Scully 1958). Novak and Long (1965), as well as Pedowitz and O'Brien (1960), concluded that 90% of the Sertoli-Leydig cell tumors cause masculinization. For Ireland and Woodruff (1976) the figure was 40%. Kurman et al. (1978) showed in their immunohistologic study of nine androblastomas that Sertoli cells, and to an even greater degree Leydig cells, contained testosterone. Estradiol and estrone were also occasionally present, most often located in the Sertoli cells. This last finding could explain the rare occurrence of an androblastoma with estrogenic clinical manifestations (Genton 1981). But although no selective venous sampling and endocrinologic studies have been performed, the possibility of conversion of produced androgens into estrogens by the peripheral fat tissue must be borne in mind.

Sertoli-Leydig cell tumors are occasionally associated with polycystic ovaries or with hyperthecosis, lesions which may both cause marked masculinization (Cruikshank and Chapler 1974; Katz et al. 1977; Aiman et al. 1978; Braithwaite et al. 1978).

Resumption of menses is likely to occur 1 month after removal of the tumor. The hair usually returns to a female distribution, but voice changes and hypertrophy of the clitoris, if present, may be permanent.

Table 1. Seven cases of Sertoli-Leydig cell tumors

Case	Age	Clinical findings	Operation	Gross pathology	Microscopic pathology	Follow-up
1	16	Secondary amenorrhea Virilization	Right salpingo-oophorectomy	3-cm solid grey-yellow tumor	Intermediate Granulosa-like areas	Well after 24 years. 2 normal pregnancies 8 and 11 years post-op. Voice change and hypertrophy of clitoris unchanged
2	32	Menometrorrhagia	Left oophorectomy	5-cm solid yellow tumor, multiple mucinous cysts	Intermediate Multiple mucinous cysts	Lost to follow-up
3	29	Secondary amenorrhea Galactorrhea	Right oophorectomy	2-cm solid and mucinous cysts	Undifferentiated Granulosa-like areas Mucinous cysts	Well after 11 years 1 normal pregnancy 2 years post-op.
4	26	Secondary amenorrhea Primary sterility Virilization	Left oophorectomy	3-cm solid yellow tumor	Intermediate	Well after 6 years 1 normal pregnancy 3 years post-op.
5	72	Right-sided ovarian tumor	Hysterectomy Bilateral salpingo-oophorectomy	4-mm solid tumor in left ovary. Serous cystadenofibroma in right ovary	Intermediate Hyalinization of stroma	Well after 4 years
6	59	Hirsutism	Hysterectomy Bilateral salpingo-oophorectomy	8-mm solid tumor. Marked hyperthecosis of both ovaries	Well-differentiated	Well after 4 years
7	67	Vaginal bleeding in postmenopause	Hysterectomy Bilateral salpingo-oophorectomy	13-cm solid lobulated tumor	Undifferentiated Marked adenomatous hyperplasia of endometrium	Well after 1 year

Prognosis and Treatment

There is a wide range of opinion about the clinical behavior of Sertoli-Leydig cell tumors and the reported frequencies of tumor relapse and/or metastases vary between 7% (Ireland and Woodruff 1976) and 25% (Held and Schreiner 1959). True malignant ovarian androblastomas are in fact probably rare. There seems to be no present justification for separating these neoplasms into benign and malignant subgroups according to their microscopic appearance. Obvious malignancy at operation, with local invasion and peritoneal metastases, is very uncommon.

The majority of Sertoli-Leydig cell tumors occur in relatively young women and treatment should respect the patient's desire for future pregnancies. In most instances extirpation of the neoplastic ovary is adequate. In older patients total hysterectomy and bilateral salpingo-oophorectomy may be indicated. A more radical surgery is required if any evidence of local malignancy or metastases is found at operation.

Case Reports

The findings in seven cases of Sertoli-Leydig cell tumors seen at the University Women's Hospital in Zürich from 1957 through 1980 are summarized in Table 1. All these cases have previously been reported in more detail (Held and Schreiner 1959; Genton 1978, 1980 b, 1981).

Three patients presented obvious signs of virilization; a fourth patient had only hirsuties. A 29-year-old woman complained about secondary amenorrhea and galactorrhea. One tumor, 4 mm in diameter, seemed to have no endocrine activity. The last patient had estrogenic clinical symptoms and a marked adenomatous hyperplasia of the endometrium was found.

Four tumors occurred in the left, three in the right ovary. The size of the neoplasms varied between 4 mm and 8 cm. In all cases the tumor tissue had a lobulated cut surface; the color was gray with a yellow hue. Microscopically one tumor was well differentiated, four were of intermediate type, and two poorly differentiated. Two neoplasms were associated with multiple mucinous cysts. Crystals of Reinke were observed in five cases.

Six androblastomas proved to be benign after an observation period of between 1 and 24 years. One patient was lost to follow-up. All three other women in reproductive age had normal pregnancies some years after removal of the tumor.

References

Accardo M, Condorelli B (1966) Arrhenoblastoma in due sorelle. Riv Patol Sper 7: 171–188

Aiman J, Edman CD, Worley RJ, Vellios F, MacDonald PC (1978) Androgen and estrogen formation in women with ovarian hyperthecosis. Obstet Gynecol 51: 1–9

Berendsen PB, Smith EB, Abell MR, Jaffe RB (1969) Fine structure of Leydig cells from an arrhenoblastoma of the ovary. Am J Obstet Gynecol 103: 192–199

Berger L (1923) La glande sympathicotrope du hile de l'ovaire; ses homologies avec la glande interstitielle du testicule; les rapports nerveux des deux glandes. Arch Anat Histol Embryol (Strasb) 2:255–306

Braithwaite SS, Erkman-Balis B, Avila TD (1978) Postmenopausal virilization due to ovarian stromal hyperthecosis. J Clin Endocrinol 46:295–300

Cervos-Navarro J, Tonutti E, Bayer JM (1964) Elektronenmikroskopische Untersuchungen eines androgenbildenden Leydigzelltumors. Endokrinologie 47:23–51

Cruikshank DP, Chapler FK (1974) Arrhenoblastomas and associated ovarian pathology. Obstet Gynecol 43:540–542

Fawcett DW, Burgos MH (1960) Studies on the fine structure of the mammalian testis. II. The human interstitial tissue. Am J Anat 107:245–270

Fiz G, Vital GI, Le Blanc M, Leng J, Vincendeau J, Leger H (1971) Etude d'un cas d'arrhénoblastome avec examen en ultrastructure. Bordeaux Méd 4:2145–2149

Galle PC, McCool JA, Elsner CW (1978) Arrhenoblastoma during pregnancy. Obstet Gynecol 51:359–364

Genton CY (1978) Ein Sertoli-Leydigzelltumor als Zufallsbefund bei einer 72jährigen Patientin. Zentralbl Gynaekol 100:154–156

Genton CY (1980a) Some observations on the fine structure of human granulosa cell tumors. Virchows Arch [Pathol Anat] 387:353–369

Genton CY (1980b) Ovarian Sertoli-Leydig cell tumors. A clinical, pathological and ultrastructural study with particular reference to the histogenesis of these tumors. Arch Gynecol 230:49–75

Genton CY (1981) Ovarian Sertoli-Leydig cell tumor with hyperoestrinism. Virchows Arch [Pathol Anat] 390:243–248

Goldstein DP, Lamb EJ (1970) Arrhenoblastoma in first cousins, report of two cases. Obstet Gynecol 35:444–450

Green JA, Maqueo M (1966) Histopathology and ultrastructure of an ovarian hilar cell tumor. Am J Obstet Gynecol 96:478–485

Hartz PH (1945) Giant cystic arrhenoblastoma of the ovary containing entodermal epithelium and a carcinoid. Am J Pathol 21:1167–1192

Held E, Schreiner WE (1959) Über einen Fall von Arrhenoblastom. Gynaecologia 147:402–414

Ireland K, Woodruff JD (1976) Masculinizing ovarian tumors. Obstet Gynecol Surv 31:83–111

Ishida T, Okagaki T, Tagatz GE, Jacobson ME, Doe RP (1977) Lipid cell tumor of the ovary: an ultrastructural study. Cancer 40:234–243

Janko AB, Sandberg EC (1970) Histochemical evidence for the protein nature of the Reinke crystalloid. Obstet Gynecol 35:493–503

Jenson AB, Fechner RE (1969) Ultrastructure of an intermediate Sertoli-Leydig cell tumor. A histogenetic misnomer. Lab Invest 21:527–535

Jones GS, Goldberg B, Woodreuff DJ (1967) Enzyme histochemistry of a masculinizing arrhenoblastoma. Obstet Gynecol 29:328–343

Kalderon AE, Tucci JR (1973) Ultrastructure of a human chorionic gonadotropin- and adrenocorticotropin responsive functioning Sertoli-Leydig cell tumor (type I). Lab Invest 29:81–89

Katz M, Hamilton SM, Albertyn L, Pimstone BL, Cohen BL, Tiltman AJ (1977) Virilization with diffuse involvement of ovarian androgen secreting cells. Obstet Gynecol 50:623–627

Kempson RL (1968) Ultrastructure of ovarian stromal cell tumors. Arch Pathol 86:492–507

Koss LG, Rothschild EO, Fleisher M, Francis JE Jr (1969) Masculinizing tumor of the ovary, apparently with adreno-cortical activity. A histologic, ultrastructural and biochemical study. Cancer 23:1245–1258

Kretser DM De (1967) The fine structure of the testicular interstitial cells in men of normal androgenic status. Z Zellforsch 80:594–609

Kurman RJ, Goebelsmann U, Andrade D, Taylor CR (1978) An immunohistological study of steroid localization in Sertoli-Leydig cell tumors of the ovary and testis. Cancer 42:1772–1783

Merkow LP, Slifkin M, Acevedo HF, Pardo M, Greenberg WV (1971) Ultrastructure of an interstitial (hilar) cell tumor of the ovary. Obstet Gynecol 37:845–859

Meyer R (1931) Pathology of some special ovarian tumors and their relation to sex characteristics. Am J Obstet Gynecol 22:697–713

Morris J McLean, Scully RE (1958) Endocrine pathology of the ovary. Mosby, St. Louis

Motta P (1972) Observations on the ultrastructure of the interstitial cells of the human ovary. Anat Anz 130:1–17

Murad TM, Mancini R, George J (1973) Ultrastructure of a virilizing ovarian Sertoli-Leydig cell tumor with familial incidence. Cancer 31:1440–1450

Novak ER, Long JH (1965) Arrhenoblastoma of the ovary. A review of the ovarian tumor registry. Am J Obstet Gynecol 92:1082–1093

Pedowitz P, O'Brien FB (1960) Arrhenoblastoma of the ovary. Obstet Gynecol 16:62–77

Pick L (1905) Über Adenome der männlichen und weiblichen Keimdrüse bei Hermaphroditismus verus und spurius. Berl Klin Wochenschr 42:502–509

Ramzy I, Bos C (1976) Sertoli cell tumors of ovary. Light microscopic and ultrastructural study with histogenetic considerations. Cancer 38:2447–2456

Reinke F (1896) Beiträge zur Histologie des Menschen. I. Über Kristalloidbildungen in den interstitiellen Zellen des menschlichen Hodens. Arch Mikrosk Anat Entwicklungsmech 47:34–44

Roth LM, Clearly RE, Rosenfield RL (1974) Sertoli-Leydig cell tumor of the ovary with an associated mucinous cystadenoma. An ultrastructural and endocrine study. Lab Invest 31:648–657

Rüttner JR (1957) Zur Morphologie und Histogenese des Arrhenoblastoms unter Berücksichtigung der Hormonanalyse des Tumorgewebes. Schweiz Z Pathol Bakteriol 20:59–68

Scully RE (1977) Ovarian tumors. A review. Am J Pathol 87:686–720

Serov SF, Scully RE (1973) Histological typing of ovarian tumors. International histological classification of tumours No. 9. WHO, Geneva

Teilum G (1958) Classification of testicular and ovarian androblastoma and Sertoli cell tumors. A survey of comparative studies with consideration of histogenesis, endocrinology and embryological theories. Cancer 11:769–782

Teilum G (1971) Special tumors of ovary and testis and related extragonadal lesions. Comparative pathology and histological identification. Munksgaard, Copenhagen

Ueda G, Yamasaki M, Sato Y, Hiramatsu K, Kurachi K (1976) Light and electron microscopic study of an intermediate Sertoli-Leydig cell tumor with a review of literature in Japan. Acta Obstet Gynecol Jpn (Engl Ed) 23:14–22

Warner NE, Friedman NB, Bomze EJ, Masin F (1960) Comparative pathology of experimental and spontaneous androblastomas and gynoblastomas of the gonads. Am J Obstet Gynecol 79:971–988

Ovarian Tumours of the Germinal Epithelium

F. A. LANGLEY [1]

Introduction

This paper is largely concerned with exploring our rather scanty knowledge of the natural history of the common epithelial tumours of the ovary and indicating the bearing this has on the investigation of their aetiology.

Natural history, in this context, properly begins with morphogenesis. The generally accepted view is that most of the common epithelial tumours of the ovary arise from the serosa, or germinal epithelium, of the ovary; but this theory cannot be regarded as satisfactorily explaining the origin of all the neoplasms. In the embryo, cells or groups of cells have many possible fates (prospective potencies). Needham (1942) has stated that "competence is the state of reactivity on the part of the embryo enabling it to respond to a given morphogenetic stimulation by determination and differentiation in a given direction", and he considered that some competences persist in adult tissues, although they are not normally expressed. Suitable stimulation may reveal these latent competences.

The coelomic cavity results from the confluence of cavities in the lateral mesodermic plates. The mesoderm bounding the coelomic cavity forms the mesothelial lining of the peritoneal cavity, parts of which become specialised to form the germinal epithelium and the epithelium of the nephrogenital ridge. Epithelium from the nephrogenital ridge gives rise to the mullerian (paramesonephric) duct from which the endocervical epithelium, endometrium, and the epithelium of the fallopian tube are derived. It also gives rise to wolffian (mesonephric) structures, including the trigone of the bladder. Thus germinal epithelium might retain competence to express such morphological patterns under suitable metaplastic or neoplastic stimulation. Metaplastic transformation of the ovarian serosa to tubal type, or more rarely, endocervical type epithelium is well documented (Numers 1965; Towers 1956). Whilst in pregnancy and under the influence of steroid hormones a decidual reaction may occur on the surface of the ovary, although whether the decidua arises from the germinal epithelium or underlying connective tissue is uncertain. Such changes support Needham's concept and indicate that the ovarian serosa retains competence in the adult to differentiate into epithelium commonly found in the uterus and oviduct. Parallel to such metaplasia of germinal epithelium, tubal (ciliated), mucinous, clear cell and hobnail cell metaplasia may be found in the endo-

1 Department of Histopathology, St. Mary's Hospitals, GB–Manchester

metrium (Hendrickson and Kempson 1980) and endometrial metaplasia occasionally occurs in the fallopian tube.

Likewise, there is similarity between the tumours of the endocervix, endometrium and fallopian tube and those of the ovary, although they occur with differing relative frequencies. Thus mucinous carcinomas occur in the endocervix, the endometrium and the ovary. Clear cell tumours of mesonephroid type may occasionally be seen in the endometrium and papillary carcinomas with psammoma bodies resembling serous ovarian carcinomas of the ovary may sometimes be found in the endometrium. Further, there is the large group of endometrioid ovarian tumours resembling endometrial carcinomas. Moreover, it is not unusual to see a mixture of patterns in the same mullerian tumour, although one usually predominates (Abell 1966; Anderson 1972; Cariker and Dockerty 1954).

Mesothelial tumours of the peritoneum are uncommon and likewise they constitute a rare group of ovarian tumours. However, their occurrence suggests retention of mesothelial competence by the germinal epithelium.

When considering common epithelial tumours of the ovary it is easy to overlook the significant component of connective tissue which is especially conspicious in the adenofibromas and Brenner tumours. This probably originates from the thin subserosal zone of fibrous tissue which arises from the coelomic mesenchyma at the same time as the germinal epithelium (Ober 1979). Nothing is known about the mechanism of response of this connective tissue to proliferating germinal epithelium. Usually it appears merely to support the epithelium but, in some tumours, it probably provides a malignant stromal component, whilst in others it may become steroidogenic and occasionally in mucinous tumours it may contain sarcoma-like nodules (Pratt and Scully 1979 a, b).

Serous Tumours

In the normal ovary invaginations of the serosa into the underlying stroma are of common occurrence and may become more frequent as the ovary contracts with age. Frequently the mouths of these invaginations become closed and inclusion cysts are formed, lined by indifferent cuboidal epithelium or by tubal epithelium. More rarely these cysts have a mucinous lining. Enlargement of these cysts by proliferation and secretion gives rise to an adenofibroma and, if a few cysts dilate disproportionately, to a cystoma (Scott 1942). From time to time small papillae, covered by tube-like epithelium, form on the surface of the ovary and these may sometimes be associated with psammoma bodies. Such structures may be regarded as precursors of surface papillomas, although it has been suggested that they might arise by implantation of fragments of epithelium of the fallopian tube (Glazunow 1937; Barzilai 1949). A few serous cysts are associated with Brenner tumours and probably have the same origin.

Grossly benign serous tumours may form adenofibromas, cystomas or surface papillomas but combinations of these types are frequent. Malignant tumours may present in any one of these forms but they are more frequently semi-solid.

Generally, three types of cells are identifiable in the epithelium of benign tumours; these include the ciliated cells, the non-ciliated cells and the basal, or peg cells, as in the fallopian tube. The epithelium of malignant tumours shows some resemblance to tubal epithelium both at the light and electron optical level, but often with marked cytological abnormalities (Roberts et al, 1970; Fenoglio 1980). Sometimes the origin of these carcinomas from benign tumours is made evident by the concomitant presence of benign and malignant epithelium. In about 8% of cystadenomas some of the epithelium shows cytological features of malignancy, but without stromal invasion. Such tumours are described as borderline tumours, or tumours of low malignant potential, and probably correspond to in situ carcinomas in other locations.

Mucinous Tumours

Mucinous tumours are a heterogeneous group, comprising at least three types (Langley et al. 1972). First, there are those tumours which are associated with teratomas and probably represent an excessive development of gastro-intestinal epithelium. Second, there are mucinous cystadenomas associated with Brenner tumours and their histogenesis is that of the Brenner tumour. The third and largest group of mucinous tumours is also heterogeneous. At the electron optical level the epithelium of most of these tumours resembles that of the endocervix but some 20% of these tumours are lined by an epithelium containing argyrophilic, argentaffin and goblet cells (Fenoglio 1980; Fox et al. 1964; Klemi 1978; Masson 1956), and occasionally Paneth cells can be seen (Janovski and Paramanandhan 1973). The simple hypothesis is that the tumours lined by endocervical type epithelium arise from germinal epithelium by a process of metaplasia. There is no proof of this but it is supported by: (a) the occasional records of the occurrence of such metaplasia (Akagi 1928; Numers 1965; Towers 1956), and (b) the occasional finding of mucinous inclusion cysts. The tumours containing intestinal type epithelium may arise as monophyletic teratomas or by a metaplastic process. The metaplastic view is supported by the occasional finding of endometrioid elements in mucinuous tumours and the observation that intestinal epithelium may be found in the inflamed reproductive tract and in normal and neoplastic epithelium of the cervix (Fox et al. 1964; Azzopardi and Hou 1965).

According to Fenoglio (1980) the borderline mucinous tumours always contain both intestinal and endocervical type cells and the areas of atypia are always confined to the intestinal-like epithelium. Mucinous cystadenocarcinomas are mainly composed of immature intestinal cells, whilst endocervical cells are seen only in the well-differentiated tumours (Fenoglio et al. 1975). Fenoglio (1980) has suggested that the relatively high proportion of mucinous cystadenomas composed solely of endocervical cells may account for the lower incidence of malignancy in mucinous neoplasms compared with serous tumours.

Carcinoembryonic antigen (CEA), first identified in the plasma of patients with colonic adenocarcinoma, was initially believed to be a specific product of fetal gut and of tumours of endodermal origin (Gold and Freedman 1965a, b). Although CEA is now known to be present in the plasma in a wide range of benign and malignant conditions, it might have been hoped that immunoperoxidase staining would distinguish those ovarian tumours of gastrointestinal type from the others. Heald et al. (1979), in an examination of 30 mucinous tumours, found it was not possible to distinguish the two types of epithelium by this method. However, all the mucinous carcinomas and mucinous tumours of borderline malignancy stained positively, but staining in the borderline tumours occurred both in the proliferating and non-proliferating areas. Significant staining was also found in 30% of the benign tumours, suggesting that these tumours, in a biochemical sense, were already of borderline malignancy.

Endometrioid Tumours

The most characteristic and common member of this group is the endometrioid adenocarcinoma, which closely resembles the adenocarcinoma of the endometrium, but benign and borderline forms occur, often as adenofibromas (Roth et al., 1981), and carcinosarcomas and mixed mesenchymal tumours are regarded as belonging to this group.

Endometriosis is a common lesion of the ovary and it is reasonable to suppose that a neoplasm might arise in such a focus. Indeed some foci have been described showing adenomatous hyperplasia and severe atypia (Czernobilsky and Morris 1979), whilst Sampson (1925) has described adenocarcinomas arising in endometrial cysts of the ovary and laid down criteria for identifying the nature of such tumours. However, the majority of endometrioid carcinomas do not conform to Sampson's criteria, appearing to arise de novo (Scully et al. 1966), but such neoplasms may have originated in a focus of endometriosis which has not been identified or has been destroyed by the growing tumour. The histogenesis of many of these neoplasms is therefore that of endometriosis. However, some endometrioid tumours may arise from benign or borderline adenofibromas and others directly from the germinal epithelium. The frequency with which they originate from each source cannot be determined at present.

Mesonephroid Tumours

Mesonephroid tumours should more properly be termed clear cell tumours, since the term mesonephroid refers to earlier and erroneous views of their origin from the wolffian duct or its anlage (Teilum 1954; Wade-Evans and Langley 1961). The present evidence, largely adducted by Scully and Barlow (1967), indicates a mullerian morphology and a close relationship to endometrioid tumours in the following respects:

1. The frequent intermingling of mesonephroid and endometrioid carcinomas
2. The occurrence of similar clear cell areas in each tumour (caused by the accumulation of glycogen)
3. The similarity, at light and electron optical levels, to the Arias-Stella reaction (Roth 1974a)
4. The occurrence of "mesonephroid" tumours in the endometrium
5. The frequent coincidental presence of mesonephroid tumours and foci of pelvic endometriosis and the occassional apparent origin of mesonephroid tumours in such foci.

Occasionally isolated benign mesonephroid adenofibromas are seen, but, more frequently, such adenofibromas form part of an otherwise malignant tumour. Hence mesonephroid carcinomas may arise directly from the germinal epithelium, foci of endometriosis or mesonephroid adenofibromas.

Brenner Tumours

The fibrous stroma of Brenner tumours is more abundant than in any other common epithelial tumour, and occasionally it is endocrinologically active (Farrar et al. 1960). The in vitro conversion of androstenedione to oestrone and oestradiol by a Brenner tumour has been described by Shinada et al. (1973). Androgenic effects have been described by Morris and Scully (1958), whilst Hamwi et al. (1963) were able to show the in vitro production of testosterone from progesterone by a virilizing Brenner tumour.

Since the anatomical reconstructions of Plaut (1933) and Arey (1961) there has been little doubt that the epithelial elements of the cortically situated tumours are derived from the surface epithelium of the ovary. Sternberg (1963) pointed out the similarity of the Brenner epithelium to uroepithelium, and the frequent mucinous metaplasia has its counterpart in such conditions as cystitis glandularis. Ultrastructural studies by Roth (1971, 1974b) and by Cummins et al. (1973) confirm the uroepithelial structure of this tissue. Such a hypothesis implies that the germinal epithelium is still competent to develop into wolffian (mesonephric) as well as mullerian structures. This is perhaps not surprising since these two nephrogenital ridge structures have a common origin in the coelomic mesoderm. Nevertheless, some authors, Lauchlan (1966, 1972) and more recently Waxman (1979), maintain that Brenner differentiation is mullerian. Brenner tumours arising in the ovarian hilus may show continuity with the rete ovarii (Schiller 1934; Greene 1952), which is probably of wolffian origin, and hence such tumours present no histogenetic problem.

Table 1 shows that a high proportion of Brenner tumours occur in association with other ovarian neoplasms, and that just over 3% may be malignant Brenner

Table 1. Brenner tumours

	Fox et al. 1972	Manchester 1974 – 1979
Simple	37	17
With mucinous cystoma	9	9
With serous cystoma	3	2
With MCT [a]	2	0
With malignant epithelium	1	2
With borderline mucinous	0	1
Malignant Brenner	1	2
Proliferating Brenner	1	2
Total	54	35

[a] MCT, mature cystic teratoma

tumours and a similar proportion proliferating tumours. The occasional association of a teratoma with a Brenner tumour might suggest a teratomatous origin for these neoplasms, and possibly those associated with mucinous cystomas. However, the mucinous epithelium of Brenner tumours appears to differ from that of other mucinous ovarian tumours (Cummins et al., 1973). Nevertheless, the possibility exists that uroepithelium in teratomas might become neoplastic and resemble a Brenner tumour.

Later Development of Common Epithelial Carcinomas of the Ovary

Turning from the origins of individual tumours to their later development it is instructive to compare the frequency of the different types of tumour in their early and late stages. The left-hand side of Table 2 shows that in a British Medical Research Council study (1981) the proportion of unclassified tumours is approximately doubled and that of undifferentiated tumours quadrupled in stages III and IV compared with those of Stage I. The right-hand side of the table, from an Australian study, also shows a change in distribution of tumour type with advancing stage. The shift in pattern in the two studies is rather different; this is probably because the Australian diagnoses were made by one pathologist whereas the British diagnoses were based on a consensus opinion of a panel of pathologists. The British results suggest that with advancing stage the tumour patterns become less easily distinguishable, that is, in effect, become less differentiated. Parallel with this, Agrofojo et al. (1977) showed that in mucinous carcinomas the more advanced the stage the higher the mitotic rate.

The implications of these observations are not entirely clear, but two particular questions arise:

1. Are Stage III and IV tumours more aggressive from their onset, or may slower growing tumours become more aggressive with the development of a new clone of malignant cells? This question can probably only be answered by taking sequential biopsies, which is unethical.
2. Are the constituent cells of these tumours which lack morphologically distinctive features part of the proliferating compartment of the tumour, or are they cells which have failed to differentiate further?

A partial answer to the second question may be obtained by looking at the functional aspects of cellular differentiation. Epithelial ovarian tumours may secrete a wide range of hormones and non-hormonal antigens. Some of these may arise from the presence of teratomatous elements in the tumour or inclusion of elements of the APUD system but such hypotheses do not account for the production of parathormone-like substances and pregnancy-associated or other antigens (Table 3). The origin of such substances can probably be explained on the random de-repression hypothesis. This assumes that most genes are inactivated, or repressed, in differentiated tissue. De-repression or deletion of a portion of the genome might thus allow ectopic production of these substances. This is very like Needham's (1942) concept that adult tissue may retain morphological competence to develop in vari-

Table 2. A comparison of Stage I with Stages III and IV

	United Kingdom		Australia (Russell)	
	Stage I [a] (%)	Stages III and IV [b] (%)	Stage I (%)	Stages III and IV (%)
Serous	15.2	28.3	24.7	70.6
Mucinous	37.0	7.8	10.8	3.8
Endometrioid	17.4	6.7	36.6	15.0
Mesonephroid	6.5	7.2	19.4	3.8
Unclassified	17.4	33.3	1.1	0.6
Undifferentiated	4.3	16.7	4.3	6.3
Mixed	2.2	0	3.2	0
No. of patients	38	180	93	160

[a] A parallel series of cases diagnosed by the same panel of pathologists, but not included in the late trial
[b] Medical Research Council trial of late cases

ous ways open to it in fetal life. Differentiation requires the inhibition of competence, but in metaplasia and neoplasia the competences may cease to be inhibited and express themselves again. Thus coelomic epithelium gives rise to peritoneal mesothelium and nephrogenital ridge structures including the ovary and kidney. There is some morphological similarity between some tumours of these organs, and on occasion they may also express functional similarities by the production of parathormone-like substances in mesotheliomas and ovarian and renal carcinomas.

Histochemical methods of identifying these various hormones and antigens are not yet sufficiently well developed to enable us to correlate function with morphology. However, Crowther et al. (1979) found raised plasma levels of trophoblastic specific proteins in ten of 37 patients with surface epithelial tumours of the ovary. One tumour was stage II, four stage III and five stage IV. Thus it is possible that the more aggressive tumours are also the more functionally undifferentiated, but other interpretations are possible (Buckley and Fox 1979). Combining those observations, there seems to be a parallelism between functional and morphological immaturity and proliferative activity.

Table 3. Some ectopic hormones and antigens produced by ovarian carcinomas

Hormones	Placental and other antigens	
ACTH-like (Brown and Lane 1965)	See Crowther et al. 1979; Seppälä 1980	
Hypercalcaemia (Plimpton and Gelhorn 1956; Rivett and Robinson 1972)	hCG	
	hLP	
	SP_1	
Hypoglycaemia (Porter and Frantz 1956; O'Neil and Mikuta 1970)	OCAA	see Bhattacharya and Barlow 1973
	OCAA-1	
Gastrin (Cocco and Conway 1975)	CEA (Heald et al. 1979)	

Age Distribution

Table 4 shows some interesting differences in the mean ages of patients with epithelial ovarian neoplasms in three countries. The Australian and American figures are very similar, but in Indian women the tumours occur appreciably earlier. A number of possible explanations for these differences can be offered, especially the effect of differences in the structure of the populations. However, the wide age range in the individual tumours in Australia raises the question whether the mean is a valid statistic. Figures 1–4 show the age distribution curves of patients with serous, mucinous, endometrioid and mesonephroid tumours in Manchester in recent years. The curves for benign mucinous tumours and serous carcinomas have an approximately normal (gaussian) shape but the others are skew, rising fairly abruptly and declining more slowly, and in these it is unlikely that the mean provides an adequate statistic.

The shape of these curves resembles that of the case incidence curve in an epidemic when there is a single source of infection. Armenian and Lilienfeld (1974) analysed the case incidence curves of several neoplastic diseases following exposure to aetiological agents at specific times such as thyroid adenomas, cancers following childhood exposure to radiation, bronchial carcinomas in asbestos workers and bladder tumours in dyestuff workers. These all fitted a "long-normal" distribution curve. A similar curve represents the day-by-day mortality in rats following adrenalectomy (Langley et al. 1956). In such curves when the logarithm of the cumulative frequency (probit) is plotted against the logarithm of time, a straight line is obtained. This mathematical transformation was applied to our observations, after correcting for the change in population structure with age (*Population Estimates* 1977). For endometrioid and mesonephroid tumours straight lines were obtained (Fig. 5) but serous carcinomas showed considerable deviation from linearity in younger women, and mucinous tumours deviated in older women (Fig. 6).

These observations suggest a similarity in carcinogenic mechanism in endometrioid and mesonephroid tumours, possibly associated with some single event such as the change in hormonal status, perhaps at the menopause. This similarity in carcinogenic mechanism parallels the similarity in histogenesis of these two tumours. These observations also suggest that such a carcinogenic mechanism does not apply to the serous or mucinous carcinomas, each of which may have its own

Table 4. Common epithelial tumours of the ovary

		Russell 1979 (Sydney) (yrs)	Madan et al. 1978 (Aligarh) (yrs)	Cramer and Cutler 1974 (United States) (yrs)
Serous	Benign	44.7 (16 – 80)	32.1	
	Borderline	47.8 (21 – 78)		
	Malignant	55.7 (24 – 78)	50.0	56.3
Mucinous	Benign	43.6 (13 – 78)	30.6	
	Borderline	48.5 (20 – 52)		
	Malignant	52.4 (21 – 72)	40.0	54.2

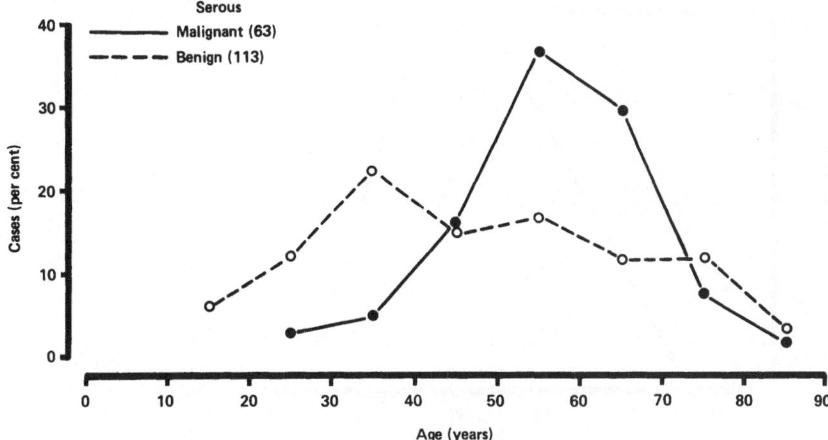

Fig. 1. Age distribution of serous ovarian tumours in Manchester

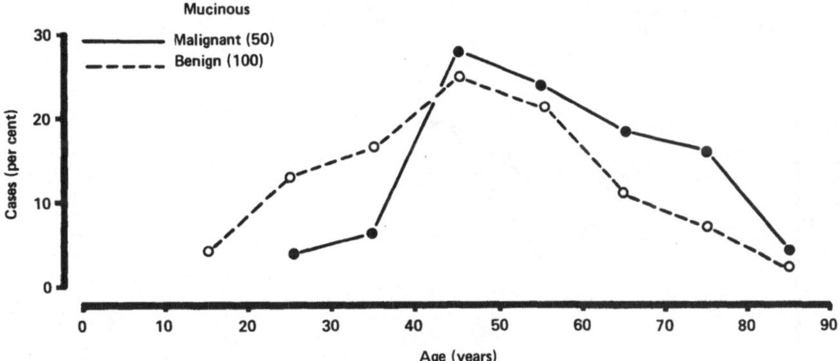

Fig. 2. Age distribution of mucinous tumours in Manchester

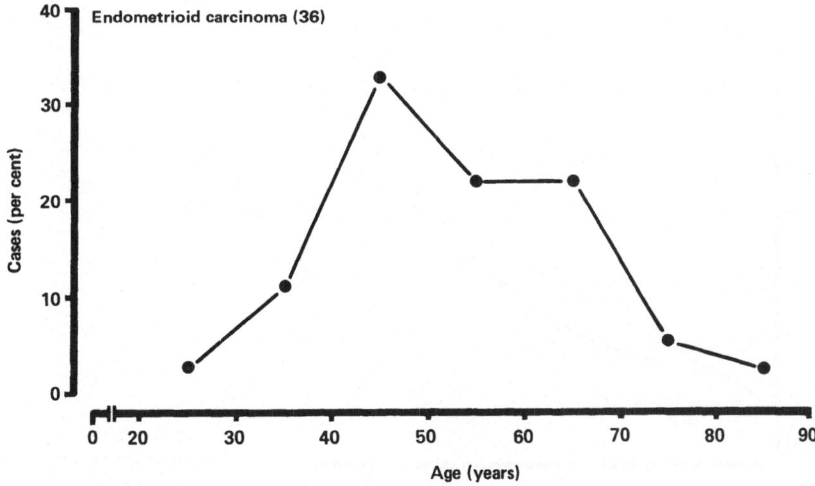

Fig. 3. Age distribution of endometrioid carcinomas in Manchester (36)

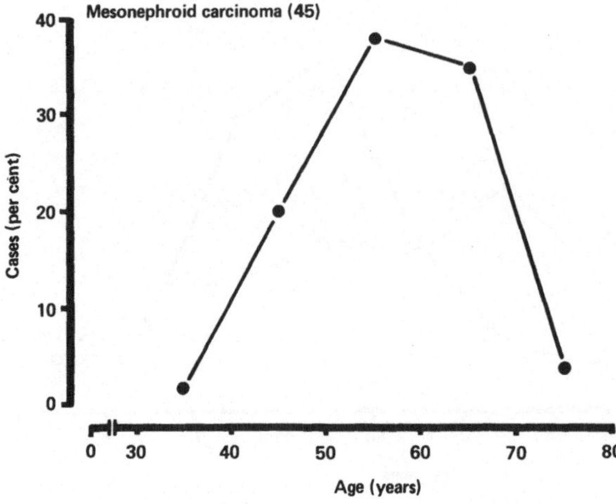

Fig. 4. Age distribution of mesonephroid carcinomas in Manchester (45)

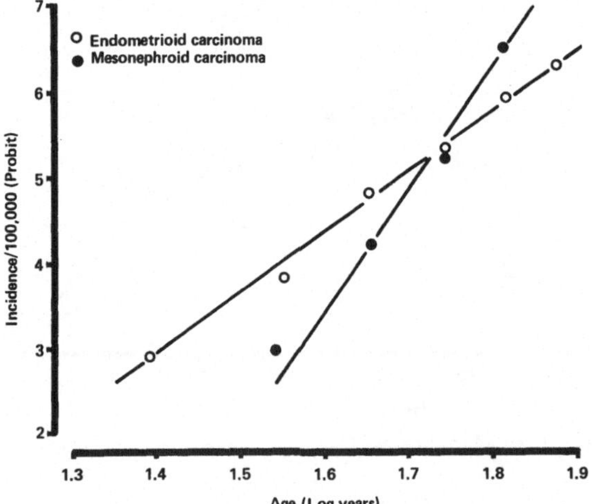

Fig. 5. Age against relative incidence of endometrioid and mesonephroid carcinomas. Log-normal transformation

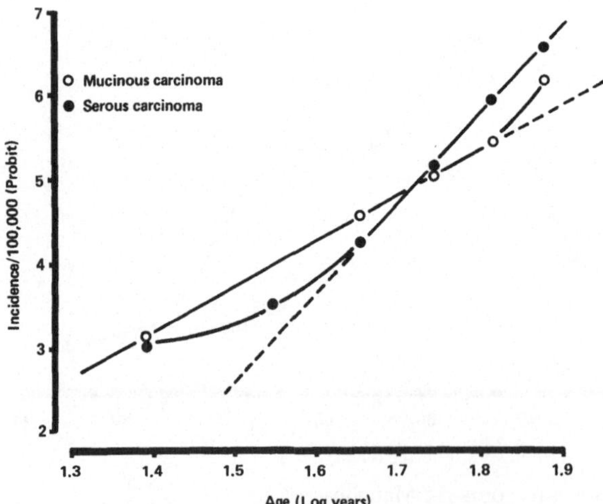

Fig. 6. Age against relative incidence of serous and mucinous carcinomas. Log-normal transformation

mechanism or mechanisms. Indeed in view of the cellular heterogeneity and differences in histogenesis of the various types of mucinous tumour it is unlikely that carcinogenesis would conform to a single pattern.

Some Epidemiologic Considerations and the Need for Quality Control

Since among the common epithelial tumours of the ovary: (a) histogenesis varies from one type of neoplasm to another, and (b) the carcinogenic mechanisms also vary, it is probable that the aetiological factors and agents also differ with tumour type. For example, what conditions determine that a tumour should show mullerian rather than wolffian differentiation or a serous rather than an endometrioid pattern? These questions can be investigated by epidemiological methods but such studies require close attention to histological quality control as well as careful planning.

Tables 5 and 6 show the variations in frequency of the different types of common epithelial tumour of the ovary in different geographic locations. The greatest difference is the relatively high frequency of benign tumours in India and California compared with Australia and Manchester. The variations in frequency of the individual benign tumours are probably the result of slightly differing diagnostic criteria or of sample variations, except for California where the proportion of benign serous tumours is twice that elsewhere. Table 6 shows greater variation in the relative frequencies of the different malignant tumours at each location. The Manchester diagnoses are based on a consensus opinion, whilst the Australian diagnoses are those of one person. If the serous and "other" cancers are added together in each of these two series the percentages are rather similar: 56.2% for Manchester and 62.4% for Australia. The "other" tumours in Manchester include a large proportion of unclassified tumours, many of which are papillary and might well have been termed serous by a single pathologist. However, the high proportion of serous carcinomas in California is still outside the range of diagnostic variation.

The proportions of the different types of tumour vary with the ethnic composition of the population. Weiss and Peterson (1978) reported the frequency of ovarian cancer in four different racial groups in the United States. Japanese, Chinese, Hispanic and black women had rates of epithelial tumours that were 19%–42% less than those of white women. Although these differences were mainly due to a lower frequency of serous and "papillary" tumours, all but the Chinese women had a decreased prevalence of mucinous tumours. Hispanic and black women also had lower rates of endometrioid and clear cell malignancies. The frequency of non-epithelial ovarian tumours showed little relation to race. Such ethnic variations, if confirmed, may afford aetiological clues, but confirmation requires strict attention to histological criteria and consistency in their use.

Table 7 compares the difference in frequency of some common epithelial tumours in Manchester in two consecutive periods. Those for 1956–1971 are taken from the records of St. Mary's Hospital and the diagnoses are of one pathologist and his team. Those for 1974–1979 are taken from five hospitals (including St. Mary's Hospital) and the diagnoses are consensus opinions. The most marked change is the

Table 5. The proportions of different types of common epithelial tumours in various centres

	Australia 1979 (Russell) (%)	Manchester 1974 – 1979 (%)	India 1972 (Ramachandran et al.) (%)	California 1968 (Bennington et al.) (%)
Benign	55.8	59.7	70.0	79.2
– Serous	22.7	29.2	29.6	62.3
– Mucinous	29.3	22.1	26.2	15.2
– Brenner	1.8	3.1	1.3	1.7
– Other	2.0	4.7	12.9	0
Borderline	14.4	9.2	–	–
Malignant	29.8	31.2	29.9	20.9
No. of patients	1000	778	620	360

Table 6. The proportions of different types of malignant common epithelial tumours in various centres

	Australia 1979 (Russell) (%)	Manchester 1974 – 1979 (%)	India 1972 (Ramachandran et al.) (%)	California 1968 (Bennington et al.) (%)
Serous	54.7	32.9	34.4	72.0
Mucinous	5.7	14.2	11.8	13.3
Endometrioid	21.8	17.1	2.7	6.7
Mesonephroid	10.1	11.2	1.1	0
Brenner	0	1.3	0	0
Other	7.7	23.3	50	8.0
No. of patients	298	240	186	75

Table 7. Common epithelial ovarian tumours in Manchester

	St. Mary's Hospital (1956 – 1971)	Five hospitals (1974 – 1979)
Benign	75.9	59.7
– Serous	38.8	29.2
– Mucinous	34.5	22.1
– Brenner	2.6	3.1
– Other	0	4.7
Borderline	–	9.2
Malignant	24.1	31.2
No. of patients	843	778

fall in the relative proportion of benign tumours, affecting both the serous and mucinous tumours but especially the latter. There are several factors which may have caused this change:

1. Variation in diagnostic criteria
2. Change in population structure
3. Proportion of referred cases
4. Therapy
   a) Contraceptive pill
   b) Conservation of ovaries
5. Decline in parity.

These need to be investigated but prior to such a study it is necessary to determine whether the diagnostic criteria used in the earlier study were the same as in the later.

Summary

1. Although some common epithelial tumours of the ovary originate as monophyletic teratomas, most arise from the germinal epithelium of the ovary either by mullerian differentiation (including origin from foci of endometriosis) or by wolffian differentiation.
2. Mechanisms of carcinogenesis vary with the type of neoplasm.
3. In the later development of ovarian carcinomas stage III and IV tumours are more aggressive and less well differentiated than stage I tumours.
4. Since morphogenesis varies with the type of tumour, it is probable that aetiological factors and agents also vary. To study this epidemiologically requires good histological control, so that the tumours are not merely classed as benign or malignant as in many international tabulations but by their individual histological types.

Acknowledgements. I would like to thank Mrs. M. A. Green for preparing the manuscript, and the Department of Medical Illustration, Manchester University and Mrs. Linda Chawner for preparing the illustrations.

References

Abell MR (1966) The nature and classification of ovarian neoplasms. Can Med Assoc J 94:1102–1124

Agrofojo A, Gibbs ACC, Langley FA (1977) Histological discrimination of malignancy in mucinous ovarian tumours. Histopathology 1:431–443

Akagi Y (1928) Die Heterogenen der Kinderovarien. Arch Gynecol 134:290–424

Anderson MC (1972) Endometrioid tumour of the ovary with mucinous and serous components. Am J Obstet Gynecol 113:686–950

Arey LB (1961) The origin and form of Brenner tumor. Am J Obstet Gynecol 81:743–751

Armenian HK, Lilienfield AM (1974) The distribution of incubation periods of neoplastic diseases. Am J Epidemiol 99:92–100
Azzopardi JG, Hou LT (1965) Intestinal metaplasia with argentaffin cells in cervical adenocarcinoma. J Pathol Bact 90:686
Barzilai G (1949) Atlas of ovarian tumors. Grune & Stratton, New York
Bennington J, Ferguson BR, Haber SL (1968) Incidence and relative frequency of benign and malignant ovarian neoplasms. Obstet Gynecol 32:627–632
Bhattacharya M, Barlow JJ (1973) Immunologic studies of human serous cystadenocarcinoma of ovary. Demonstration of tumor-associated antigens. Cancer 31:588–595
Brown H, Lane M (1965) Cushing's and malignant carcinoid syndromes from ovarian neoplasms. Arch Intern Med 115:490–494
Buckley CH, Fox H (1979) An immunohistochemical study of HCG secretion by large bowel adenocarcinoma. J Clin Pathol 32:368–372
Cariker M, Dockerty MB (1954) Mucinous systomadenomas and mucinous cystadenocarcinomas of the ovary. Cancer 7:302–310
Cocco AE, Conway SJ (1975) Zollinger-Ellison Syndrome with ovarian mucinous cystadenocarcinoma. N Engl J Med 295:485–486
Cramer DW, Cutler SS (1974) Incidence and histopathology of malignancies of the female genital organs in the United States. Am J Obstet Gynecol 118:443–460
Crowther ME, Grudzinkas JG, Poulton IA, Gordon YB (1979) Trophoblastic proteins in ovarian carcinoma. Obstet Gynecol 53:59–61
Cummins PA, Fox H, Langley FA (1973) An ultrastructural study of the nature and origin of the Brenner tumour of the ovary. J Pathol 110:167–176
Czernobilsky B, Morris WJ (1979) A histologic study of ovarian endometriosis with emphasis on hyperplastic and atypical change. Obstet Gynecol 53:318–323
Farrer HK, Elesh R, Libretti J (1960) Brenner tumors and estrogen production. Obstet Gynecol Surv 15:1
Fenoglio CM (1980) Overview article: Ultrastructural features of the common epithelial tumours of the ovary. Ultrsatructural Pathology 1:419–444
Fenoglio CM, Ferenczy A, Richart RM (1975) Mucinous tumors of the ovary. Ultrastructural studies of mucinous cystadenomas with histogenetic considerations. Cancer 36:1709–1722
Fox H, Kazzaz B, Langley FA (1964) Argyrophil and argentaffin cells in the female genital tract and in ovarian mucinous cysts. J Pathol Bact 88:479–488
Fox H, Agrawal K, Langley FA (1972) The Brenner tumour of the ovary. J Obstet Gynecol Br Commonw 79:661–665
Glazunow M (1937) Histologie und Histogenese der sog. cilioepithelialen (serosen) Cystome der Ovarien. Arch Gynecol 164:358
Gold P, Freedman SO (1965 a) Demonstration of tumor-specific antigens in human colonic carcinomata by immunological tolerance and absorption techniques. J Exp Med 121:439–462
Gold P, Freedman SO (1965 b) Specific carcinoembryonic antigens in the human digestive system. J Exp Med 122:467–481
Greene RR (1952) The diverse origins of Brenner tumors. Am J Obstet Gynecol 64:878–898
Hamwi GJ, Byron RC, Besch PG, Vorys N, Teteris MJ, Uller JC (1963) Testosterone synthesis by a Brenner tumor. Part I. Clinical evidence of masculinization during pregnancy. Am J Obstet Gynecol 80:1015–1020
Heald J, Buckley CH, Fox H (1979) An immunohistochemical study of the distribution of carcinoembryonic antigen in epithelial tumours of the ovary. J Clin Pathol 32:918–926
Hendrickson MR, Kempson RL (1980) Surgical Pathology of the Uterine Corpus, chapt 7. Saunders, Philadelphia
Janovski NA, Paramanandhan TL (1973) Ovarian Tumors. Major problems in obstetrics and gynecology, vol 4. Saunders, Philadelphia
Klemi PS (1978) Pathology of mucinous ovarian cystadenomas. l. Argyrophil and argentaffin cells and epithelial mucosubstances. Acta Pathol Microbiol Scand [A] 86:465–470
Langley FA, Lodge KV, Woodcock AS (1956) The survival of rats after adrenalectomy. Br J Exp Pathol 37:350–356

Langley FA, Cummins PA, Fox H (1972) An ultrastructural study of mucin secreting epithelia in ovarian neoplasms. Acta Pathol Microbiol Scand [A] [Suppl 233] 80:76–86

Lauchlan SC (1966) The histogenesis and historelationships of Brenner tumors. Cancer 19:1628–1634

Lauchlan SC (1972) The secondary Müllerian system. Obstet Gynecol Surv 27:133–146

Madan A, Tyagi SP, Moshin S, Hameed F, Rizvi (1978) Incidence of ovarian tumours in Aligarh with particular reference to histological typing. J Obstet Gynecol India 28:827–832

Masson P (1956) Tumeurs Humaines, 2e éd, p 714. Maloine, Paris

Medical Research Council Study on Chemotherapy in Advanced Ovarian Cancer (1981) Br J Obstet Gynecol 88:1174–1185

Morris JM, Scully RE (1958) Endocrine pathology of the ovary. Henry Kimpton, London

Needham (1942) Biochemistry and morphogenesis. Cambridge University Press, Cambridge

Numers C von (1965) Observations of metaplastic changes in the germinal epithelium of the ovary and on the etiology of endometriosis. Acta Obstet Gynecol Scand 44:107–116

Ober WB (1979) Carcinosarcoma of the ovary. Case report, review of literature and comment on subcoelomic mesenchyme. Am J Diagn Gynecol 1:73–81

O'Neil RI, Mikuta JJ (1970) Hypoglycaemia associated with serous cystadenocarcinoma of the ovary. Obstet Gynecol 35:287–289

Plaut A (1933) Der sogenannte „Tumor ovarii Brenner". (Fibroepithelioma mucinosum benignum ovarii). Arch Gynecol 153:97–126

Plimpton CH, Gelhorn A (1956) Hypercalcemia in malignant disease without evidence of bone destruction. Am J Med 21:750–759

Population Estimates (1977) Office of Population Censuses and Surveys, Series PP1 No 2. H. M. Stationery Office, London

Porter MR, Frantz VK (1956) Tumors associated with hypoglycemia–pancreatic and extrapancreatic. Am J Med 21:944–961

Pratt J, Scully RE (1979a) Sarcomas in ovarian mucinous tumors. Cancer 44:1327–1331

Pratt J, Scully RE (1979b) Ovarian mucinous tumors with sarcoma-like mural nodules. Cancer 44:1332–1344

Ramachandran G, Harilal KR, Chinnamma KK, Thangavelu M (1972) Ovarian neoplasms – a study of 903 cases. J Obstet Gynecol India 22:309–315

Rivett JD, Robinson SM (1972) Hypercalcaemia associated with an ovarian carcinoma of mesonephromatous type. J Obstet Gynecol Br Commonw 72:1047–1052

Roberts DK, Marshall RB, Wharton JT (1970) Ultrastructure of ovarian tumors. I. Papillary serous cystadenocarcinoma. Cancer 25:947–958

Roth LM (1971) Fine structure of the Brenner tumor. Cancer 27:1482–1488

Roth LM (1974a) Clear cell adenocarcinoma of the female genital tract. Light and electron microscopic study. Cancer 33:990–1001

Roth LM (1974b) The Brenner tumor and the Walthard cell rest. Lab Invest 31:15–23

Roth LM, Czernobilsky B, Langley FA (1981) Endometrioid tumor with squamous metaplasia and fibrous stroma of low malignant potential. Cancer 48:1838–1849

Russell P (1979) The pathological assessment of ovarian neoplasms. 1: Introduction to the common "epithelian" tumours and an analysis of benign "epithelial" tumours. Pathology 11:5–26

Sampson JA (1925) Endometrial carcinoma of the ovary arising on endometrial tissue in that organ. Arch Surg 10:1–72

Schiller W (1934) Zur Histogenese der Brennerschen Ovarialtumoren. Arch Gynecol 157:65–83

Scott RB (1942) Serous adenofibromas and cystadenofibromas of the ovary. Am Obstet Gynecol 43:733–751

Scully RE, Barlow JF (1967) "Mesonephroma" of the ovary. Cancer 20:1405–1417

Scully RE, Richardson GS, Barlow JF (1966) The development of malignancy in endometriosis. Clin Obstet Gynecol 9:384–411

Seppälä M (1980) Markers for neoplastic ovarian cells, in Biology of ovarian neoplasia. In: Murphy ED, Beamer WG (eds) U.I.C.C. Technical report series 50. U.I.C.C., Geneva

Shinada T, Tsukui J, Matsumoto S (1973) Estrogen synthesis by Brenner tumors. Am J Obstet Gynecol 116:408–411

Sternberg WH (1963) In: Gray HG, Smith DE (eds) The Ovary. Williams & Wilkins, Baltimore (International Academy of Pathology. Monograph No 3, chapt 11.)
Teilum G (1954) Histogenesis and classification of mesonephric tumors of the female and male genital system and relation to benign so-called adenomatoid tumors (mesotheliomas). Acta Pathol Microbiol Scand- [A] 1954, 34:431–451
Towers RP (1956) A note on the origin of the pseudomucinous cystadenoma of the ovary. J Obstet Gynecol Emp 63:253–254
Wade-Evans T, Langley FA (1961) Mesonephric tumors of the female genital tract. Cancer 14:711–725
Waxman M (1979) Pure and mixed Brenner tumors of the ovary. Cancer 43:1830–1839
Weiss NS, Peterson AS (1978) Racial variations in the incidence of ovarian carcinomas in U.S. Am J Epidemiol 107:91–95

Problems in the Differential Diagnosis of Common Epithelial Carcinomas of the Ovary

R. E. SCULLY [1]

Introduction

In 1973 the World Health Organization (WHO) published its "blue book", *Histological Typing of Ovarian Tumours* [11]. Each tumor was defined, with a description of its characteristic features, but a detailed discussion of problems in differential diagnosis was beyond the scope of the monograph. In the 8 years since its publication, a number of difficulties in the application of the classification have become evident. These difficulties require continuous exploration and discussion to ensure uniformity of diagnosis among pathologists, thus providing the most reliable pathologic basis for epidemiologic studies and comparision of the treatment results of various institutions. This article will discuss problems in the differentiation of common epithelial carcinomas from one another, as well as from several ovarian tumors within other categories.

Borderline Tumors vs Invasive Carcinomas

Tumors of borderline malignancy (carcinomas of low malignant potential) are characterized by: (a) stratification of the neoplastic epithelial cells, often accompanied by their detachment as cellular clusters, as well as nuclear abnormalities greater than those encountered in clearly benign tumors, and (b) a lack of "destructive" invasion of the adjacent stroma.

The criteria used to differentiate serous borderline from invasive tumors differ to some extent from those used to distinguish analogous tumors in the mucinous category, and, therefore, the tumors of these two cell types will be discussed separately. Serous borderline tumors are characterized by the presence of noninvasive neoplastic epithelial cells that show varying amounts of cytologic and architectural atypicality, ranging from minimal degrees to carcinoma in situ. So far, various authors have not been able to correlate the grade of atypicality with the prognosis (Santesson 1969, personal communication) [4]. The major problem that confronts the pathologist in his attempt to distinguish borderline from invasive serous tumors is the recognition of destructive invasion. Borderline tumors are often characterized

1 Massachusetts General Hospital, Harvard Medical School, Department of Pathology, Boston, Massachusetts 02114, USA

by an extensive but orderly downgrowth of glandular and tubular structures, sometimes containing papillae, into the stromal component of the neoplasm. The stroma in these areas of pseudoinvasion, however, does not differ in appearance from the stroma elsewhere in the specimen. In contrast, true invasion is typically irregular and disorderly and is often accompanied by a desmoplastic stromal response. On rare occasions, microinvasion of the stroma or lymphatic invasion is encountered in serous tumors that are otherwise characteristic of borderline malignancy. Such tumors should be placed in a separate category until their clinicopathologic features have been established by an investigation of an adequate number of cases.

Peritoneal "implants" may occur in cases of serous borderline tumors, and typically have the cytologic and architectural features of borderline neoplasia. In rare cases the implants have the microscopic features of serous carcinoma. Sometimes they are seen in the form of small mature glandular structures of tubal type, the presence of which has been designated "endosalpingosis". Controversy exists as to whether these so-called implants are true neoplastic deposits or pseudoimplants, i.e., independent foci of proliferation of the peritoneal lining cells. It appears impossible to resolve this question in the great majority of cases. Exceptionally, a borderline tumor of serous type is diffusely distributed on the pelvic peritoneum with no greater involvement of the ovarian surfaces than of other sites. In such cases a multifocal origin from the peritoneum is the most probable explanation for the distribution of the tumor. Regardless of whether the implants of serous borderline tumors are considered to be metastases or separate primary foci of neoplasia, the pathologist should not alter his diagnosis because of their presence, as the prognosis in such cases remains unusually good, and patients with implants of benign or borderline nature may live for decades even in the absence of therapy.

Mucinous borderline tumors may be quite difficult to distinguish from true carcinomas if one relies only on the presence or absence of invasion as the differential feature. The reason for this problem is that mucinous neoplasms often grow in the form of small glands distributed throughout the stroma, and if these are lined by atypical cells it may be impossible to tell whether they have invaded the stroma without exciting a response on its part, or are merely proliferating within it. To obviate this difficulty, Hart and Norris [3] devised a more elaborate set of criteria for distinguishing borderline and invasive mucinous malignancy: if there is obvious invasion, a diagnosis of carcinoma is made; if invasion is absent or equivocal, the differentiation is made on the basis of the height of the atypical neoplastic epithelial cells; stratification of four or more of them in any area warrants the diagnosis of carcinoma, even in the absence of demonstrable invasion. Using such criteria, these investigators demonstrated a striking difference in the actuarial 10-year survival for the two forms of mucinous malignancy (59% for stage 1 carcinomas in contrast to 96% for stage 1 borderline tumors). Later Hart [2] stated that a cribriform pattern was an additional feature that warranted the diagnosis of carcinoma. As in cases of serous neoplasia, the presence of peritoneal implants or pseudomyxoma peritonei should not deter one from making a diagnosis of borderline malignancy if the primary tumor shows the appropriate diagnostic features.

Common epithelial tumors of other cell types that belong morphologically in the borderline group (endometrioid, clear cell) are so rare that the validity of their existence as clinicopathologic entities has not been established.

Serous vs Mucinous Tumors

The terms "serous" and "mucinous" are not entirely appropriate for the types of tumor they designate, and are occasionally misleading. Some serous neoplasms produce large quantities of thick mucinous material, whereas a number of mucinous tumors secrete only thin, watery mucinous fluid or secrete it only at a cellular level. The serous tumors that are most apt to produce substantial amounts of mucin are those in the borderline category. Although the designation "seromucinous" has been used for such tumors, the WHO prefers to classify them within the serous category. The essential difference between serous tumors that secrete mucin and mucinous neoplasms is that the mucin in the former is almost entirely extracellular, with only small quantities visible in the apical portion of the cytoplasm of the neoplastic cells. In contrast, the great majority of mucinous tumors are characterized by the presence of considerable amounts of mucin within significant numbers of the neoplastic cells. In exceptional cases, however, only occasional mucin-filled goblet cells are encountered among mucin-free neoplastic cells.

Serous vs Endometrioid Carcinomas

Serous carcinomas have a variety of characteristic patterns that facilitate their recognition in most cases. These include a delicate, often complex papillarity, sometimes with the formation of glomerulus-like structures, glandular spaces that are irregular and often slit-like, and solid areas ranging from diffuse masses to small regular nests separated by a desmoplastic stroma. Psammoma bodies are characteristic but not specific features, and are often absent. Endometrioid carcinomas, in contrast, are characterized in differentiated areas by the presence of regular tubular glands lined by stratified non-mucin-containing epithelium. Occasionally strips of cells resembling endocervical epithelium are encountered in small foci. Cytologically benign or malignant squamous differentiation is often present and may provide an important diagnostic clue. The squamous element may appear in the form of solid nests or masses of cells with small spindle-shaped nuclei. Occasionally an endometrioid carcinoma is highly papillary, creating a problem in differentiation from a serous papillary adenocarcinoma. The papillarity, however, is broader and more regular in the former, and other diagnostic features of endometrioid carcinoma are typically present. Some common epithelial carcinomas, particularly those in the more poorly differentiated categories, have features that are intermediate between those of the serous and endometrioid carcinoma. In our opinion, these tumors should be placed in the former category to permit more valid clinicopathologic and epidemiologic characterization of the relatively new entity of endometrioid carcinoma.

Endometrioid vs Mucinous Carcinomas, Primary and Metastatic

Endometrioid carcinomas, like serous tumors, may secrete mucin, but, again, except for its occasional presence in small foci of endocervical type epithelium, it is almost entirely extracellular within the lumens of the glands. Occasional well-differentiated endometrioid adenocarcinomas are of the mucin-rich type, in which the glandular spaces are distended with thick mucin. When mucin is present only within scattered goblet cells in a mucinous carcinoma, it can resemble an endometrioid carcinoma, at least on low-power examination. The performance of mucin stains, which facilitates the identification of intracellular globules, is helpful in the differential diagnosis in such cases. Metastatic adenocarcinoma from the large intestine, the most common form of metastatic carcinoma that presents as an ovarian mass, may be particularly difficult to distinguish from an endometrioid carcinoma because it typically contains considerably less intracellular mucin than primary mucinous adenocarcinomas of the ovary. In general, for a comparable degree of glandular differentiation, metastatic intestinal adenocarcinomas show more extensive necrosis and have more poorly differentiated glandular lining cells than endometrioid carcinomas. They also lack the squamous component so frequently encountered in the latter.

Primary vs Metastatic Mucinous Carcinomas

The ultimate criterion for distinguishing a primary from a metastatic mucinous adenocarcinoma of the ovary is the demonstration of a primary extraovarian carcinoma by operative or radiologic means. In the absence of such evidence, the distribution of the tumor on exploration provides suggestive evidence of its origin. Metastatic carcinomas from the stomach are bilateral in approximately four-fifths of cases, and metastatic carcinomas from the large intestine in about two-thirds of cases [10]. In contrast, primary mucinous carcinomas of the ovary are bilateral in only 10% of cases [5]. On gross examination metastatic carcinomas from the large intestine are frequently cystic, with most of the cysts lined by necrotic tumor; occasional cysts, however, may be thin-walled and have a smooth lining. Krukenberg tumors (signet-ring cell carcinomas), most of which are of gastric origin, are typically solid and often extensively necrotic and hemorrhagic, but rarely contain numerous thin-walled cysts, simulating a primary mucinous cystic tumor. On low-power microscopic examination, metastatic carcinomas are often present as multiple discrete or confluent nodules, and are frequently seen within vessels, whereas primary carcinomas show these features much less commonly. The best microscopic criterion for establishing a diagnosis of primary mucinous cystadenocarcinoma is the coexistence of benign and borderline neoplasia with the carcinomatous component. It must be emphasized, however, that cysts lined by well-differentiated, benign-appearing mucinous epithelium are rarely encountered also within metastatic adenocarcinomas from the large intestine and Krukenberg tumors. Although it has been claimed that the presence of goblet cells in an ovarian mucinous carcinoma excludes a metastatic origin, we have encountered such cells in a number of metastatic adenocarcinomas from the large intestine, and do not consider their presence or absence a reliable diagnostic criterion.

Endometrioid vs Sertoli Cell Carcinoma

Testicular Sertoli cell tumors are generally easy to recognize because of their distinctive tubular pattern and the rarity of similar patterns in other forms of testicular neoplasia. In the ovary, however, a number of carcinomas, particularly those of endometrioid type, may also have a tubular architecture, creating problems in differential diagnosis. If any of the other characteristic patterns of the Sertoli-Leydig cell tumor are present in a specimen under consideration, the diagnosis is obvious. Also, if the tubules contain significant amounts of intracellular lipid and the tumor is estrogenic, a diagnosis of lipid-rich Sertoli cell tumor ("folliculome lipidique") is warranted. In the absence of these findings, differentiation from an endometrioid carcinoma may be difficult or even impossible. In addition to typical large tubular glands, an endometrioid carcinoma can form small glands mimicking the tubules of the well-differentiated Sertoli cell tumor (Pick's tubular adenoma), elongated thin tubular glands, and winding solid tubules resembling atrophic testicular tubules that have lost their germ cells. Luteinization of the stroma of an endometrioid carcinoma, sometimes accompanied by estrogenic manifestations, may enhance its resemblance to a Sertoli-Leydig cell tumor. The presence somewhere in the specimen of typical endometrioid carcinoma, squamous differentiation, and/or intraluminal mucin, however, generally permits identification of the tumor as endometrioid.

Clear Cell Carcinoma

Clear cell carcinomas are usually among the most easily recognized forms of common epithelial carcinoma because of their content of: (a) large polyhedral or rounded clear cells containing glycogen and resembling the clear cells of a renal cell carcinoma, and/or (b) distinctive hobnail cells lining cysts and tubules that may contain multiple papillae. Occasional patterns and cell types of the clear cell carcinoma may, however, create problems in differential diagnosis, particularly when they characterize the major component of a specimen. The most common of the deviant patterns, the adenofibromatous, is characterized by small cysts typically lined by flattened epithelium and separated by varying amounts of fibromatous stroma. The presence of these cysts led to the original designation of tumors having this pattern as parvilocular cystomas [8]. High-power examination of the cysts reveals the flattened, hobnail or clear cell character of their lining cells. When a parvilocular pattern is present, careful sampling almost always discloses typical clear cell carcinoma elsewhere in the specimen. In the occasional case in which the tumor appears to be entirely or almost entirely parvilocular, a designation of atypical clear cell adenofibroma or adenofibroma of borderline malignancy is suggested, but not enough experience has accumulated with rare tumors of this type to allow characterization of their biologic behavior. Occasionally the clear cell carcinoma is partly composed of large cells with abundant eosinophilic cytoplasm growing in cords or lining glandular spaces. Rarely this pattern and cell type characterize the major component of the tumor. Another unusual appearance of the clear cell carcinoma that may create confusion is one in which solid nests and masses of predominant clear cells contain scattered cells with intracytoplasmic mucin, which may have a targetoid appearance, and peripheral compressed nuclei. These cells resemble signet-ring cells, and tumors containing them have occasionally been confused with Krukenberg tumors.

Several other types of tumor can be confused with clear cell carcinoma. The endodermal sinus tumor (yolk sac tumor) and the clear cell carcinoma were considered variants of one another at the time of their initial description [7], but are rarely confused nowadays, due to the important contributions of Teilum, who first clearly distinguished them [12]. Not only do these two types of tumor have a different age distribution, but their microscopic patterns and cell types differ so widely in the great majority of cases that the differential diagnosis is not a problem. Occasionally, however, some of the features characterizing one of these tumors may be seen in the other. For example, intracytoplasmic hyaline bodies are sometimes encountered in the clear cell carcinoma, and glandular structures lined by clear cells full of glycogen are rarely observed in endodermal sinus tumors.

An occasional clear cell carcinoma has a complex papillary pattern simulating that of certain serous carcinomas, but the characteristic appearance of the neoplastic cells enables one to identify it as belonging in the clear cell category. Sometimes one encounters a tumor with features intermediate between those of a clear cell carcinoma and an endometrioid carcinoma, the cells of which may also contain cytoplasmic glycogen. Only when the material is present in relatively large amounts is a diagnosis of clear cell carcinoma justified. The finding of tumors intermediate in appearance between these two types of neoplasia is not surprising in view of the close histogenetic relation between them [9]. Clear cell carcinomas can also secrete considerable mucin into the lumens of tubules and cysts and should not be confused with mucinous carcinomas under such circumstances.

Very rarely a renal cell carcinoma presents as a metastatic ovarian mass. When a clear cell carcinoma is composed entirely of clear cells, it may be impossible to exclude a metastatic renal cell carcinoma on histologic grounds alone, but when other patterns and cell types characteristic of the former are also present, a diagnosis of clear cell carcinoma can be established; renal cell carcinomas do not secrete mucin at a light microscopic level and rarely, if ever, contain hobnail cells. Clear cell carcinomas composed exclusively of clear cells may also be confused with dysgerminomas, however. The former typically contain polyhedral cells with eccentric nuclei and the latter, rounded cells with central nuclei; likewise infiltration of the stroma by lymphocytes and the occasional presence of stromal granulomas are characteristic of the dysgerminoma, but absent in the clear cell carcinoma. Finally, clear cell carcinomas typically occur in women older than those with dysgerminomas.

Brenner Tumors

There is still controversy whether the proliferating Brenner tumor, which typically contains cysts lined by mitotically active transitional type epithelium, has been correctly designated a tumor of borderline malignancy in view of the great rarity or absence of a malignant behavior in the reported cases. In one instance, however, a tumor that was interpreted as borderline on the basis of its microscopic features was associated with the later development of hepatic metastases [6]. Unfortunately, many of the cases in the literature have been reported without adequate follow-up, and further experience with tumors of this type is necessary before resolving the dispute. The distinction between a borderline and a malignant Brenner tumor may be difficult because, like mucinous neoplasms, Brenner tumors are characterized by epithelial elements scattered throughout a stromal component. We now consider the degree of atypicality of the neoplastic cells as well as the presence or absence of invasion in differentiating these two forms of neoplasia. If the tumor cells are cytologically malignant, we exclude a diagnosis of borderline malignancy even though stromal invasion may not be clearly demonstrable. It must be emphasized that before diagnosing a malignant Brenner tumor one should demonstrate a benign Brenner component within the specimen. A failure to fulfil this diagnostic requirement has often resulted in the misinterpretation of endometrioid adenoacanthomas and adenosquamous carcinomas and undifferentiated carcinomas having a transitional appearance as malignant Brenner tumors. Very rarely a transitional cell carcinoma of the urinary bladder or ureter metastasizes to the ovary and simulates a borderline or malignant Brenner tumor. In addition to helpful clinical information, the presence or absence of a benign Brenner component provides a clue to the differential diagnosis.

Undifferentiated Carcinoma

Probably the great majority of undifferentiated carcinomas of the ovary are common epithelial carcinomas, mostly of very poorly differentiated serous or endometrioid type. The category of undifferentiated carcinoma, according to WHO, includes tumors with minimal differentiation. Therefore the presence of mucin droplets or pools, psammoma bodies or rare glands does not exclude the diagnosis. Rare small-cell undifferentiated carcinomas, encountered mainly during the second to fourth decades and often associated with paraneoplastic hypercalcemia [1], are probably not of common epithelial type, although their histogenesis is at present obscure.

One tumor that should not be confused with the undifferentiated carcinoma is the diffuse granulosa cell tumor. This distinction is of great importance because of the striking differences between these tumors, particularly in regard to their prognosis and therapy. The best criterion for distinguishing them is the appearance of their nuclei. Those of the granulosa cell tumor are typically round or angular, pale, and often grooved, whereas those of the undifferentiated carcinoma are usually hyperchromatic, with coarser irregular chromatin, and rarely contain grooves; atypical mitotic figures are often encountered in undifferentiated carcinomas as well.

Mixed Carcinomas

Careful examination of many common epithelial carcinomas discloses the presence of more than one cell type, but according to the WHO definition, the identification of a mixed carcinoma requires a significant contribution of a second or even a third cell type; minor components are ignored in the choice of a diagnostic term.

Conclusion

Remarkable progress has been made in achieving uniformity of diagnosis and nomenclature of ovarian cancer on the part of pathologists, but a continuing effort to refine present diagnostic criteria and improve agreement is essential to achieve the degree of pathologic knowledge that is optimal for progress in combating this extremely lethal disease.

References

1. Dickersin GR, Kline IW, Scully RE (1982) Small cell carcinoma of the ovary with hypercalcemia. A report of 11 cases. Cancer 48: 188–197
2. Hart WR (1977) Ovarian epithelial tumors of borderline malignancy (carcinomas of low malignant potential). Hum Pathol 8:541–549
3. Hart WR, Norris HJ (1973) Borderline and malignant mucinous tumors of the ovary. Histologic criteria and clinical behavior. Cancer 31: 1031–1045
4. Katzenstein A-LA, Mazur MT, Morgan TE, Kao M-S (1978) Proliferative serous tumors of the ovary. Am J Surg Pathol 2:339–355
5. Kottmeier HL (1968) Surgical management-conservative surgery. Indications according to the type of the tumour. In: Gentil F, Junqueira AC (eds) Ovarian Cancer. Springer, Berlin Heidelberg New York (UICC monograph series, vol 11, pp 157–164)
6. Prat-Thomas HR, Kreutner A Jr, Underwood PB, Dowdeswell RH (1976) Proliferative and malignant Brenner tumors of ovary. Report of 2 cases, one with Meigs' syndrome, review of literature and ultrastructural comparisons. Gynecol Oncol 4: 176–193
7. Schiller W (1939) Mesonephroma ovarii. Am J Cancer 35: 1–21
8. Schiller W (1943) Parvilocular tumors of the ovary. Arch Pathol 35:391–413
9. Scully RE, Barlow JF (1967) "Mesonephroma" of ovary. Tumor of Müllerian nature related to the endometrioid carcinoma. Cancer 20: 1405–1417
10. Scully RE, Richardson GS (1961) Luteinization of the stroma of metastatic cancer involving the ovary and its endocrine significance. Cancer 14:827–840
11. Serov SF, Scully RE, Sobin LH (1973) International histological classification of tumours, No 9. Histological typing of ovarian tumours. WHO, Geneva
12. Teilum G (1950) "Mesonephroma ovarii" (Schiller). An extra-embryonic mesoblastoma of germ cell origin in the ovary and the testis. Acta Pathol Microbiol Scand 27:249–261

Die Bedeutung verschiedener morphologischer Parameter für die Prognose des Ovarialkarzinoms

G. Breitenecker [1], W. Bartl [1] und V. Scheiber [2]

Einleitung

Während die Mortalität des Zervixkarzinoms in den vergangenen Jahren in Österreich ständig abnahm, ist die des Ovarialkarzinoms etwa gleichgeblieben, so daß diese beiden Karzinome heute etwa die gleiche Mortalität aufweisen [2]. Dieser Trend ist auch in anderen Industriestaaten zu beobachten. So ist in den USA die Mortalität des Ovarialkarzinoms bereits seit Anfang der 70er Jahre höher als die des Zervixkarzinoms [8]. Es ist daher verständlich, wenn zunehmend verstärkte Anstrengungen zu Verbesserung der Therapie des Ovarialkarzinoms unternommen werden. Dazu gehören ein aggressiveres operatives Vorgehen mit möglichst weitgehender Tumorentfernung, Second-look-Operationen und neue Formen der Strahlen- und Chemotherapie [7, 9, 19]. Um den Erfolg neuer Therapieformen objektiv beurteilen zu können, ist eine differenzierte Klassifikation und Beschreibung der Tumoren unter Berücksichtigung der bekannten prognostischen Faktoren nötig, da nur so verschiedene Patientenkollektive miteinander verglichen werden können.

Es erscheint heute hinreichend belegt, daß neben dem klinischen Stadium das Ausmaß des bei der Operation zurückgelassenen Tumorgewebes von entscheidender prognostischer Bedeutung ist [8, 19]. Darüber hinaus scheinen aber auch morphologische Parameter des Tumorgewebes prognostische Aussagekraft zu besitzen [6, 12, 15, 17]. Ziel der vorliegenden Studie war es daher, an einem retrospektiv nachuntersuchten Kollektiv zu prüfen, welche Wertigkeit den verschiedenen morphologischen Parametern für die prognostische Beurteilung von Ovarialkarzinomen zukommt.

Material und Methoden

Es wurden die histologischen Schnitte von 122 malignen epithelialen Ovarialtumoren ausgewertet, die in den Jahren 1968–1977 an der II. Universitäts-Frauenklinik operiert wurden, also vor der Einführung der heute geübten Therapieformen mit Second-look-Operationen und kombinierter Strahlen-Chemo-Therapie.

---

1 II. Frauenklinik der Universität Wien, Spitalgasse 23, A-1090 Wien
2 Institut für medizinische Statistik und Dokumentation der Universität Wien, A-1090 Wien

Die Ovarialkarzinome wurden nach folgenden Gesichtspunkten beurteilt:

1. Histologische Klassifikation (*Typing*), entsprechend den Empfehlungen der WHO [16].
2. Ausbreitung des Tumors (*Staging*), nach der histopathologischen pTNM-Klassifikation der UICC [23].
3. Morphologische Parameter der Gewebs- und Zellreife (*Grading*)
   a) histologischer Differenzierungsgrad (hoch – mäßig – undifferenziert),
   b) zytologischer Differenzierungsgrad, modifiziert nach Broders [4],
   c) Mitoseindex.

Typing und Grading durch den Pathologen (G.B.) erfolgte ohne Kenntnis des klinischen Stadiums, des Verlaufs und der Überlebenszeit der Patientinnen.

Statistische Berechnungen

Die an jeder Patientin erhobenen Merkmale wurden vorerst auf Unabhängigkeit geprüft: Waren zwei untersuchte Merkmale Meßdaten, so wurde der Pearson-Korrelationskoeffizient berechnet; war nur ein Faktor eine Messung, wurde eine einfache Varianzanalyse durchgeführt; in den übrigen Fällen wurde der χ^2-Test auf Unabhängigkeit angewandt. Für jeden der möglichen Einflußfaktoren wurde ein Vergleich der Überlebenskurven sowohl mit dem Test nach Breslow [3] als auch mit dem Test von Mantel [11] durchgeführt. Bildeten die Stufen des untersuchten Einflußfaktors eine Ordnung, wurde der Trendtest von Tarone [22] sowohl für den Test nach Breslow, als auch für den Mantel-Test gerechnet.

Da das Stadium eine besonders deutliche Auswirkung auf die Sterbekurve hatte, wurde das jeweilige Stadium als Stratifizierungsvariable oder Kovariable berücksichtigt und die erwähnten Analysen für die anderen Einflußfaktoren unter Elimination des Einflusses des Stadiums nochmals durchgerechnet.

Für die Durchrechnung wurde ein von Schemper [13] entwickeltes Programmpaket verwendet.

Unabhängig von dem oben angeführten Kollektiv wurden unter Anwendung der Peroxidase-Antiperoxidase-Methode nach Sternberger et al. [20] Paraffinschnitte von 71 epithelialen Ovarialtumoren verschiedener Dignität (benigne, Borderlinelesions, maligne) auf CEA und 45 Fälle mittels einer modifizierten „Mixed-cell"-Agglutinationsreaktion auf Blutgruppeneigenschaften untersucht [5].

Darüber hinaus werden an unserer Klinik seit kurzer Zeit in Gefrierschnitten maligner Ovarialtumoren Östrogen- und Progesteronrezeptoren fluoreszenzoptisch mittels Steroidkonjugaten nachgewiesen [1, 10].

Ergebnisse

Etwa ein Viertel der Karzinome befanden sich im Stadium I, ein weiteres Viertel im Stadium II und etwa die Hälfte der Fälle in den Stadien III und IV (Tabelle 1). Das Durchschnittsalter in den verschiedenen Stadien war nicht signifikant unterschiedlich ($p=0{,}71$).

Tabelle 1. Ovarialkarzinome II. UFK Wien 1968 bis 1977

Stadium			
FIGO	TNM	n	%
I	T_1	34	27,9
II	T_2	28	23,0
III	T_3	48	39,3
IV	M_1	12	9,8
		122	100,0

In Übereinstimmung mit den Angaben in der Literatur [14] stellten die serösen Karzinome die überwiegende Mehrheit, gefolgt von den muzinösen und undifferenzierten bzw. unklassifizierbaren Karzinomen, während die endometrioiden und klarzelligen Karzinome relativ selten zu beobachten waren. Die fünf klarzelligen Karzinome mußten wegen der geringen Fallzahl aus der statistischen Untersuchung ausgeschieden werden (Tabelle 2, oben). Die verschiedenen histologischen Typen waren auf die Stadien nicht signifikant unterschiedlich verteilt ($p = 0{,}3$).

Die Aufteilung der Fälle auf die verschiedenen Gradingparameter bzw. das Stadium geht aus Tabelle 2 (unten) und Tabelle 3 hervor. Dabei erwies sich auch hier die Verteilung als statistisch nicht signifikant unterschiedlich ($p = 0{,}1–0{,}8$).

Tabelle 2. Beziehung von histologischem Typ und histologischem Differenzierungsgrad zum Stadium

Histologischer Typ	Stadium								Gesamt
	I		II		III		IV		
	n	%	n	%	n	%	n	%	$p = 0{,}3$
Serös	27	31,8	15	17,7	35	41,2	8	9,4	85
Muzinös	3	20,0	6	40,0	5	33,3	1	6,7	15
Endometrioid	2	33,3	2	33,3	1	16,7	1	16,7	6
Undifferenziert	0	0	3	27,3	6	54,6	2	18,2	11
	32		26		47		12		117
Histologischer Differenzierungsgrad	n	%	n	%	n	%	n	%	$p = 0{,}8$
G 1	17	31,5	12	22,2	19	35,2	6	11,1	54
G 2	12	28,6	8	19,1	19	45,2	3	7,1	42
G 3	5	19,2	8	30,8	10	38,5	3	11,5	26
	34		28		48		12		122

Tabelle 3. Beziehung von zytologischem Differenzierungsgrad und der Zahl der Mitosen zum Stadium

Zytologischer Differenzierungsgrad	Stadium I		II		III		IV		Gesamt
	n	%	n	%	n	%	n	%	p=0,5
B 1+2	16	40,0	8	20,0	12	30,0	4	10,0	40
B 3	13	22,8	13	22,8	26	45,6	5	8,8	57
B 4	5	20,0	7	28,0	10	40,0	3	12,0	25
	34		28		48		12		122
Mitosen	n	%	n	%	n	%	n	%	p=0,1
unter 10	6	31,6	4	21,1	8	42,1	1	5,3	19
11-20	18	45,0	9	22,5	8	20,5	5	12,5	40
21-30	7	22,6	5	16,1	17	54,8	2	6,5	31
31-40	3	12,5	7	29,2	11	45,8	3	12,5	24
über 40	0	0	3	37,5	4	50,0	1	12,5	8
	34		28		48		12		122

Hingegen war ein statistisch signifikanter Zusammenhang zwischen histologischem Typ und histologischem bzw. zytologischem Differenzierungsgrad feststellbar: Muzinöse Tumoren waren häufiger hoch differenziert als endometrioide, seröse und undifferenzierte (in dieser Reihenfolge) (Tabelle 4).

Die verschiedenen Gradingparameter zeigten zueinander eine statistisch signifikante Beziehung (Tabelle 5).

Die stärkste Abhängigkeit der Überlebenszeit der Patientinnen bestand erwartungsgemäß vom *Stadium* (Abb. 1). 85% der Frauen im Stadium I der Erkrankung überlebten 3 Jahre, 73% 5 Jahre. Im Stadium II lebten nach 3 Jahren noch 43% der Frauen, nach 5 Jahren nur noch 21%. Die Patientinnen des Stadiums III erreichten nur in 6%, die des Stadiums IV in keinem Fall die Dreijahresgrenze. Insgesamt überlebten 43% der Patientinnen 3 Jahre und 30% 5 Jahre, 6 Patientinnen sind verschollen.

Einen statistischen Unterschied der Überlebensraten von Patientinnen mit serösen, muzinösen und endometroiden Karzinomen konnten wir in unserem Material nicht nachweisen, lediglich Patientinnen mit *undifferenzierten Karzinomen* zeigten eine signifikant schlechtere Überlebensrate (Abb. 2).

Signifikante Unterschiede der Überlebenszeit waren hingegen in Abhängigkeit vom *histologischen Differenzierungsgrad* zu erkennen. Während Patientinnen mit hochdifferenzierten Karzinomen (G 1) in 52% bzw. 43% die Drei- bzw. Fünfjahresgrenze erreichten, betrugen diese Prozentsätze bei mäßig differenzierten Karzinomen (G 2) 31% bzw. 19%, während Patientinnen mit undifferenzierten Karzinomen (G 3) nur in 6% 5 Jahre überlebten (Abb. 3).

Tabelle 4. Beziehung von histologischem Differenzierungsgrad, zytologischem Differenzierungsgrad und Zahl der Mitosen zum histologischen Typ

	Histologischer Typ								Gesamt
	serös		muzinös		endo-metrioid		undifferen-ziert		
Histologischer Differenzierungsgrad	n	%	n	%	n	%	n	%	p=0,0004
G 1	37	43,5	11	73,3	3	50,0	0	0	51
G 2	31	36,5	4	26,7	2	33,3	3	27,3	40
G 3	17	20,0	0	0	1	16,7	8	72,7	26
Zytologischer Differenzierungsgrad									p=0,05
B 1+2	25	29,4	9	60,0	3	50,0	1	9,1	38
B 3	41	48,2	5	33,3	3	50,0	5	45,5	54
B 4	19	22,4	1	6,7	0	0	5	45,5	25
Mitosen									p=0,03
unter 10	12	14,1	5	33,3	2	33,3	0	0	19
11 – 20	25	29,4	5	33,3	2	33,3	4	36,4	36
21 – 30	27	31,8	1	6,7	0	0	3	27,3	31
31 – 40	16	18,8	3	20,0	2	33,3	2	18,2	23
über 40	5	5,9	1	6,7	0	0	2	18,2	8
	85	100	15	100	6	100	11	100	117

Tabelle 5. Beziehung von zytologischem Differenzierungsgrad und Zahl der Mitosen zum histologischen Differenzierungsgrad

	Histologischer Differenzierungsgrad						Gesamt
	G 1		G 2		G 3		
Zytologischer Differenzierungsgrad	n	%	n	%	n	%	p=0,0001
B 1+2	32	59,3	4	9,5	4	15,4	40
B 3	21	38,9	26	61,9	10	38,5	57
B 4	1	1,9	12	28,6	12	46,2	25
Mitosen							p=0,01
unter 10	14	25,9	4	9,5	1	3,9	19
11 – 20	22	40,7	12	28,6	6	23,1	40
21 – 30	6	11,1	15	35,7	9	34,6	30
31 – 40	10	18,5	7	16,7	7	26,9	24
über 40	2	3,7	4	9,5	3	11,5	9
	54	100	42	100	26	100	122

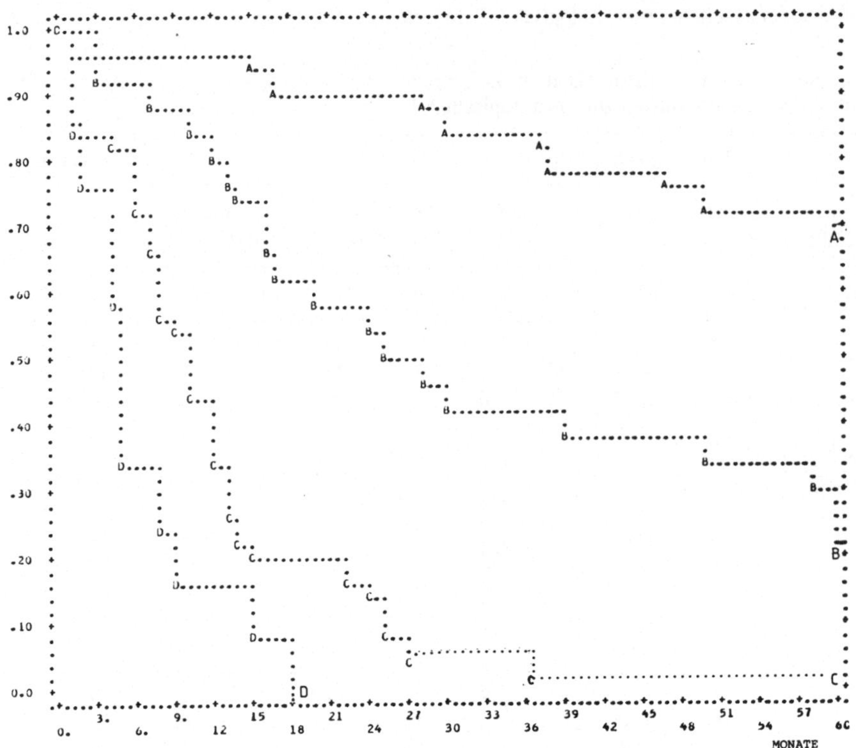

Abb. 1. Abhängigkeit der Überlebenszeit vom Stadium. p = 0,0000. *A* = Stadium I, *B* = Stadium II, *C* = Stadium III, *D* = Stadium IV

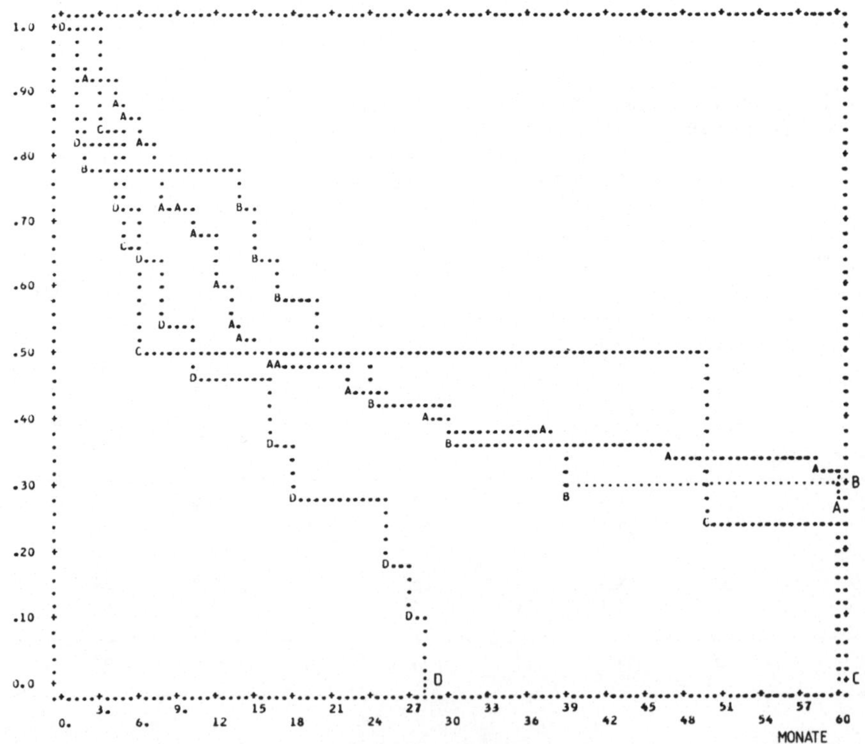

Abb. 2. Abhängigkeit der Überlebenszeit vom histologischen Typ. p = 0,2 (n.s.). *A* = serös, *B* = muzinös, *C* = endometrioid, *D* = undifferenziert

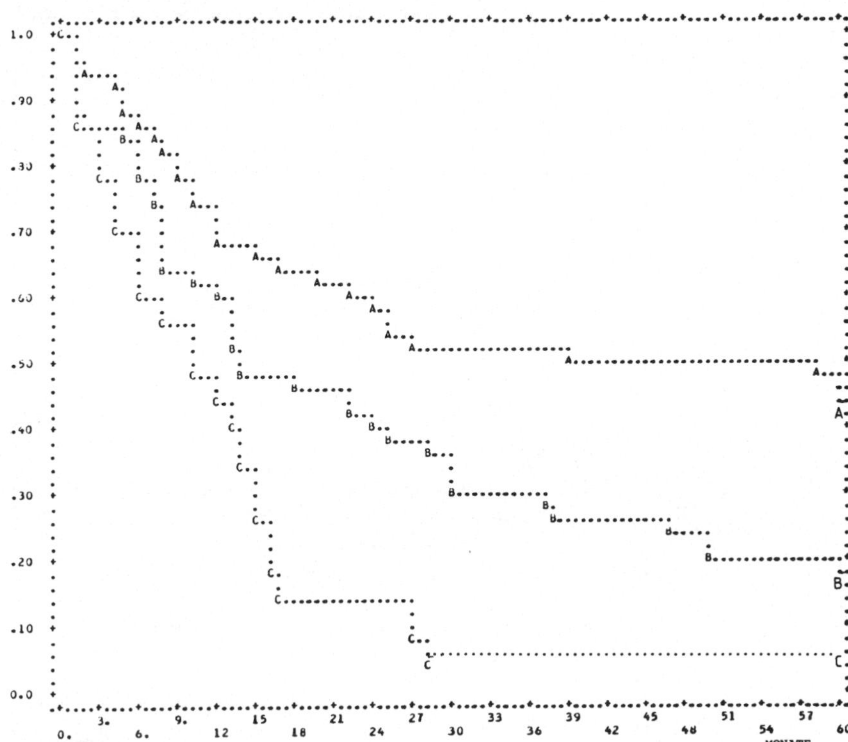

Abb. 3. Abhängigkeit der Überlebenszeit vom histologischen Differenzierungsgrad. p = 0,0004. *A* = hoch differenziert, G 1, *B* = mäßig differenziert, G 2, *C* = undifferenziert, G 3

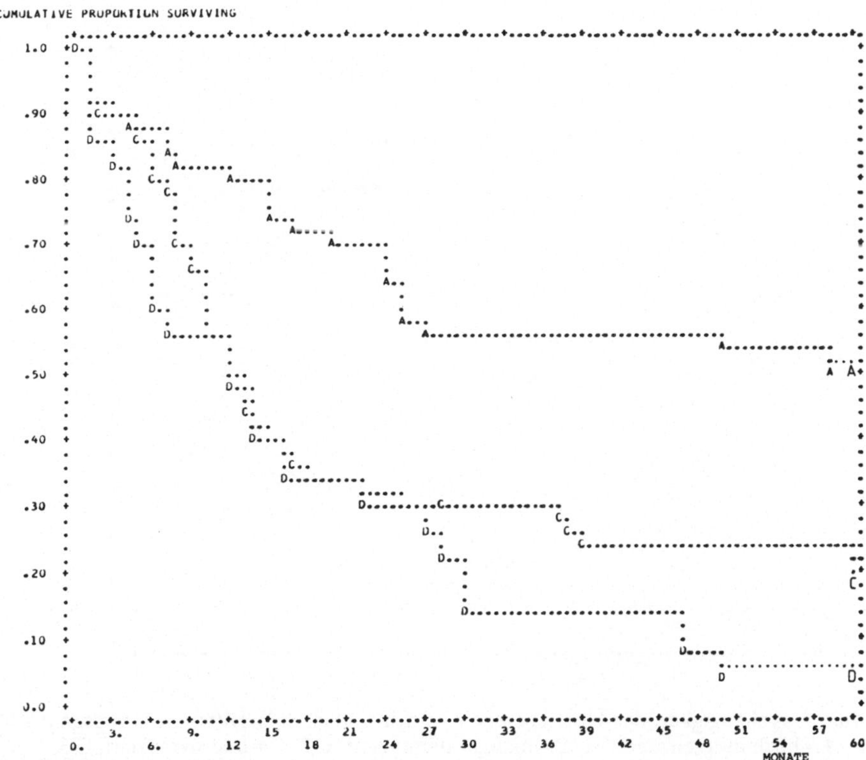

Abb. 4. Abhängigkeit der Überlebenszeit vom zytologischen Differenzierungsgrad (Broders). p = 0,0006. *A* = Broders 1–2, *C* = Broders 3, *D* = Broders 4

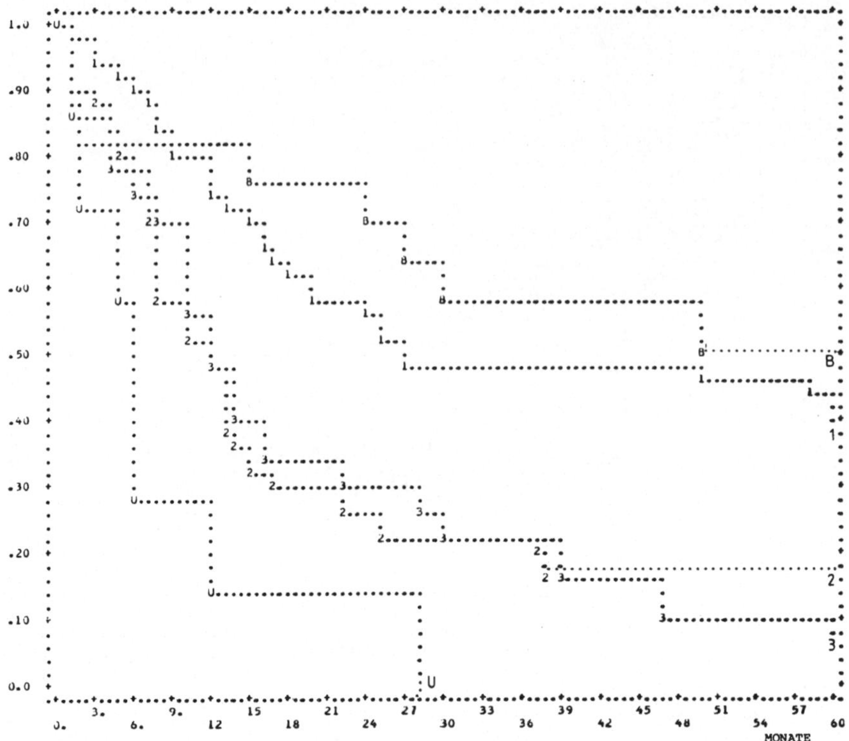

Abb. 5. Abhängigkeit der Überlebenszeit vom Mitoseindex. p = 0,0001. *B* = bis 10 Mitosen/10 Gesichtsfelder, *1* = 11–20 Mitosen/10 Gesichtsfelder, *2* = 21–30 Mitosen/10 Gesichtsfelder, *3* = 31–40 Mitosen/10 Gesichtsfelder, *U* = über 40 Mitosen/10 Gesichtsfelder

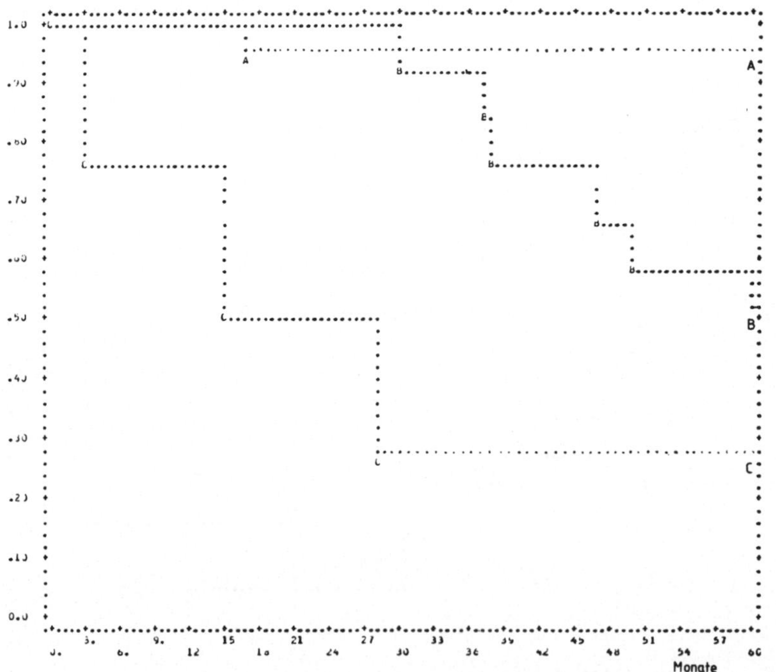

Abb. 6. Abhängigkeit der Überlebenszeit vom histologischen Differenzierungsgrad (Stadium I). *A* = hoch differenziert, G 1, *B* = mäßig differenziert, G 2, *C* = undifferenziert, G 3

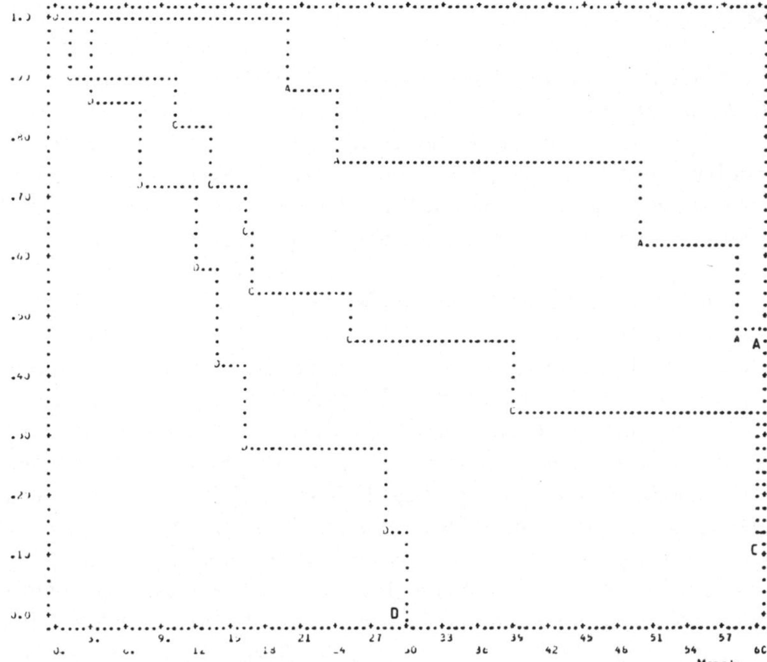

Abb. 7. Abhängigkeit der Überlebenszeit vom zytologischen Differenzierungsgrad (Stadium II). *A* = Broders 1–2, *C* = Broders 3, *D* = Broders 4

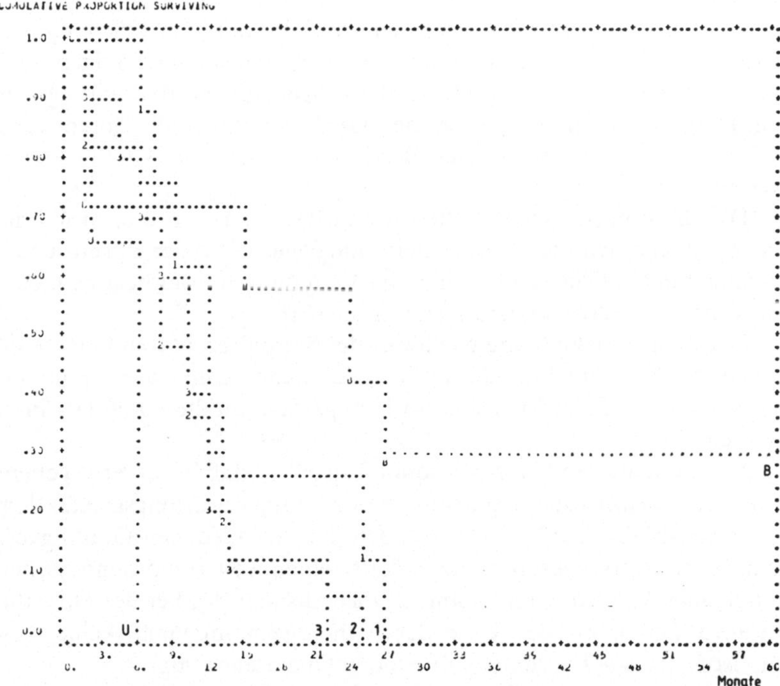

Abb. 8. Abhängigkeit der Überlebenszeit vom Mitoseindex (Stadium III). *B* = bis 10 Mitosen/10 Gesichtsfelder, *1* = 11–20 Mitosen/10 Gesichtsfelder, *2* = 21–30 Mitosen/10 Gesichtsfelder, *3* = 31–40 Mitosen/10 Gesichtsfelder, *U* = über 40 Mitosen/10 Gesichtsfelder

Ähnlich signifikante Unterschiede bestanden in Abhängigkeit vom *zytologischen Differenzierungsgrad.* Wegen der geringen Fallzahl der Fälle von Broders 1, die vorwiegend bei in diesem Kollektiv nicht enthaltenen „Borderline-lesions" gesehen werden, wurden die Gruppen 1 und 2 zusammengefaßt. Während Patientinnen mit zytologisch hochdifferenzierten Karzinomen in der Hälfte der Fälle die Fünfjahresgrenze erreichten, waren es nur 6% der Frauen mit anaplastischen Karzinomen (Abb. 4).

Auch der *Mitoseindex* hat signifikante prognostische Bedeutung. Die Patientinnen mit Karzinomen mit bis zu 20 Mitosen/10 Gesichtsfelder überlebten durchschnittlich länger als jene mit Tumoren mit 21–40 Mitosen, während Patientinnen mit über 40 Mitosen in keinem Fall länger als 2,5 Jahre überlebten (Abb. 5).

Da die verschiedenen Gradingparameter zur Stadienverteilung keine statistisch gesicherte Beziehung aufwiesen, waren die Abhängigkeiten der Überlebenszeit vom histologischen und zytologischen Differenzierungsgrad sowie vom Mitoseindex auch innerhalb der einzelnen Stadien nachweisbar. Als Beispiele seien angeführt: Die Abhängigkeit der Überlebenszeit vom histologischen Differenzierungsgrad im Stadium I (Abb. 6), die Abhängigkeit der Überlebenszeit vom zytologischen Differenzierungsgrad im Stadium II (Abb. 7) und die Abhängigkeit der Überlebenszeit vom Mitoseindex im Stadium III (Abb. 8). Dabei zeigte sich, daß Tumoren mit günstigen Gradingparametern eines fortgeschritteneren Stadiums gleiche oder sogar bessere Überlebensraten aufwiesen als solche mit weniger fortgeschrittenem Stadium, aber histologisch und zytologisch undifferenzierten, mitosereichen Karzinomen.

Das CEA konnten wir bei serösen Ovarialtumoren in 22% der gutartigen, hingegen in 78% der „Borderline-lesions" und in allen malignen Tumoren nachweisen, was möglicherweise in Zukunft bei der prognostischen Beurteilung von Grenzfällen von Bedeutung sein könnte. Bei den muzinösen Ovarialtumoren war hingegen bei 86% der gutartigen und in allen Borderline-Fällen und Karzinomen CEA nachzuweisen.

Die Blutgruppeneigenschaften waren bei gutartigen und proliferierenden serösen Zystadenomen nicht vermindert, hingegen bei 12 der 13 serösen Zystadenokarzinome. Ein ähnlicher Unterschied im Verteilungsmuster bei den muzinösen Tumoren konnte jedoch nicht gefunden werden [21].

Der fluoreszenzoptische Nachweis der Steroidrezeptoren brachte in einigen Fällen ein positives Ergebnis, das mit biochemischen Untersuchungsmethoden gut korrelierte. Unsere Fallzahlen sind noch zu gering, um diese Befunde interpretieren zu können.

Zusammenfassend läßt sich somit feststellen, daß bei einer gegebenen Therapieform die wesentlichste prognostische Bedeutung erwartungsgemäß dem Staging zukommt, daß aber darüber hinaus auch die verschiedenen Gradingverfahren hochsignifikante Aussagekraft besitzen. Über einen weiteren prognostischen Faktor von entscheidender Bedeutung, nämlich das Ausmaß des bei der Operation zurückgelassenen Tumorgewebes, kann der Pathologe naturgemäß keine Aussage treffen, hier ist die exakte Beurteilung durch den Operateur nötig.

Die Bedeutung des Nachweises von CEA, Blutgruppensubstanzen und Steroidhormonrezeptoren in histologischen Schnitten kann derzeit noch nicht abschließend beurteilt werden.

Literatur

1. Boehm M, Binder M, Czerwenka K, Kolb R, Jakesz R, Reiner G, Spona J (1980) Ein fluoreszenzoptischer Nachweis der Oestrogen- und Progesteronrezeptoren bei menschlichen Mammatumoren. Vergleich mit der DCC-Methode. Bull S.S.C.C./S.G.K.C. 21/3:39–41
2. Breitenecker G (1980) Mortalität und Morbidität des Ovarialkarzinoms in Österreich. Gynaekol Rundsch [Suppl 2] 20:109–112
3. Breslow NE (1970) A generalized Kruskal-Wallis test for comparing K samples subjects to unequal patterns of censorship. Biometrika 57:579–594
4. Broders AC (1926) Grading and practical application. Arch Pathol Lab Med 2:376–381
5. Denk H, Tappeiner G, Davidovits A, Eckersdorfer R, Holzner JH (1974) Carcinoembryonic antigen and blood substances in carcinomas of the stomach and colon. J Nat Cancer Inst 53:993–938
6. Dyson JL, Beilby JOW, Steele SJ (1971) Factors influencing survival in carcinoma of the ovary. Br J Cancer 25:237–249
7. Griffiths CT, Parker LM, Fuller AF (1979) Role of cytoreductive surgical treatment in the management of advanced ovarian cancer. Cancer Treat Rep 63:235–240
8. Heyden S (1972) Klinische Epidemiologie des Krebses. Thieme, Stuttgart
9. Janisch H, Gerstner G (1980) Die Stellung der Second-look-Operation nach Radiochemotherapie beim fortgeschrittenen Ovarialkarzinom. Wien klin Wochenschr 92:310–314
10. Lee SH (1979) Simultaneous detection of estrogen and progesterone receptors in breast cancer cells. Fed Proc 38/3 (2):913
11. Mantel N (1966) Evaluation of survival data and two rank order statistics arising in its consideration. Cancer Chemother Rep 50:163–170
12. Ozols RF, Garvin AJ, Costa J, Simon RM, Young RC (1979) Histologic grade in advanced ovarian cancer. Cancer Treat Rep 63 (2):255–263
13. Schemper M (1981) Verfahren und Programme zur Auswertung zensierter Daten. Arbeitsunterlage der Arbeitsgruppe Biometrie und Dokumentation Chir Univ Klinik, Wien
14. Scully RE (1970) Recent progress in ovarian cancer. Human Pathol 1:73–98
15. Scully RE (1979) Tumors of the ovary and maldeveloped gonads. Atlas of tumor pathology, Fasc 16. AFIP
16. Serov SF, Scully RE, Sobin LH (1973) Histological typing of ovarian tumours. International Histological Classification of Tumours, 9. WHO, Geneva
17. Sievers S, Dallenbach-Hellweg G, Susemihl D, Pohl R (1981) Die Prognose der malignen Ovarialtumoren in Abhängigkeit vom histopathologischen Befund. Geburtshilfe Frauenheilkd 41:10–14
18. Smith JP, Day TG (1979) Review of ovarian cancer at the University of Texas Systems Cancer Center, M.D. Anderson Hospital and Tumor Institute. Am J Obstet Gynecol 135 (7):984–993
19. Smith JP, Schwartz PE (1980) Second look laparotomy and prognosis related to extend of residual disease. In: Therapeutic progress in ovarian cancer, testicular cancer and the sarcomas, Boerhaave Series vol 16:77
20. Sternberger LA, Hardy PH Jr, Cuculis JJ, Meyer HG (1970) The unlabelled antibody enzyme method of immunohistochemistry. Preparation and properties of soluble antigen-antibody (horseradish perioxidase-antihorseradish perioxidase) and its use in identification of spirochetes. J Histochem Cytochem 18:315–333
21. Szalay S, Frimmel H, Bartl W, Breitenbecker G, Genk H, Janisch H (1980) Karzinoembryonales Antigen (CEA) und Blutgruppenantigene A, B in Paraffinschnitten epipthelialer Ovarialtumoren. Gynaekol Rundsch [Suppl 2] 20:148–150
22. Tarone RE (1975) Test for trend in life table analysis. Biometrika 62:679–682
23. UICC (1979) TNM-Klassifikation der malignen Tumoren. Springer, Berlin Heidelberg New York

Diskussion

Der Zervixabstrich stellt im Rahmen der gynäkologischen Vorsorgeuntersuchung im wesentlichen eine Methode zur Diagnostik des Zervixkarzinoms und seiner Vorstadien dar. Ovarialkarzinome werden in Zervixabstrichen nur selten diagnostiziert. Herr Prof. Geiger (Köln) hat die wichtigsten Gesichtspunkte dazu bereits zusammengefaßt. Die Häufigkeit, mit der Ovarialkarzinome im Zervixabstrich nachgewiesen werden, kann auf etwa einen Fall pro 20 000 Zervixabstriche geschätzt werden. Das typische Zellbild beim Ovarialkarzinom im Zervixabstrich zeigt einen sauberen Präparathintergrund und Tumorzellen mit oft ausgeprägter zytoplasmatischer Vakuolisation. Innerhalb der Vakuolen finden sich keine Leukozyten, wie dies bei Endometriumkarzinomen oft beobachtet wird. Besonders der saubere Präparathintergrund gilt als Hinweis auf Ovarialkarzinome. Ein weiterer Fall mit sehr ähnlichem Zellbild wie bei den zuvor gezeigten Diapositiven zeigt die differentialdiagnostischen Schwierigkeiten: Die in diesem Fall vorliegenden vakuolisierten Tumorzellverbände bei sauberem Präparathintergrund stammten aus einem Sigmakarzinom mit Peritonealkarzinose.

Auch in Kollektiven von an einem Zervixabstrich zytologisch nachgewiesenen Ovarialkarzinomen ist der Nachweis von Psammomkörperchen selten. Sie gelten dann in besonderem Maße als Hinweis auf ein Ovarialkarzinom. Der saubere Präparathintergrund war in unseren beiden demonstrierten Fällen ein wesentlicher Grund, den Verdacht auf ein Ovarialkarzinom zu äußern.

Fall 1: An zahlreichen Stellen finden sich isolierte oder in Gruppen gelagerte Psammomkörperchen. Diese liegen teils frei, teils sind sie innerhalb von Verbänden gelagert. Die begleitenden Tumorepithelien weisen in diesem Fall keine sicheren Atypien auf. Deshalb konnten wir diesen Fall nur als Pap. III mit Verdacht auf Ovarialkarzinom einstufen. Histologisch fand sich ein seröses papilläres Adenokarzinom des Ovars mit Psammomkörperchen.

Die Diagnose wurde vor jetzt genau 3 Jahren bei einer 43jährigen Patientin durch den Zervixabstrich bei der Vorsorgeuntersuchung gestellt. Die Patientin ist nach der Operation und Nachbestrahlung beschwerdefrei und ohne Anhalt für ein Rezidiv.

Fall 2: Bei der nächsten Patientin wurde wegen der im Diapositiv gezeigten Psammomkörperchen ebenfalls der Verdacht auf ein Ovarialkarzinom geäußert. Auch hier ein sauberer Präparathintergrund, einzelne Tumorzellgruppen zeigen ein deutlich vakuolisiertes Zytoplasma und stark vergrößerte Zellkerne mit prominenten Nukleolen. In diesem Fall war die Einstufung als Pap. V unproblematisch.

Die 73jährige Patientin wies in der Computertomographie einen großen Genitaltumor auf. Die Patientin ist jedoch ohne histologische Abklärung verstorben.

Das hier als letztes gezeigte Zellbild ist nicht ein Zervixabstrich, sondern ein nach Pappenheim gefärbtes Pleurapunktat einer 44jährigen Patientin, die vor 4 Jahren wegen eines serösen papillären Zystadenokarzinoms des linken Ovars operiert wurde. Solche zilientragende Tumorzellen sind ein sehr seltener Befund, der auch einen wichtigen Hinweis auf ein Ovarialkarzinom als Primärtumor darstellt. Im vorliegenden Fall wurden im Pleuraergußmaterial ebenfalls Psammomkörperchen gefunden.

Dallenbach-Hellweg:

Es sollte vielleicht darauf hingewiesen werden, daß Psammomkörperchen auch in Endometriumkarzinomen und ganz vereinzelt in endozervikalen Karzinomen auftreten, also nicht etwa für das Ovarialkarzinom spezifisch sind.

Schenck:

Ja, da stimmen wir zu. Psammomkörperchen im Zervixabstrich bei Endometriumkarzinomen wurden beschrieben, allerdings wesentlich seltener als bei Ovarialkarzinomen. Ich sollte vielleicht noch darauf hinweisen, daß Psammomkörperchen im Zervixabstrich ganz selten auch bei Patientinnen ohne Malignome beschrieben wurden, darunter auch bei Patientinnen mit Intrauterinpessaren. Eine zytologische Tumoridagnose muß deshalb immer auf dem Nachweis von Tumorzellen beruhen. Psammomkörperchen im Zervixabstrich sind ein Hinweis auf Malignität und Ovarialkarzinome, aber keineswegs ein Beweis.

Digital Picture Analysis of Borderline Papillary Serous Cystadenomas of the Ovary

F. Dallenbach and D. Komitowski [1]

Introduction

As numerous authors explain in the recent literature (Barber 1978; Blanco et al. 1977; Czernobilsky 1977; Fox and Langley 1976; Gati et al. 1978; Hart 1977; Honoré 1980; Itskovitz et al. 1979; Julian and Woodruff 1972; Katzenstein et al. 1978; Klemi and Nevalainen 1978; Malkasian et al. 1975; Osadchaia 1980; Rini and Woodruff 1975; Russell and Merkur 1979; Ueda et al. 1980), and as several of the contributors to these proceedings have restated, borderline malignant epithelial tumors of the ovary may often prove difficult to recognize and diagnose histologically, since they show many but not all morphological features of malignancy. The recognition of these features is an exercise in subjective analysis, the success of which depends on the experience, knowledge, skill, diligence, and perhaps alertness of the examiner.

In a search to try to find objective qualities that might make it easier to distinguish borderline tumors from invasive adenocarcinomas, we turned our attention to the new systems of digital picture analysis (Andrews and Hunt 1977; Bartels 1979; Eriksson et al. 1977; Erozan et al. 1979; Fisher 1971; Fukunaga 1972; Komitowski and Zinser 1980; Pratt 1978; Rosenfeld and Kak 1976; Rosenfeld and Weszka 1976; Voss et al. 1981). Figure 1 schematically explains the various instruments we used and how they are interconnected to collect, store, retrieve, and analyze the data we obtained from our measurements. In our system a television camera on the microscope projects the image of the stained tissue section to the picture analyzer, a screen with 550 000 points that measure light intensity, each of which can be varied in 64 shades of gray. Thereby, darker regions can be distinguished from lighter regions, and differences in size, shape, and through the use of conversion factors also in volume, can be determined. The data obtained can be stored in the computer, enabling qualities to be compared or related in virtually unlimited combinations.

Material and Methods

For our studies we compared ten borderline tumors with ten invasive papillary cystadenocarcinomas and two cystadenomas. Between six and eight blocks of tissue

1 Institut für experimentelle Pathologie des Deutschen Krebsforschungszentrums, D-6900 Heidelberg

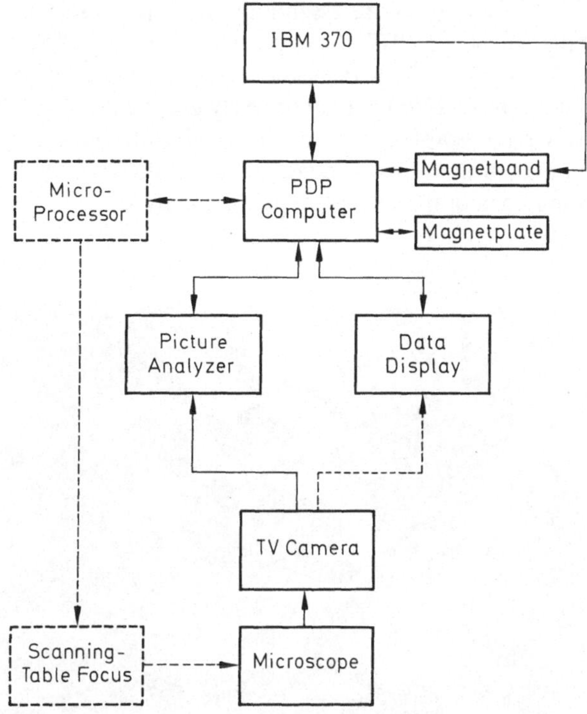

Fig. 1. Schematic layout of different pieces of equipment and their interconnections and for digital picture analysis

were available for study from each tumor, and multiple sections 5 μm thick from each block were stained using: hematoxylin-eosin, the Masson trichrome method, Foote's silver method for reticulum fibers, the Feulgen for nuclei, and the PAS method, in order to bring out in better contrast different components of the tissues.

The qualities we selected to measure are as follows:

1. Growth pattern
   a) Papillary – simple or complex
   b) Glandular, cystic
   c) Microfollicular
2. Epithelium
   a) Single-layered
   b) Stratified
   c) Tufted
3. Cellular characteristics
   a) Pleomorphism – nuclear, cytoplasmic
   b) Hyperchromasia
   c) Mitoses
   d) Loss of polarity
4. Stroma

These criteria are essentially those proposed or recommended by other authors (Blanco et al. 1977; Chenevart and Gloor 1980; Czernobilsky 1977; Elahi et al. 1967; Hart 1977; Katzenstein et al. 1978; Pomerance et al. 1966; Scully 1970; van Orden et al. 1966), and are merely grouped differently for our convenience. Figure 2 is a photograph of one of the borderline tumors we studied. In Fig. 3 are photographs of the mirror-image picture of the encircled area of Fig. 2, as it appeared on the screen of the television picture analyzer.

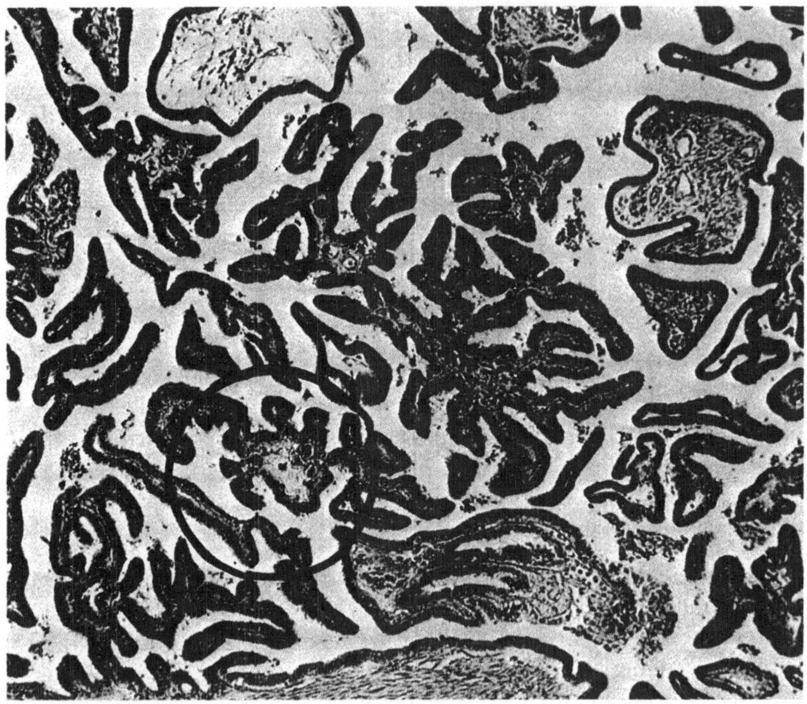

Fig. 2. A low-power view of a well-differentiated, noninvasive papillary serous cystadenocarcinoma (borderline type). H & E, ×80

Although many have stressed the importance of mitoses in evaluating malignant qualities, we ignored them in these studies because their number can be influenced by so many factors beyond our control (Fox and Langley 1976):

1. Cooling of tumor after resection before samples taken for histologic study
2. Compromised blood-supply in large tumors
3. Hormones
4. Circadian biorhythm
5. Geometric artefacts
6. Proper identification.

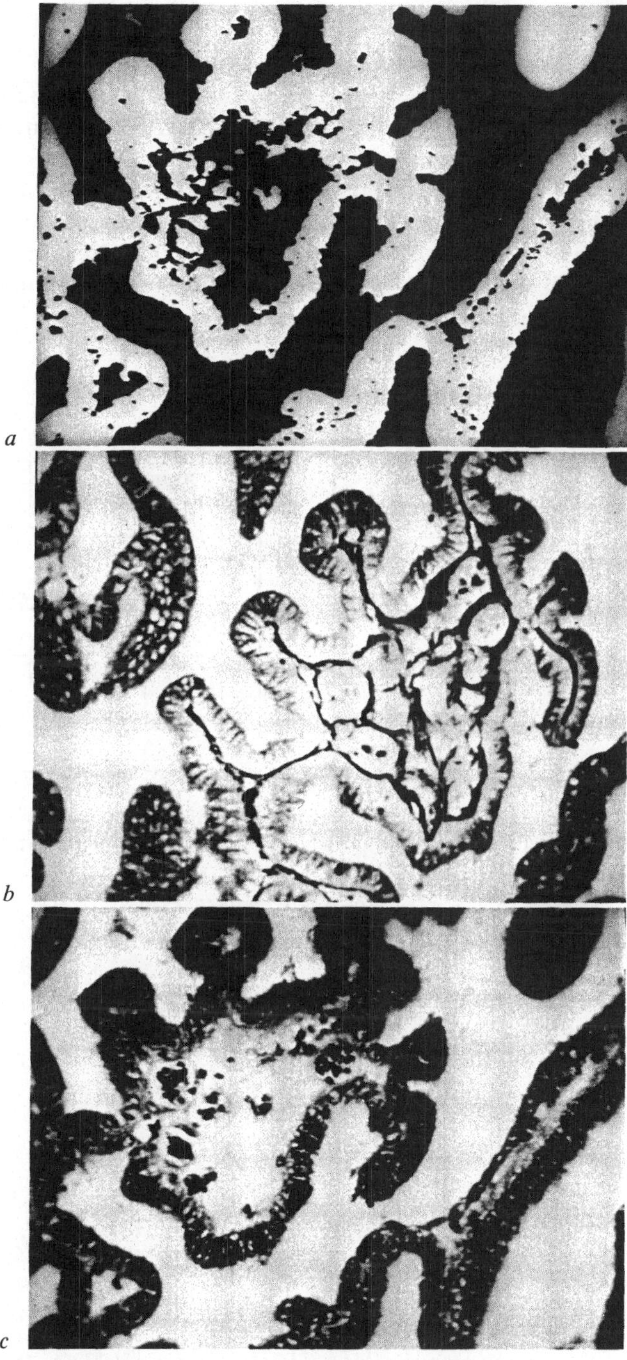

Fig. 3a–c. Photographs of the mirror-images of the highly magnified encircled area of Fig. 2 taken of the picture on the screen of the television analyzer. *a* H & E stained section at high intensity for gray-white differentiation. ×340 *b* same area as in *a*, section stained with Foote's silver method for reticulum fibers. ×340 *c* same area as in *a* and *b*, section stained with Masson's trichrome method. Gray-white differentiation of moderate intensity. ×340

Results

Our results were as follows: As was to be expected the three classes of tumors differed, sometimes greatly, sometimes insignificantly, and sometimes in ways we had failed to anticipate. As shown in Fig. 4, the area covered by the epithelium of borderline tumors varied more than that of carcinomas; the epithelium of the cystadenomas occupied the least area. The density of the epithelial cells (Fig. 4), that means the stratification, was greatest in the carcinomas, and varied greatly. Collagen fibers (Fig. 5) were consistently least abundant in carcinomas, but some borderline tumors also contained only a few such fibers. Reticulum fibers (Fig. 6) were

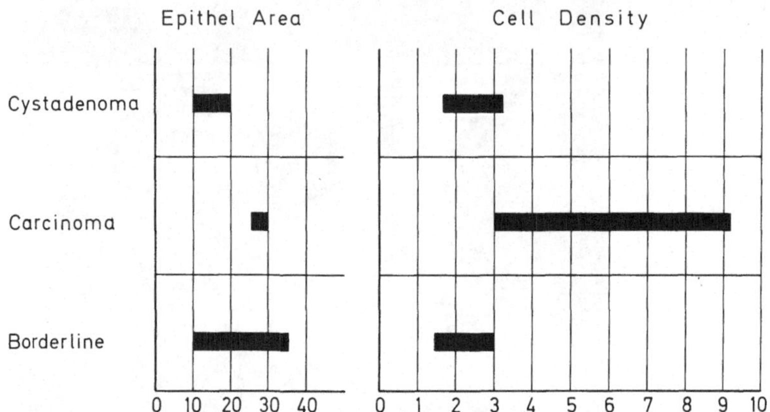

Fig. 4. Comparison of the measurements of the areas occupied by the epithelia or the cell density (cell stratification) in each class of tumor. Numerical units relative but nonspecific

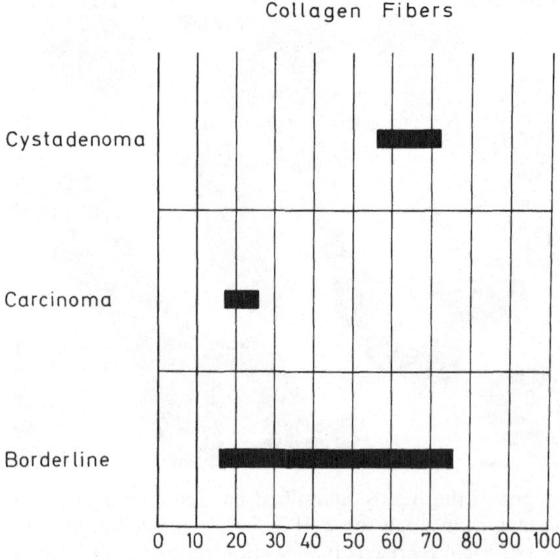

Fig. 5. Variations in the quantity of collagen fibers in the three classes of tumors. Numerical units relative, nonspecific

more plentiful in the carcinomas than in borderline tumors, but most abundant in the cystadenomas. The nuclei of carcinomatous cells (Fig. 7) revealed the greatest variations in size, total area occupied, and shape. In general the nuclei of the cells of the borderline tumors were small and more uniform than those of the carcinomas. That result suggested that borderline tumors might represent a clone or race of cells,

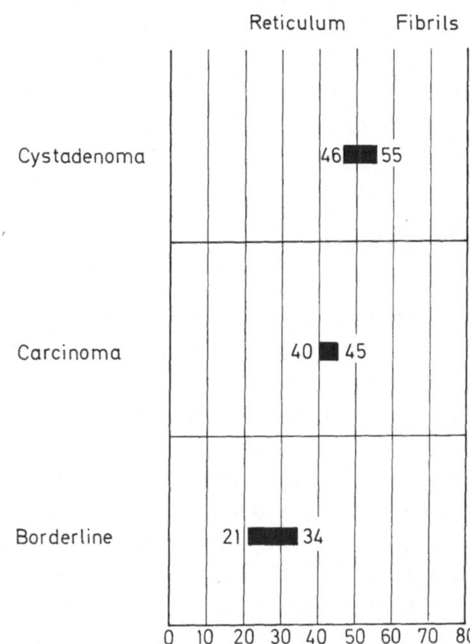

Fig. 6. Variations in the quantity of reticulum fibers measured in the three classes of tumors stained with Foote's silver method. Numerical units relative, nonspecific

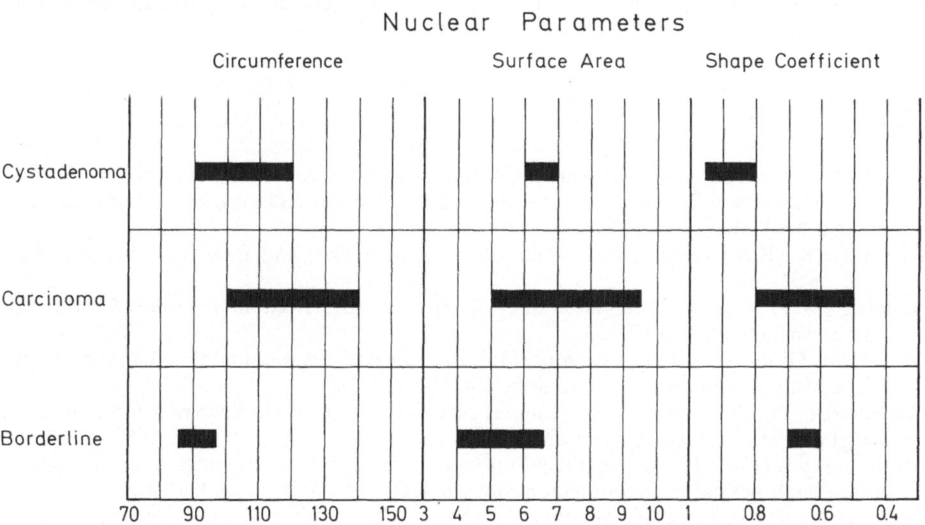

Fig. 7. Variations in nuclear qualities – circumference, surface area, and volume (shape coefficient) – in the three classes of tumor. Numerical units relative, nonspecific

which although accelerating in their growth potentialities, had not as yet lost controls that kept them from becoming pleomorphic. From his measurements of DNA in nuclei of borderline ovarian papillary cystadenomas, Sachs (1975) believed nuclear pleomorphism represented a reliable criterion for the presence of aneuploidy, and by extending that thought "for the diagnosis of malignancy in proliferating and nonproliferating papillary cystomas". In their chromosome studies, Knörr-Gärtner et al. (1977) reported that all their borderline tumors cultured in vitro revealed an abnormal stemline and a more or less marked tendency for polyploidy. They suggested, however, that the initiation of malignant transformation at the chromosome level escaped histologic detection until the abnormal cell line with polyploidy became established (outnumbered the euploidic cells).

Conclusion

We should like to summarize our studies as follows: Although we found no hallmark features enabling us to distinguish borderline malignant tumors from invasive carcinomas as yet (Katzenstein et al. 1978), we believe the objective technique of quantitative analysis we have used can be refined to advantage, and should be pursued for several reasons. Such studies will provide quantitative values for the process of malignant transformation, helping us thereby to understand what that change really is. These studies will also provide quantitative values for many words we use loosely, such as hyperplasia, neoplasia, anaplasia, and stratification, telling us what these words mean and how we ought better to apply them.

The hardware, that is the equipment for making such measurements, is available. We need only to work out the appropriate system of analysis, to select and improve the algorithms for analyzing multicolor and multicellular images for quantifying histopathologic states (Preston and Dekker 1980; Komitowski and Zinser 1980).

References

Andrews HC, Hunt BR (1977) Digital image restoration. Prentice-Hall, Englewood Cliffs, N.J.

Auer GU, Caspersson TO, Wallgren AS (1980) DNA content and survival in mammary carcinoma. Anal Quant Cytol 2:161

Barber HRK (1978) Ovarian carcinoma, etiology, diagnosis, and treatment. Masson, New York, pp 51–56

Bartels P (1979) Numerical evaluation of cytologic data: III. Selection of features for discrimination. Anal Quant Cytol 1:153

Blanco AA, Gibbs ACC, Langley FA (1977) Histological discrimination of malignancy in mucinous ovarian tumours. Histopathology 1:431

Chenevart P, Gloor E (1980) Cystadénomes séreux et muqueux de l'ovaire à la limite de la malignité. Schweiz Med Wochenschr 110:531

Czernobilsky B (1977) Primary epithelial tumors of the ovary. In: Blaustein A (ed) Pathology of the female genital tract. Springer, Berlin Heidelberg New York, pp 456–463

Elahi EH, Long ME, Frick HC, Sommers SC (1967) Long-term survival in disseminated ovarian carcinoma. Am J Obstet Gynecol 99:522

Eriksson O, Westman-Naeser S, Stenkvist B, Bengtsson E, Holmquist J (1977) A computerized recording system for cytoplathologic diagnoses. Acta Cytol (Baltimore) 21:266

Erozan YS, Pressman NJ, Donovan PA, Gupta PK, Frost JK (1979) A comparative cytopathologic study of noninvasive and invasive squamous cell carcinoma of the lung. Anal Quant Cytol 1:50

Fenoglio CM, Ferenczy A, Richart RM (1976) Mucinous tumors of the ovary. II. Ultrastructural features of mucinous cystadenocarcinomas. Am J Obstet Gynecol 125:990

Fisher C (1971) The new quantimet 720. Microscopy 19:20

Fox H, Langley FA (1976) Tumours of the ovary. Heinemann Medical Books, London, pp 37–46

Fukunaga K (1972) Introduction to statistical pattern recognition. Academic Press, New York, p 288

Gáti É, Töttössy B, Sugár J (1978) Klinisch-pathologische Beziehungen der potentiell malignen Kystadenome der Eierstöcke. Zentral Gynaekol 100:978

Hart WR (1977) Ovarian epithelial tumors of borderline malignancy (Carcinomas of low malignant potential.) Hum Pathol 8:541

Honoré LH (1980) Ovarian serous cystadenofibroma of borderline malignancy: report of two cases. Gynecol Oncol 9:220

Itskovitz J, Kerner H, Brandes JM (1979) Ovarian surface papillomatosis of borderline malignancy. J Reprod Med 22:144

Julian CG, Woodruff JD (1972) The biological behavior of low grade papillary serous carcinoma of the ovary. Obstet Gynecol 40:860

Katzenstein A-L, Mazur MT, Morgan TE, Kao M-S (1978) Proliferative serous tumors of the ovary: histologic features and prognosis. Am J Surg Pathol 2:339

Klemi PJ, Nevalainen TJ (1978) Ultrastructural and histochemical observations on serous ovarian cystadenomas. Acta Pathol Microbiol Scand [A] 86A:303

Knörr-Gärtner H, Schuhmann R, Kraus H, Uebele-Kallhardt B (1977) Comparative cytogenic and histologic studies on early malignant transformation in mesothelial tumors of the ovary. Hum Genet 35:281

Komitowski D, Zinser G (1980) Automatische Bildverarbeitung in der Histopathologie-Motivation, Ziele, Probleme und Aktivitäten in der ersten Entwicklungsphase. Veröffentlichung der zentralen Histodiagnostik und Dokumentation am Institut für experimentelle Pathologie, Deutsches Krebsforschungszentrum, Heidelberg

Malkasian GD, Decker DG, Webb MJ (1975) Histology of epithelial tumors of the ovary: clinical usefulness and prognostic significance of the histologic classification and grading, chapt 3: Staging and treatment of ovarian carcinoma. In: Yarbo JW, Bornstein RS, Mastrangelo MJ (eds) Seminars in oncology, vol 2. Grune & Stratton, New York London, pp 191–201

Orden DE Van, McAllister WB, Zerne SRM, Morris JM (1966) Ovarian carcinoma. The problems of staging and grading. Am J Obstet Gynecol 94:195

Osadchaia VV (1980) Borderline mixed epithelial tumor of the ovary. Arkh Patol 42:56

Pomerance W, Moltz A, Hall JE (1966) Factors influencing survival in ovarian carcinoma. Am J Obstet Gynecol 96:418

Pratt WK (1978) Digital image processing. Wiley & Sons, New York Chichester Brisbane Toronto

Preston K, Dekker A (1980) Differentiation of cells in abnormal human liver tissue by computer image processing: a preliminary investigation into its potential application to diagnostic microscopy. Anal Quant Cytol 2:203

Rini JM, Woodruff JM (1975) A case of ovarian papillary serous carcinoma of low malignant potential. Clin Bull 5:64

Rosenfeld A, Kak A (1976) Digital picture processing. Academic Press, New York San Francisco London

Rosenfeld A, Weszka JS (1976) Picture recognition. In: Fu KS (ed) Digital pattern recognition. Springer, Berlin Heidelberg New York, pp 135–166

Russell P, Merkur H (1979) Proliferating ovarian "epithelial" tumours: a clinico-pathological analysis of 144 cases. Aust NZ J Obstet Gynecol 19:45

Sachs H (1975) Cytophotometric study of papillary ovarian cystomas: borderline cases of malignancy. In: De Watteville H, Burch PRJ (eds) Diagnosis and treatment of ovarian neoplastic alterations. Excerpta Medica, Amsterdam Oxford; Elsevier, Amsterdam Oxford New York, pp 132–133

Scully RE (1970) Recent progress in ovarian cancer. Hum Pathol 1:73

Shiromizu K (1980) Study on the biologic nature of ovarian cystadenoma of low potential malignancy. Analysis from the viewpoint of the relationship between the nuclear DNA contents and histological findings. Acta Obstet Gynecol Jpn (Engl Ed) 32:427

Ueda G, Yamasaki M, Inoue M (1980) A malignant parovarian tumor accompanied by ovarian serous cystadenoma of low potential malignancy. Acta Obstet Gynecol Jpn (Engl Ed) 32:491

Voss K, Simon H, Wenzelides K (1981) Logical classifiers for image analyses in medicine. Anal Quant Cytol 3:39

The Identification and Prognosis of Borderline Epithelial Tumors

H. J. NORRIS [1]

Introduction

There is a group of epithelial neoplasms of the ovary histologically and clinically intermediate between cystadenoma and cystadenocarcinoma. Earlier reports have emphasized the favorable prognosis of neoplasms within the group by applying to the diagnosis qualifying terms, such as "proliferative", "borderline", "potentially malignant", and "low malignant potential" [4, 11, 12, 26, 28, 29]. Others have classified them as well-differentiated or grade I carcinoma [5, 14]. The word "carcinoma", however, usually implies a poor prognosis and a need for aggressive therapy. Also, a large proportion of the proliferative tumors arise in relatively young women and to conserve reproductive function some clinicians recommend that the word "carcinoma" not be appended to the diagnosis because so few stage I tumors progress. To avoid these implications, the term "carcinoma" is abandoned in referring to proliferating neoplasms with low malignant potential. The terms "borderline", "proliferative tumor", and "tumor of low malignant potential" are used synonymously.

The low malignant potential or proliferative tumor must be recognized if meaningful data on the relative frequency, behavior, and therapeutic results of primary carcinomas of the ovary are to be obtained. The 5-year survival rate for patients with stage I carcinoma ranges from 45% to 100% [1, 19], and the survival is from 20% to 75% when all stages are included [11, 12, 21]. The tremendous variations in survival can be attributed, in large part, to the inclusion of tumors of low malignant potential in some studies of carcinoma and to their exclusion in others.

A borderline tumor has some, but not all, of the features of malignancy. The histologic assessment of atypism, mitotic activity, stratification, and detachment of cellular clusters places them between cystadenoma with cellular atypia and the well-differentiated carcinomas that demonstrate frank invasion [4, 29].

Wide variation in the histologic features may occur within ovarian epithelial tumors. Since the grade is determined from the least-differentiated area, thorough sampling is necessary. A block of tissue for microscopic examination should be taken for each 1 or 2 mm of the maximum dimension. Solid areas, the base of papillary processes, and areas that are closest to the ovarian surface should be given special attention.

1 Department of Gynecologic and Breast Pathology, Armed Forces Institute of Pathology, Washington, D.C. 20306, USA

At present there are several categories of proliferative tumors. Serous and mucinous tumors of low malignant potential have been delineated, as has the proliferative Brenner tumor (a neoplasm of unproven malignant potential and a close relative of the malignant Brenner tumor). Endometrioid and clear cell tumors of low malignant potential have also been cited, but their full clinical and pathologic profiles have yet to be established.

When strict criteria are followed, most proliferative tumors are distinct entities and easily identified. Mucinous and serous tumors of low malignant potential will be described in this section, and a summary of diagnostic features of the emergent proliferative endometrioid and clear cell tumors will be provided. Proliferative Brenner tumors and the diagnostic criteria of proliferative and malignant adenofibromas are reviewed.

Mucinous Tumors of Low Malignant Potential and Mucinous Carcinoma

Of 688 primary mucinous tumors confined to one or both ovaries at the time of initial surgery, 80% were benign cystadenomas [12]. The remaining 20% were characterized by a proliferation of malignant epithelium. Two-thirds of these were of low malignant potential and one-third were frank carcinoma. Mucinous tumors of low

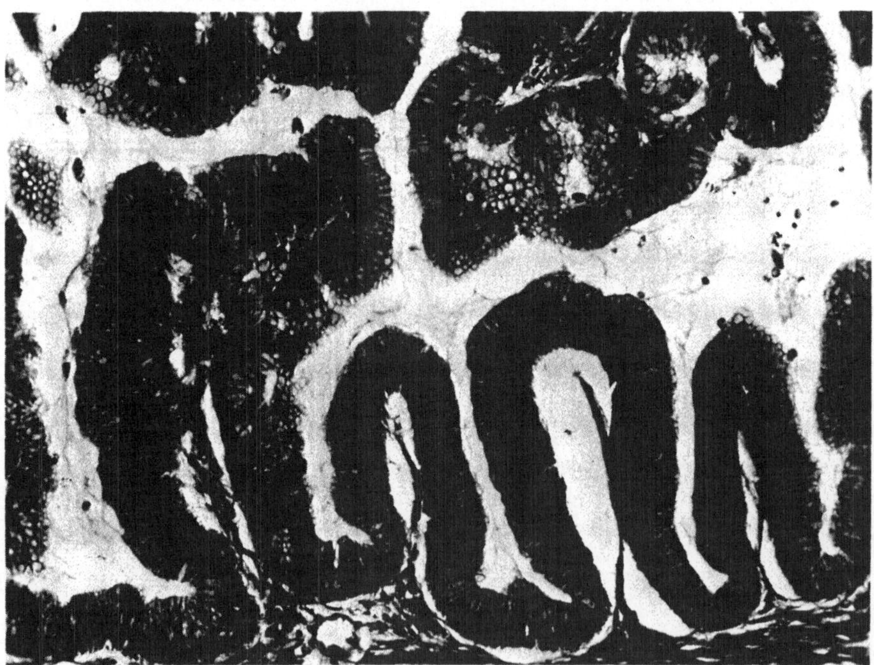

Fig. 1. A mucinous tumor of low malignant potential. Benson WL, Norris HJ (1978) Problems in gynecologic oncology. In: McCowan (ed) Gynecologic Oncology, Appleton-Century, New York. HE, ×150

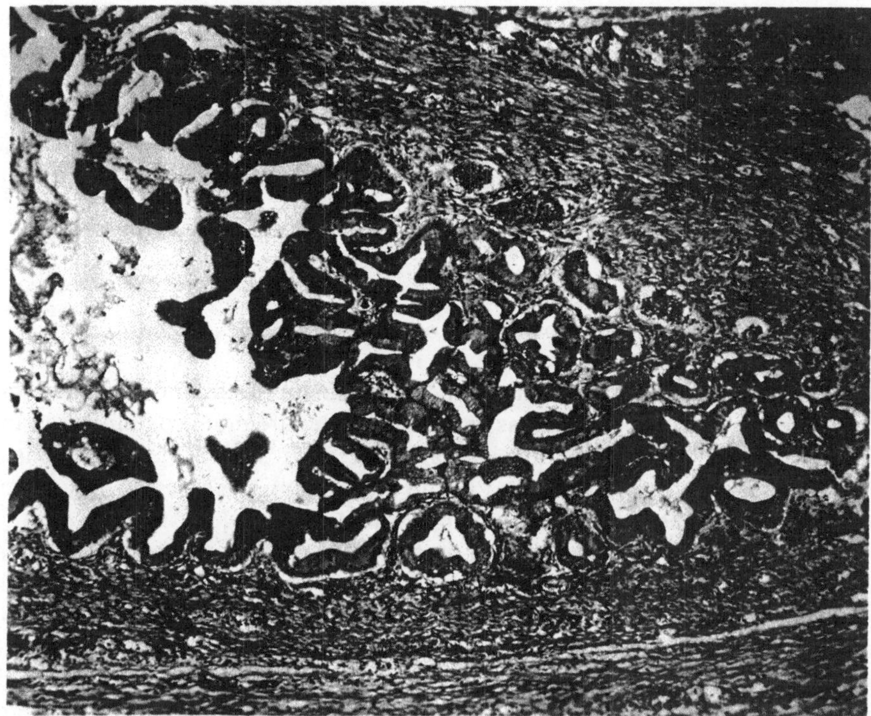

Fig. 2. A benign mucinous cystadenoma with an irregular interface with the stroma, illustrating how invasion can be simulated by benign tumors. HE, ×60

malignant potential were delineated from stage I cystadenocarcinomas by invasion and by the depth of stratification of the atypical cells.

Diagnostic Criteria of Proliferative Mucinous Tumors

Microscopically, proliferative mucinous tumors show more variation within individual neoplasms than do serous proliferative tumors. Secondary cysts and short papillary infoldings are characteristics. In some mucinous tumors, a filigree of epithelial projections is supported on delicate septa of connective tissue. Larger papillae with well-developed fibrovascular support are less frequent, but occasionally broad papillae similar to those found in serous tumors are encountered [11, 12, 26].

Instead of a single layer of well-differentiated mucinous cells as seen in mucinous cystadenomas, the cysts are lined by atypical epithelium stratified into two or three layers (Fig. 1). This proliferation of cells is usually associated with papillary infoldings, but can be found also in cysts devoid of papillae. Tangential sections of glands at times simulate a pattern of intraglandular bridging, but the presence of delicate connective tissue septa between the cells indicates that the cribriform pattern is artificial. Exfoliation of clusters of epithelial cells in a frequent finding. By definition, the nuclei show significant hyperchromatism, increased size, irregular contour, and enlarged nucleoli. The atypism is usually slight or moderate in degree.

Mitotic figures are often conspicuous and many tumors have two or more mitotic figures for every ten high-power fields (hpf) [26]. Invasion of the stroma is absent in all tumors. The glands may be closely spaced, but intervening stroma is always present. Small, seemingly isolated glands within the ovarian stroma (Fig. 2) are not regarded as evidence of invasion because the smooth contour and orderly arrangement is unlike the haphazard destructive growth pattern found in infiltrating carcinoma. Instead, the small glands in the stroma represent the formation of secondary cysts and outpouching from larger cysts.

Diagnostic Criteria of Mucinous Carcinoma

Mucinous carcinomas have a gross appearance similar to that of borderline tumors. Most are multilocular. Solid areas and firm nodules are more common than in proliferative tumors. Growth on the cortical surface is grossly visible in some instances and papillary processes are evident within the cyst in some cases [11, 12]. Mucinous carcinoma has a median diameter of approximately 16 cm [12].

Microscopically, the diagnosis of mucinous carcinoma is based on the presence of either definite invasion of the stroma, or areas where stratified atypical cells devoid of connective tissue support exceed three layers (Fig. 3). Stromal invasion usually consists of irregular cords and nests of cells haphazardly scattered in the ovarian stroma, in contrast to the smooth contour and orderly arrangement of the glands present at the periphery of borderline tumors. In addition to a destructive growth pattern, invasion is diagnosed when sheets of large glands occupy approximately half of a low-power field (2.1 mm) without intervening stroma. Invasion should be unequivocally identified before it is diagnosed and questionable areas should be ignored.

In the absence of identifiable stromal invasion, a diagnosis of carcinoma is also made when the glands contain a marked overgrowth of atypical epithelial cells. In

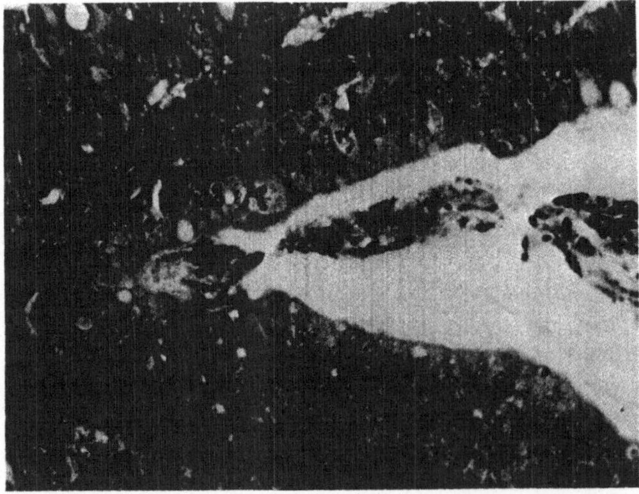

Fig. 3. Stratified atypical cells in a mucinous cystadenocarcinoma. HE, ×160

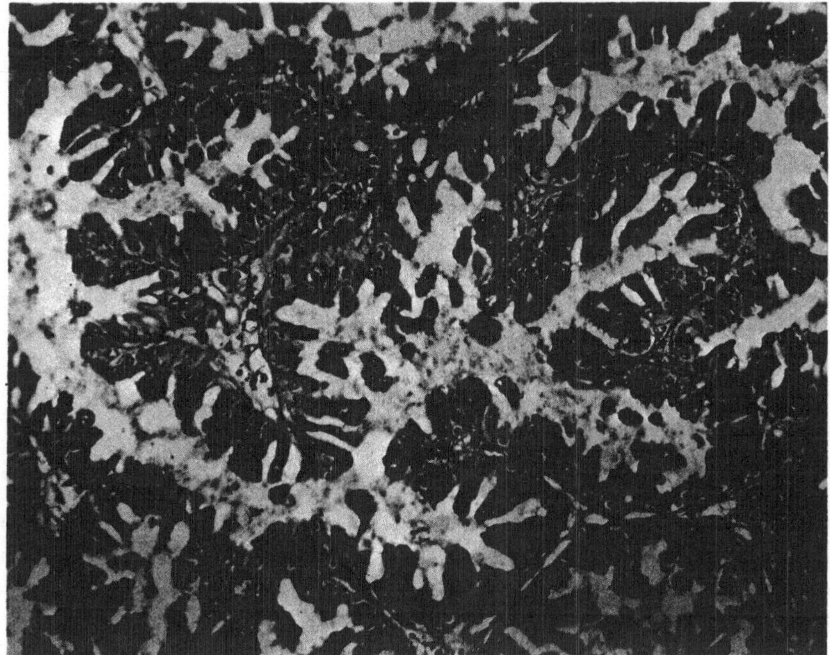

Fig. 4. A tumor of low malignant potential having cellular features intermediate between serous and mucinous cells. HE, ×200

many cases, the lining of the cyst is so thick with cellular proliferation that solid masses of epithelium obscure the glandular pattern. In other neoplasms, the glands have a cribriform appearance formed by intraglandular bridges of epithelial cells.

The stratified cells within mucinous carcinomas show moderate to marked nuclear atypism, and the degree of atypism usually exceeds that found in mucinous tumors of low malignant potential. In carcinoma, the cells are severely anaplastic at times and have large nuclei that contain multiple prominent nucleoli. The degree of nuclear atypism generally parallels the extent of the stratification of the cells. Often, carcinoma cells show little intracytoplasmic mucin. Where mucin production is scant, the appearance is that of a nonspecific adenocarcinoma (Fig. 4). In such instances, the mucinous character of the tumor can be identified in the more-differentiated portions.

Comment on Mucinous Tumors

The borderline category is much larger than was believed years ago. Russell [25] and Hart and Norris [12] found 75%–80% of the malignant mucinous tumors to be in the low malignant potential category, whereas Santesson and Kottmeier [27] and Aure et al. [1] found 52% and 40% of malignancies respectively to be in the low malignant potential category. About 6% of proliferative mucinous tumors are bilateral, whereas there is a much higher proportion of bilaterality in carcinomas [12,

26]. About 85% of proliferative mucinous tumors are stage I when first identified [12, 26]. The mean age of patients with proliferative tumors is 48 years, 4 years lower than the median age for women with carcinoma [11, 26]. Usually, mucinous carcinoma has unequivocal stromal invasion, but invasion in mucinous tumors is more difficult to assess than in serous tumors. Multilocularity may be a result of invasion or it may develop from proliferative enlargement of glands. Irregular margins, an irregular glandular-stromal interface, and lymphoplasmacytic infiltrates are early features of invasion. Leakage or dissection of mucin through the ovary is not a form of destructive growth. Rupture of a mucinous ovarian tumor with spillage of its contents into the peritoneal cavity often causes much alarm, but in a study of 16 women whose neoplasms had either ruptured during the operative procedure or had ruptured prior to surgery, only one neoplasm metastasized and none of the women developed pseudomyxoma peritonei [12]. While the survival of patients with true carcinoma is compromised when it spills, the rupture of a borderline tumor does not appear to affect the prognosis significantly.

Pseudomyxoma peritonei was present in 25% of the proliferative mucinous tumors described by Russell [26], but most reported cases of pseudomyxoma peritonei associated with an ovarian mucinous tumor indicate that the pseudomyxoma had been present at the time of initial surgery and many have also had a coexistant mucocele of the appendix [12].

Only 4% [3] of 87 patients with a mucinous tumor of low malignant potential in stage I who were followed up subsequently died of their neoplasm [12]. This survival is vastly superior to that of mucinous cystadenocarcinoma where only 45%–75% of patients with stage I tumors can be expected to survive 5 years [1, 5, 19, 21, 23]. Thus the two entities should be separated if meaningful data on frequency, behavior, and therapeutic results are to be obtained. Obviously, with such a very low recurrence rate for stage I proliferative mucinous tumors, an uninvolved contralateral ovary in a young woman can be spared and adjunctive radiotherapy or chemotherapy are not likely to improve the survival significantly.

Serous Tumors of Low Malignant Potential and Serous Carcinoma

Serous tumors are composed of epithelium resembling that of the fallopian tube. Characteristically papillary and cystic, they may arise directly on the surface of the ovary as surface papillary tumors, or from within the substance of the ovary from surface epithelial crypts, entrapped epithelium, and perhaps from epithelial differentiation by cells within the stroma which have retained the potency to develop into epithelium.

Diagnostic Criteria of Proliferative Serous Tumors

The microscopic descriptions of Katzenstein et al. [18] and Russell [25, 26] are the most vivid and detailed. Extensive, complex branching papillary fronds are lined by several layers of cells in which the cells are heaped into tufts and form buds of four or more cells lacking a supporting stalk. Generally, the extent of tufting and papillae formation is the same as in serous carcinoma [18]. Cellular atypism is present in all cases and severe in one-fourth [18]. Characterized by nuclear enlargement with pleomorphism and peripheral condensation of chromatin, the atypism can be graded [26]. The proportion with prominent nucleoli is only slightly less than in serous carcinoma [18]. Mitotic counts reveal that only 6% of cases have five or more mitotic figures in 10 hpf, which contrasts with serous carcinoma in which nearly half of tumors have more than that figure [18]. Cribriform patterns, necrosis within the tumor, and inflammation in the stroma are less frequent in serous tumors of low malignant potential than in serous carcinoma [18]. Psammoma bodies are present in 40%–66% of serous tumors of low malignant potential, a proportion similar to that in the case of serous carcinoma [18, 25]. When proliferative serous tumors are graded, 90% of the lower grades are stage 1 as compared with only 60% of the higher grades [26].

Serous tumors of low malignant potential should be distinguished from cystadenomas with atypia [18, 25]. The latter lack the complex tufting of epithelium formed by stratified atypical cells and the detachment of atypical cell clusters which characterize the serous tumor of low malignant potential (Figs. 5, 6). Cystadenomas may have atypia and focally proliferative areas [18]. None of the histologic features of degree of cell atypism, mitotic activity, cellular disorganization, cribriform pat-

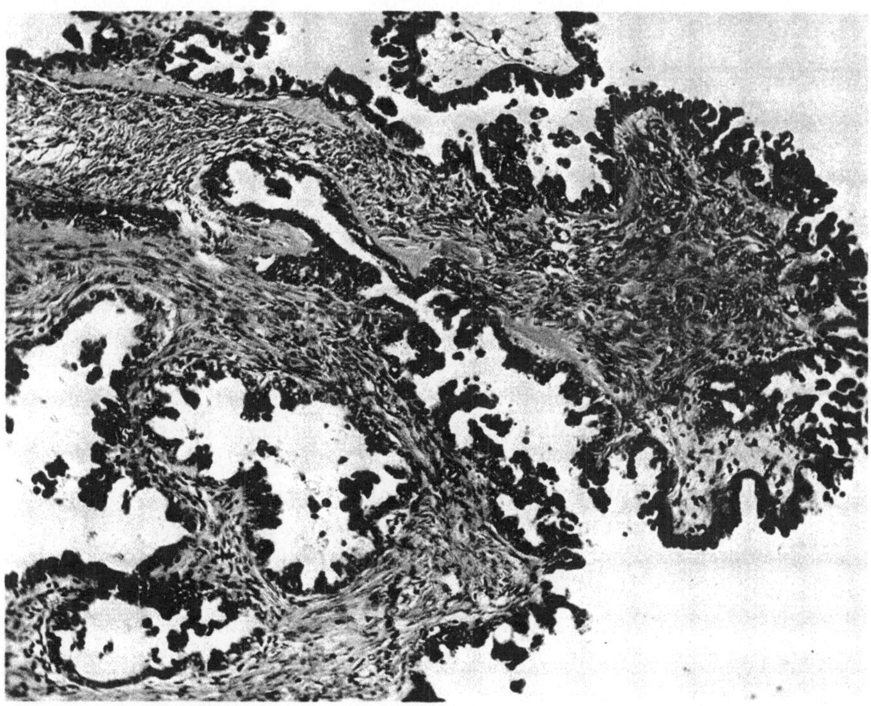

Fig. 5. Detached atypical cells and tufts identify this serous tumor of low malignant potential in a 15-year-old girl. Jenson RD, Norris HJ (1972) Epithelial tumors of the ovary in children. Arch Pathol 94:29–34. HE, ×100

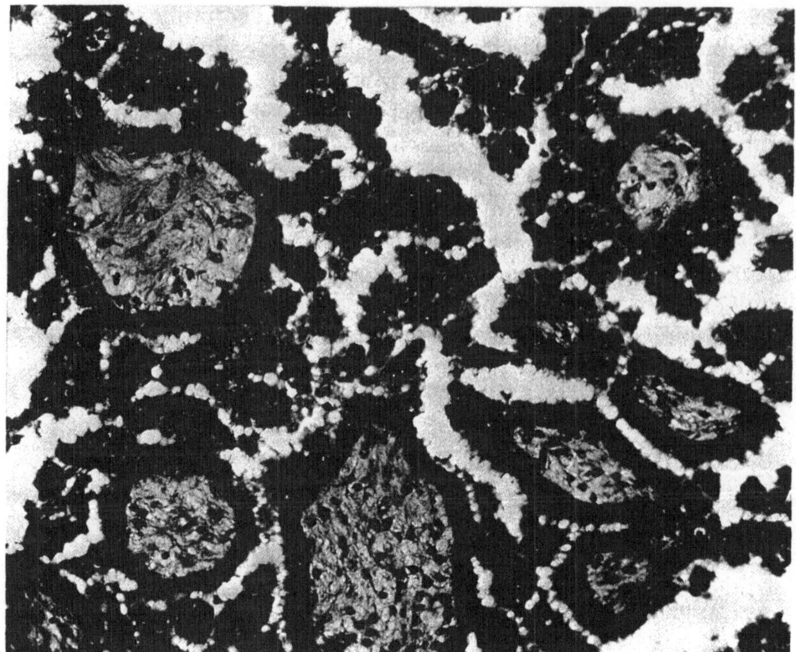

Fig. 6. Serous tumor of low malignant potential (low grade). HE, ×200

terns, tufting, papillae formation or stromal inflammation are related to the prognosis. Neoplasms which form psammoma bodies and have epithelial necrosis seem to be slightly more aggressive than those that lack, or contain lesser degrees of, these features.

Peritoneal implants of proliferative serous tumors tend to be found beneath the peritoneal surface rather than as surface deposits as in metastatic carcinoma. Metastases from borderline serous tumors invade lymph-nodal parenchyma from the peripheral nodal sinuses and serous cells may appear within lymphatics of the lungs and other organs [9]. The metastases from serous tumors of low malignant potential do not show destructive invasion and epithelial necrosis as in carcinoma [9]. Low or absent mitotic activity is characteristic of the metastases of proliferative serous tumors, and the implants usually have the same grade as the primary tumor and prominent psammoma bodies [9, 18, 26].

Distinguishing lymph node and peritoneal metastases from benign glandular inclusions may be impossible [9]. Glandular inclusions can be found in 4%–13% of patients in whom the pelvic nodes are removed for reasons other than adenocarcinoma [9, 13, 17]. The origin of the peritoneal inclusions has been ascribed to a number of causes, including müllerian metaplasia of the mesothelium of the peritoneum [3, 13, 22], a condition termed "müllerianosis" [3]. Some ascribe the epithelial inclusions to congenital rests or forms of endometriosis, the latter also being a form of müllerianosis. Benign epithelial inclusions of the peritoneum and lymph nodes are found exclusively in females [9]. When inclusions are cystically dilated, have cilia and lack atypism, cell stratification or necrosis, the epithelium in question should be regarded as benign, even if psammoma bodies are present [9, 17]. Regardless of the microscopic appearance of the primary tumor, epithelium within the peritoneum and pelvic and abdominal lymph nodes should be evaluated on its own merits because histologically benign inclusions do not progress.

Diagnostic Criteria of Serous Carcinoma

Of the histologic features of carcinoma that aid in its identification, none is as important as invasion. Characterized by irregular projections into the stroma, invasion is often associated with irregular glandular margins, inflammation, edema, and fibrosis of the stroma. Crowding of the glands and individual cell clusters within the stroma are present in carcinoma, in addition to the microscopic features described for serous tumors of low malignant potential. Mitotic activity within the epithelium of carcinoma usually exceeds 2 per 10 hfp [18].

Comment on Serous Tumors

In a study of 990 ovarian epithelial malignancies in all stages, 16% were of low malignant potential [1]. The low malignant potential tumors were equally divided between serous and mucinous types. Of the 460 serous tumors described by Russell [25, 26], 15% were in the proliferative category, a proportion similar to that found by Purola [23]. Santesson and Kottmeier [27] place a third of the serous malignancies in the proliferative category.

Patients with borderline serous tumors have a median age about 7 years younger than those with serous carcinoma [26]. Only about 15% of serous tumors of low malignant potential have spread beyond the ovary when the patients are first encountered, whereas three-fourths of serous carcinomas are stage II or higher at the time of initial surgery [1]. Bilaterality is higher in serous carcinoma and stage Ib is unusually frequent (about 20%–30% of all patients) [1, 25]. When the patients are first seen, the median tumor diameter is about 10 cm in both categories [18, 25]. Cellular atypia, stratification of cells, surface bridges, high mitotic activity, necrosis of the epithelium and cellular disorganization are more marked in serous carcinoma than in proliferative serous tumors, but these features, singularly or taken together, do not distinguish serous carcinoma from serous tumors of low malignant potential [18]. Also, all of the aforementioned features are subjective. Stratification of serous cells in especially difficult to evaluate because of the tendency of serous tumors to form buds and tufts four cells or more in thickness. In these, stratification of four or more cells does not appear to have an adverse effect on the prognosis [26].

The survival of patients with serous low malignant potential tumors far exceeds that of patients with serous carcinoma, stage for stage. Of 27 patients in stage I followed up by Katzenstein et al. [18], all were well even though two-thirds had not received therapy other than surgery. None of the 32 low-grade serous tumors described by Julian and Woodruff [14] metastasized, despite the fact that most had only surgical therapy. This is in contrast with the 5-year survival of patients with serous carcinoma in stage I which is in the order of 45%–50% [1, 2, 21, 23], and

20%–30% in the more advanced stages [1, 8, 21, 23]. Five-year survival rates of patients with stage I proliferative neoplasms of all types are at least 95% at 5 years and 85% at 15 years, to judge from the survival data offered by Aure et al. [1], Russell [26], Creasman et al. [6], Julian and Woodruff [14], and Katzenstein et al. [18]. Since so few recur, it appears that adjunctive therapy in the form of either chemotherapy or pelvic irradiation is not warranted in stage I proliferative malignancies.

Since proliferative tumors grow slowly and are often diagnosed in young patients, conservative surgery for unilateral lesions is justified, except possibly if rupture has occurred. Only one of 55 stage I proliferative tumors reviewed by the author (reported by Creasman et al. [6]) recurred and that one had ruptured intraoperatively. The patient subsequently died of carcinomatosis. In this instance, the tumor had been incompletely examined microscopically.

Less Common Proliferative Tumors

Endometrioid Tumors of Low Malignant Potential

Endometrioid tumors of low malignant potential are neoplasms that resemble hyperplastic epithelial proliferations in the endometrium. Endometrioid ovarian tumors are more commonly associated with an endometriosis in the same ovary or elsewhere in the pelvis than other ovarian epithelial tumors [28]. In the past, endometrioid tumors were recognized because of their good differentiation and squamous metaplasia, features which highlight their resemblance to endometrial carcinoma. In recent years, there has been an increasing tendency to recognize less well-differentiated varieties of endometrial carcinoma. At the same time, a group of benign and proliferative endometrioid tumors is emerging, but endometrioid tumors of low malignant potential make up only a small proportion of endometrioid tumors. Benign endometrioid tumors, not directly arising within endometrioitic cysts, are especially rare. Investigators have found that only 4%–19% of endometrioid tumors are in the low malignant potential category [1, 25, 27]. Quite rare compared to serous and mucinous proliferative tumors, only one 1 (2%) of 55 stage I proliferative tumors reviewed by the author [6] was endometrioid in nature.

Endometrioid tumors of low malignant potential are characterized by crowded irregular glands of endometrial type. The proliferation often has the structure of endometrial hyperplasia or atypical hyperplasia (Fig. 7). Best illustrated by Russell [26], much of the architecture is similar to endometrial hyperplasia except that the intervening stroma is more fibrous (Fig. 8, 9) or nonspecific rather than like endometrial stroma [15]. Complex branches, stratification of cells, squamous metaplasia (Fig. 9), and irregular cystic spaces are characteristic. The stroma is usually more prominent than in serous and mucinous tumors of low malignant potential, since the neoplasms are partly solid or microcystic [15, 26]. In some, it appears that the proliferative epithelial component may have arisen in a cystadenofibroma [7, 15]. Invasion into the stroma is difficult to recognize. Most of the epithelial periphery is expansile, forming cysts with a smooth or rounded contour. About a quarter have associated pelvic endometriosis and endometrial carcinoma is present in at least 10% of cases [26].

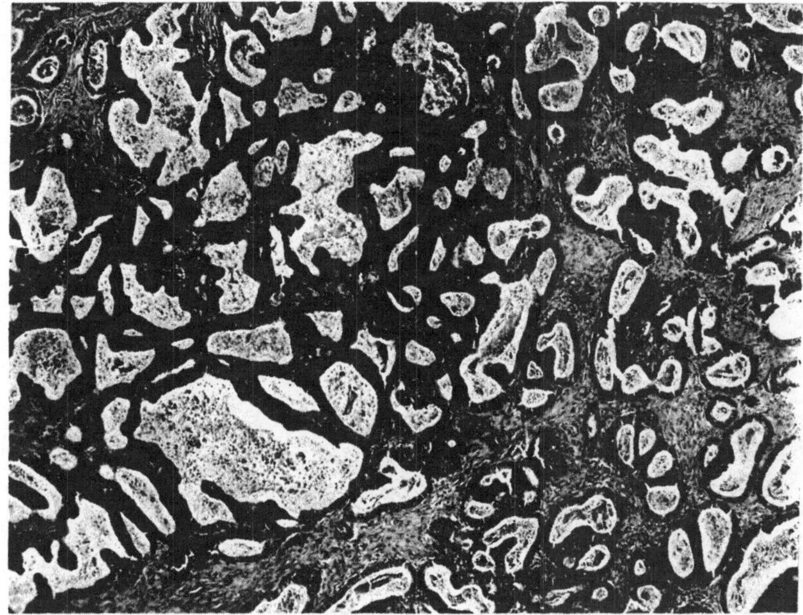

Fig. 7. Endometrioid tumor of low malignant potential. Note resemblance to endometrial atypical hyperplasia. HE, ×43

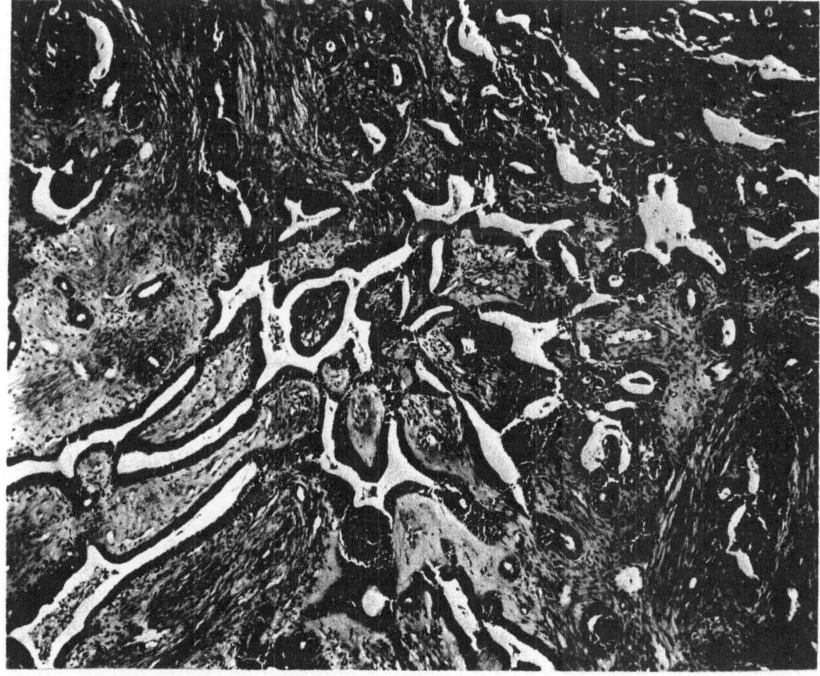

Fig. 8. A benign or low-grade proliferative endometrioid tumor. HE, ×60

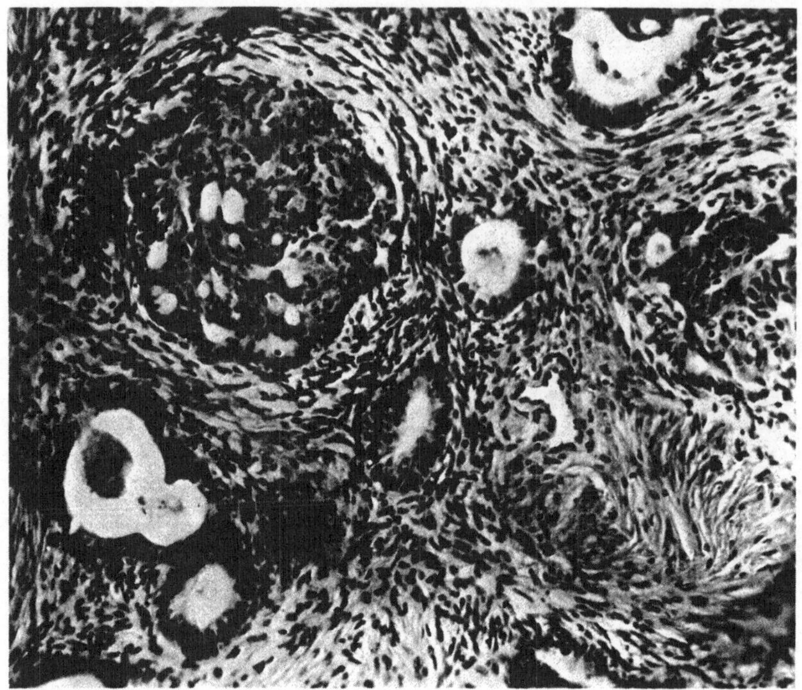

Fig. 9. Low-grade proliferative endometrial tumor. Benson WL, Norris HJ (1978) Current problems in gynecologic pathology. In: McGowan L (ed) Gynecologic Oncology. Appleton-Century, New York. HE, × 160

Clear Cell Tumors of Low Malignant Potential

Clear cell tumors of low malignant potential are very rare. The only description has been set forth by Russell [26] who placed 8% of clear cell (mesonephroid) malignancies in the proliferative category. He described three cases in which dense fibrous stroma resembling the stroma of a cystadenofibroma was the basic supporting structure. A rare clear cell cystadenofibroma was described by Kao and Norris [16]. Recognition of a proliferative clear cell tumor is difficult because the hobnail cells lining tubules and clear cell differentiation can be confused with bland areas within a fully malignant clear cell carcinoma. Such areas may be misleading in a tumor that has not been well sampled. Most of the glands are deeply embedded in stroma and may actually represent invasion, a point that supports the view that a borderline category of clear cell tumor of low malignant potential is not well grounded at present.

Proliferative Brenner Tumors

The category proliferative Brenner tumors was described by Roth and Sternberg [24], and later amplified by Miles and Norris [20] and Hallgrimsson and Scully [10]. None have metastasized and it may be that the proliferative Brenner tumor is wholly benign. It is likely, however, that some do have low malignant potential and that the follow-up studies conducted in the past may have relied too much on the follow-up behavior as a basis for the classification, rather than on the histology.

Proliferative Brenner tumors differ from malignant Brenner tumors by the formation of broad papillary processes of transitional epithelium resembling transitional papillomas and low-grade papillary carcinomas of the bladder. Destructive stromal invasion is not present, but cystic spaces lined by masses of epithelium may occur. Proliferative Brenner tumors are rare and usually develop in elderly women. Their clinical and pathologic features have been described elsewhere in detail and contrasted with malignant Brenner tumors [10, 20, 24]. For an unequivocal diagnosis, some require the coexistence of a benign Brenner tumor, whereas others accept the diagnosis simply if there is the typical proliferation of epithelium of a urothelial or transitional cell type.

Cystadenofibromas with Atypism and Malignant Potential

Cystadenofibromas containing a degree of epithelial atypism comparable to that seen in serous tumors of low malignant potential have been described [7, 15]. Representing less than 10% of cystadenofibromas, cystadenofibromas with epithelial atypism have clinical features and gross appearance similar to ordinary cystadenofibromas, except that the median age of the patients with cystadenofibromas containing atypism is about 10 years older than patients with ordinary cystadenofibromas [15]. This raises the possibility that cystadenofibromas with epithelial atypism may evolve from ordinary cystadenofibromas.

Cystadenofibromas with mild to moderate epithelial atypism and little or no cellular stratification should be thought of as benign tumors. Those with more advanced cellular atypism along with stratification of cells, glandular differentiation, papillary processes, epithelial tufts, and detachment of clusters of atypical cells from their lining site, correspond histologically to a serous tumor of low malignant potential. It is not clear whether cystadenofibromas having cellular atpyia will show progression in a significant number of cases, because few patients with it have been followed up. It appears that cystadenofibromas with epithelial atypism probably have less aggressive potential than serous tumors of low malignant potential having the same epithelial histology [15].

Only about 30 malignant adenofibromas (adenofibrocarcinoma) have been described [7]. They are solid neoplasms with minor cystic areas, and some have been bilateral. A diagnosis of carcinoma in a cystadenofibroma should be reserved for cytologically malignant tumors in which stromal invasion or metastasis can be demonstrated.

References

1. Aure JC, Hoeg K, Kolstad P (1971) Clinical and histological studies of ovarian carcinoma. Obstet Gynecol 37:1–9
2. Barber HRK, Sommers SC, Snyder R, Kwon TH (1975) Histologic and nuclear grading and stromal reactions as indices for prognosis in ovarian cancer. Am J Obstet Gynecol 121:759–807

3. Bassis M (1960) An embryologically derived classification of ovarian tumors. J Am Med Assoc 174:170–174
4. Classification and staging of malignant tumors in the female pelvis (1971) Acta Obstet Gynecol Scand 50:1–7
5. Cariker M, Dockerty MB (1954) Mucinous cystadenomas and mucinous cystadenocarcinomas of the ovary. Cancer 7:302–310
6. Creasman WT, Park R, Norris HJ, DiSaia PJ, Morrow CP, Hreshchyshyn MM, Sall S, Blessing JA. Stage I borderline ovarian tumors. Obstet Gynecol 59:93–96
7. Czernobilsky B (1977) Cystadenoma, adenofibroma, and malignant adenofibroma of the ovary. Pathol Annu 12 (1):201–206
8. Decker DG, Malkasian GD, Taylor WF (1975) Prognostic importance of histological grading in ovarian carcinoma. Natl Cancer Inst Monogr 42:9–11
9. Ehrmann RL, Federschneider JM, Knapp RC (1980) Distinguishing lymph node metastases from benign glandular inclusions in low grade ovarian carcinoma. Am J Obstet Gynecol 136:737–746
10. Hallgrimsson J, Scully RE (1972) Borderline and malignant Brenner tumors of the ovary. Acta Pathol Microbiol Scand [Suppl 233] 80A:56–66
11. Hart WR (1977) Ovarian epithelial tumors of borderline malignancy (carcinomas of low malignant potential). Hum Pathol 8:541–549
12. Hart WR, Norris HJ (1973) Borderline and malignant mucinous tumors of the ovary. Histologic criteria and clinical behavior. Cancer 31:1031–1045
13. Hsu YK, Parmley TH, Rosenshein NB, Bhagavan BS, Woodruff JD (1980) Neoplastic and non-neoplastic mesothelial proliferations in pelvic lymph nodes. Obstet Gynecol 55:83–88
14. Julian CG, Woodruff JD (1972) The biological behavior of low-grade papillary serous carcinoma of the ovary. Obstet Gynecol 40:860–867
15. Kao GF, Norris HJ (1978) Cystadenofibromas of the ovary with epithelial atypism. Am J Surg Pathol 2:357–363
16. Kao GF, Norris HJ (1979) Unusual cystadenofibromas: endometrioid, mucinous, and clear cell types. Obstet Gynecol 54:729–736
17. Karp LA, Czernobilsky B (1969) Glandular inclusions in pelvic and abdominal para-aortic lymph nodes. Am J Clin Pathol 52:212–217
18. Katzenstein AA, Mazur MT, Morgan TE, Kao M (1978) Proliferative serous tumors of the ovary. Histologic features and prognosis. Am J Surg Pathol 2:339–355
19. Malloy JJ, Dockerty JJ, Welch JS, Hunt AB (1965) Papillary ovarian tumors. I. Benign tumors and serous and mucinous cystadenocarcinoma. Am J Obstet Gynecol 93:867–879
20. Miles PA, Norris HJ (1972) Ovarian adenocarcinoma of mesonephric type. Cancer 30:1074–1081
21. Nieminin U, Purola E (1970) Stage and prognosis of ovarian cystadenocarcinomas. Acta Obstet Gynecol Scand 49:49–55
22. Parmley TH, Woodruff JD (1974) The ovarian mesothelioma. Am J Obstet Gynecol 120:234–241
23. Purola E (1963) Serous papillary ovarian tumours: A study of 233 cases with special reference to histological type of tumour and its influence in prognosis. Acta Obstet Gynecol Scand [Suppl 3] 42:7
24. Roth LM, Sternberg WH (1971) Proliferating Brenner tumors. Cancer 27:687–693
25. Russell P (1979) The pathological assessment of ovarian neoplasms. I: Introduction of the common 'epithelial' tumours and analysis of benign 'epithelial' tumours. Pathology 11:5–26
26. Russell P (1979) The pathological assessment of ovarian neoplasms. II. The proliferating 'epithelial' tumors. Pathology 11:251–289
27. Santesson L, Kottmeier HL (1968) General classification of ovarian tumors. In: Gentil F, Junquerira AC (eds) Ovarian Cancer. Springer, Berlin Heidelberg New York (UICC Monograph Series, vol 11, pp 1–8)
28. Scully RE (1978) Tumors of the ovary and maldeveloped gonads. Atlas of tumor pathology, Fasc 16, 2nd Ser. Armed Forces Institute of Pathology, Washington, D.C. pp 32–33
29. Serov SF, Scully RE (1973) Histological typing of ovarian tumours (International histological classification of tumours, No 9.) WHO, Geneva

Facultative Malignant Ovarian Tumors (Tumors of Borderline Malignancy)

An Immunohistochemical, Cytophotometric, and Electron Microscopic Study

M. Dietel [1]

Abstract

Epithelial ovarian tumors of borderline malignancy (BOTs) have a significantly better prognosis compared to malignant ovarian tumors (MOTs), and the application of differentiated therapeutical regimes is possible. This emphasizes the importance of discrimination between the two tumor types. The histological differential diagnosis is sometimes difficult. Another consideration concerns the possibility of a continuous transformation from benign to borderline and finally to malignant ovarian tumors.

In this investigation 464 malignant ovarian tumors were examined, and 13.8% were classified as BOTs. The incidence of BOTs was observed to be 20 years earlier than that of MOTs. Immunohistochemical determination of the carcinoembryogenic antigen (CEA) revealed a higher CEA positivity in MOTs (70%) than in BOTs (10%) at a dilution of 1 : 1000 of the CEA antiserum. Regarding the individual case, a differentiation between BOTs and MOTs was not possible, based on the appearance of CEA. The nuclear DNA content was determined by cytophotometry. BOTs showed a DNA distribution mainly in the diploid region with few values around the 4n region. Carcinomas consisted predominantly of cells with heteroploid nuclei. The DNA distribution patterns were characteristic for each individual tumor examined. Electron microscopic examinations were not helpful in the differentiation between BOTs and MOTs.

The results presented support the possibility of a continuous conversion from benign to borderline and to malignant ovarian tumors. Regarding the morphological diagnosis of the individual case, only the DNA measurement is a useful but arduous means of supplementing light microscopy. CEA determination and electron microscopy were of limited value.

Introduction

It is generally accepted that about 10%–20% of epithelial lesions of the ovary show a histologic appearance intermediate between clearly benign and unquestionably malignant (Lingeman 1974; Hart 1977; Scully 1979). In these cases a proliferation

1 Pathologisches Institut, Universitäts-Krankenhaus Eppendorf, Martinistr. 52, D-2000 Hamburg 20

of the surface epithelium and cellular abnormalities develop, indicating some malignant potential. The necessity of defining the group of borderline ovarian tumors (BOTs) as precisely as possible is emphasized by clinical long-term follow-up studies (Aure et al. 1971; Yaker and Benirschke 1975; Tobias and Griffiths 1976; Smith and Day 1979). They document a different prognosis for borderline and for malignant ovarian tumors (MOTs). The first group shows a 5-year survival rate of 95%, the second one of only 30% (Scully 1970; Sommers and Long 1972). Thus, on the basis of histologic diagnosis different therapeutical approaches can be applied, and may exclude patients with tumors of the borderline group from radical treatment (Munnell 1969; Scully 1970).

The characterization of borderline tumors given by the WHO (Serov et al. 1973) leaves room for interpretation. In the WHO classification the terms "tumors of borderline malignancy" and "carcinomas of low malignant potential" are used interchangeably, indicating some difficulties in the assessment of the capacity for malignant change.

Regarding morphology, the boundary line between borderline and malignant lesions is in some cases vague. The criteria defined by WHO refer to the "stratification of epithelial cells, detachment of cellular clusters from their sites of origin, mitotic activity, and lack [sic] of stromal invasion". The assessment of these criteria depends to a considerable extent on the subjective interpretation of the observer.

The vagueness of the definition and description of borderline tumors is understandable, since the cancerization of ovarian epithelial tumors is possibly a continuous process involving numerous intermediate steps. A sharp distinction and precise differentation is very difficult, if not impossible. On the basis of this unsatisfactory situation two questions appear to be of importance:

1. Is there indeed a continuous transformation from benign to borderline and finally to malignant tumors with intermediate stages of cancerization?
2. Are modern morphological methods helpful in the determination of the malignant potential of borderline ovarian tumors?

In the present study we compared borderline and malignant forms of ovarian tumors with regard to statistical data on the incidence, the distribution pattern of the carcinoembryogenic antigen (CEA), the nuclear DNA content, and the electron microscopic appearance.

Material and Methods

During the last 10 years 464 malignant epithelial tumors of the ovary have been diagnosed in the Department of Gynecologic Pathology, University Hospital of Hamburg. All cases have been reclassified independently by two pathologists, using the classification and the light microscopic criteria defined by WHO (Serov et al. 1973).

CEA determination was carried out on formalin-fixed tissue specimens using the triple layer method (unlabeled antibody enzyme method) described by Sternberger (1979). The following steps are necessary (Dietel et al. 1980; Caselitz et al. 1981):

1. Blocking of the endogene peroxidase by H_2O_2 (0.38% in PBS, pH 7.4)
2. Preincubation with normal goat serum, 1 : 30 (Nordic, Tilburg)

3. Incubation with the first antiserum, anti-CEA 1:200 and 1:1000 (Dakopatts, Copenhagen) from rabbit
4. Incubation with the second antiserum, goat antirabbit IgG, 1:30 (Nordic)
5. Incubation with a peroxidase-antiperoxidase complex from rabbit, 1:60 (Nordic)
6. Exposure to diaminobenzidine (0.05% in 0.05 M tris-HCL buffer plus 0.01% H_2O_2) (Sigma, Munich)
7. Postfixation with 1% osmium tetroxide.

The specificity was controlled: (a) by replacing the first antiserum with normal rabbit serum, (b) by replacing the second antiserum with normal rabbit serum, or (c) by omitting diaminobenzidine or H_2O_2.

For DNA determination, formalin-fixed specimens were stained by the procedure of Feulgen for cytophotometric measurement of the nuclear DNA content. The plug technique was used after focusing cell nuclei (Swift and Rasch 1956). The DNA content was determined at 570 μm using a Leitz microspectrophotometer MPV I (Würthner et al. 1972; Sachs et al. 1974).

The electron microscopic methods applied have been described previously (Dietel et al. 1980).

Results

Statistical Data

Of the 464 malignant ovarian tumors examined, 64 (13.8%) showed a borderline character and 400 were diagnosed as malignant. Figure 1 shows that 9.4% of the BOT group were found in patients aged within the first three decades. This rate of incidence is somewhat higher than that of MOTs, of which 8.5% were diagnosed in patients up to the age of 30. In those between 30 and 40 years the diagnostic rate of BOTs increased dramatically to 31%, while MOTs represented only 16.7% during

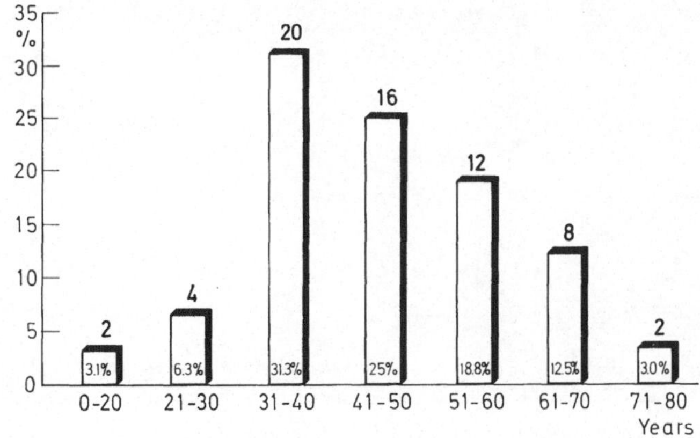

Fig. 1. Age distribution of common epithelial tumors of the ovary with borderline malignancy (n = 64)

the fourth decade (Fig. 2). From 40 up to 80 years a continuous decrease in BOTs was found. In contrast, the incidence of MOTs increased until the sixth decade (Fig. 2). Thus the majority of the BOT group was diagnosed 20 years earlier than the majority of the MOT group. During the postmenopausal phase both types appeared at an equal rate.

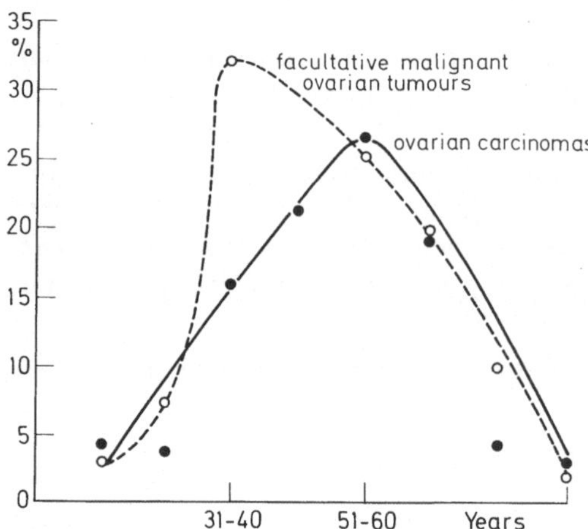

Fig. 2. Comparison of the age distribution of ovarian tumors of borderline malignancy (n=64) with clearly malignant ovarian tumors (n=400)

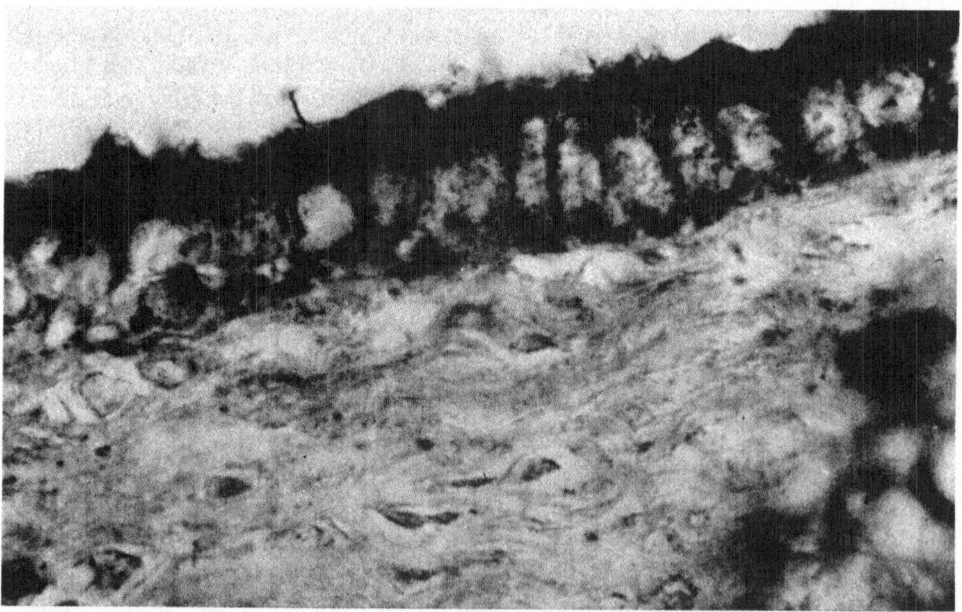

Fig. 3. Immunohistochemical CEA demonstration in the proliferating surface epithelium of mucinous borderline ovarian tumor. Apical concentration of the precipitates. No CEA is present in the stroma cells. ×400

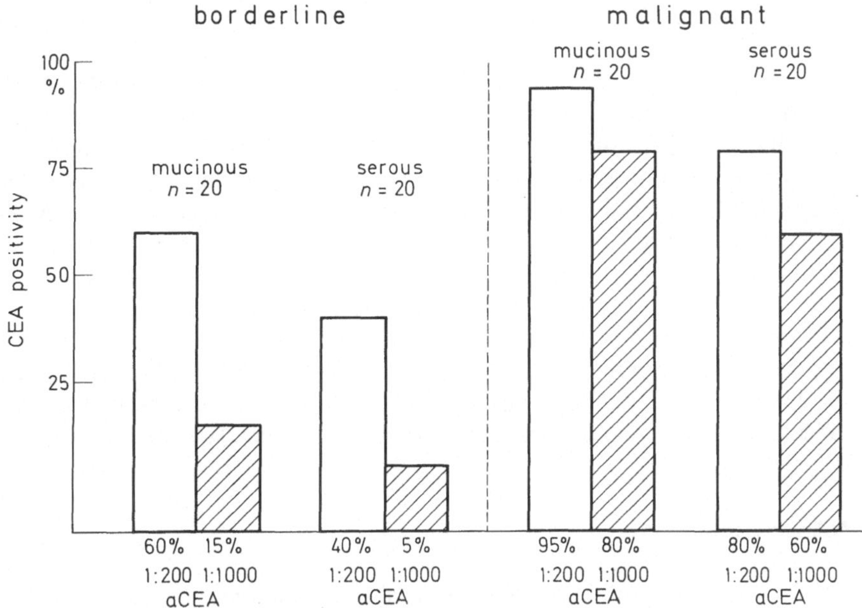

Fig. 4. Immunohistochemical determination of CEA in borderline ovarian tumors of serous (n=20) and mucinous (n=20) character compared to the CEA content of serous (n=20) and mucinous (n=20) carcinomas at different dilutions of the antiserum

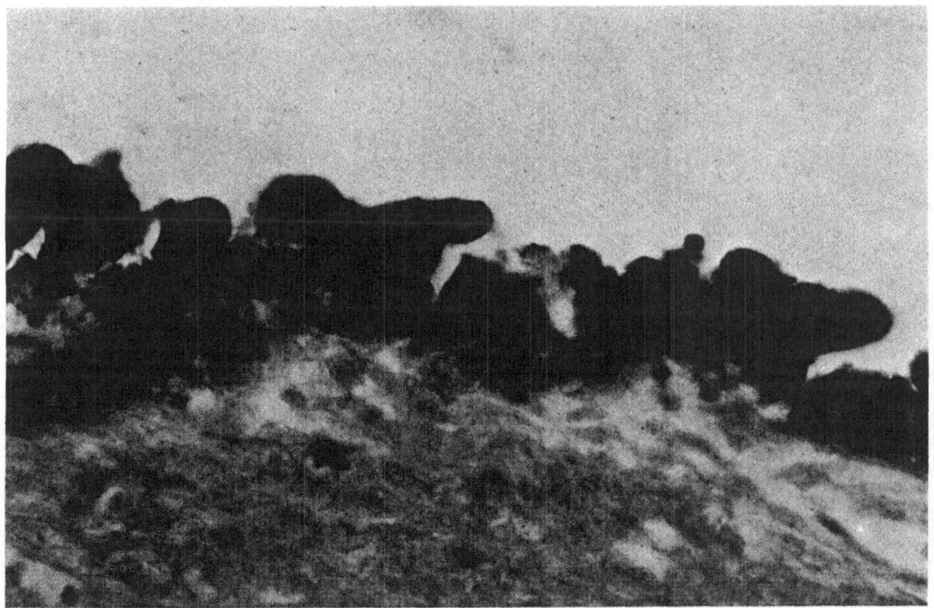

Fig. 5. Immunohistochemical CEA demonstration in the proliferating surface epithelium of serous borderline ovarian tumor. High content of the precipitates in the cytoplasm. Nuclei are free of CEA. No CEA can be found in the stroma cells. ×300

CEA Demonstration

The presence of CEA (Fig. 3) could be shown in 60% of mucinous BOTs at a dilution of 1:200 of the CEA antiserum and in 15% at a 1:1000 dilution (Fig. 4). In serous BOTs the CEA precipitates (Fig. 5) appeared about 15% less (Fig. 4). Mucinous malignant lesions presented a CEA positivity (Fig. 6) in 95% at a 1:200 and in 80% at a 1:1000 dilution (Fig. 4). Serous carcinomas were slightly less CEA-positive (Fig. 7): 80% at 1:200 and 60% at 1:1000 (Fig. 4). If the average CEA positivity of BOTs and MOTs was compared at identical dilutions of the antiserum, the statistical differences were obvious (Fig. 8). At an antiserum dilution of 1:200, 50% of BOTs and 87.5% of MOTs contained CEA precipitates. The difference was even more pronounced if a higher dilution was applied: at 1:1000 10% of BOTs and 70% of MOTs were CEA-positive (Fig. 8). These results were obtained by simultaneous application of an identical antiserum under standardized experimental conditions.

DNA Determination

In BOTs with mild proliferations of the surface epithelium, the cytophotometrically determined DNA content showed predominantly diploid (2n) values (Fig. 9). Only a few cells contained slightly heteroploid nuclei with DNA values around the 4n region of the histogram. There was no support for a malignant potential.

Borderline tumors with focally increased proliferations of the epithelium, pronounced papillary projections, multilayering of the cells, and a disturbed polarity with atypical nuclei, but lacking in invasive growth, revealed a more atypical DNA pattern (Fig. 10). The maximum of the mean DNA content was not as clear as in the BOTs group with mild proliferations (cf. Fig. 9). Some values were determined in

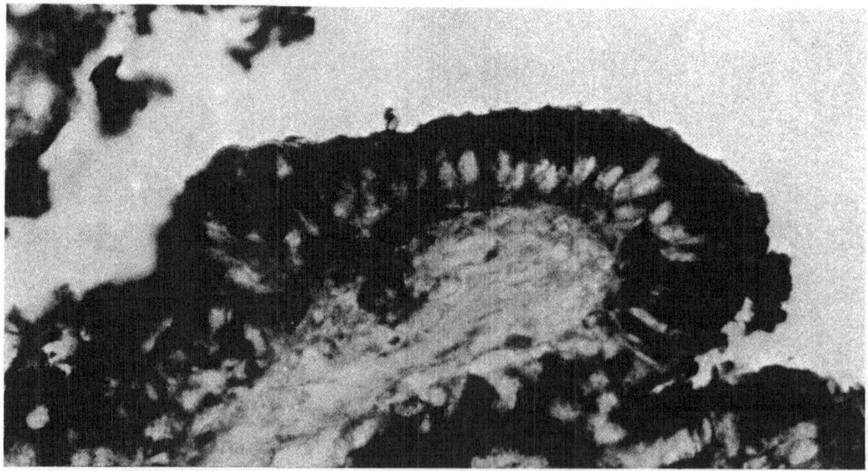

Fig. 6. Irregularly distributed CEA in a mucinous carcinoma; microinvasion of epithelial cells can be found at the basal layer. Concentration of the CEA precipitates is developed at the apical border. ×300

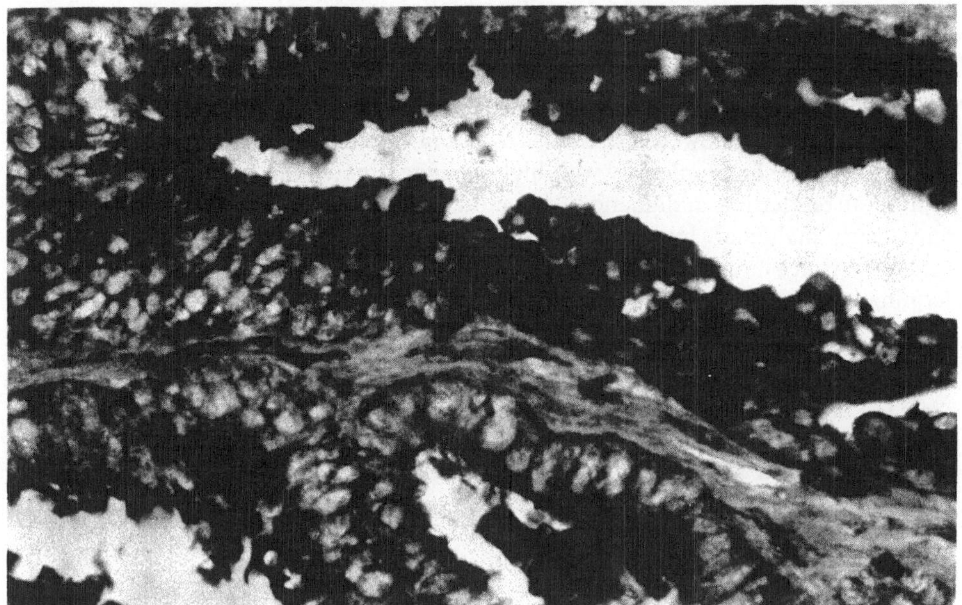

Fig. 7. High content of CEA precipitates in serous ovarian carcinomas. Different distribution of the CEA in the more highly differentiated areas (*top*) and in the less-differentiated region (*bottom*). In the stroma microinvasion of epithelial cells containing CEA. ×300

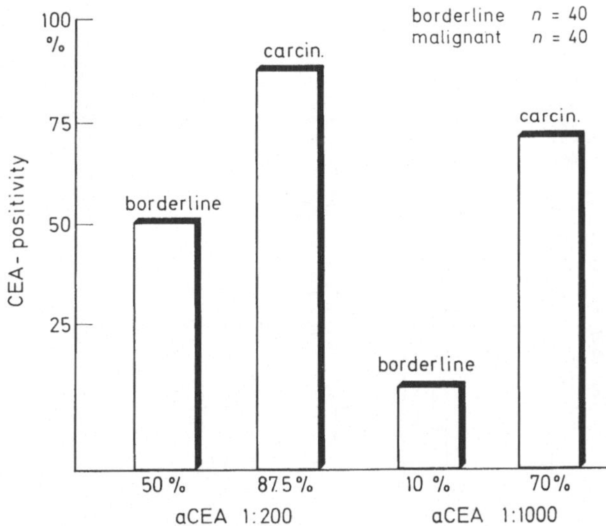

Fig. 8. Immunohistochemical demonstration of CEA in epithelial ovarian tumors. Direct comparison between borderline (n=40) and malignant (n=40) forms with regard to the CEA positivity at different dilutions of the antiserum

the hypo- or hyperploid region of the histogram, indicating some malignant potential.

The measurements of the average DNA content in the MOTs group resulted in a heteroploid grouping of the values (Fig.11). A diploid maximum was not observed. Most of the nuclei showed a broad distribution between 4n and 8n and more, indicating a severe heteroploidity with high malignant potential. In summary, ovarian tumors of borderline malignancy with mild proliferation or distinct proliferation, and clearly malignant tumors, each contained typical amounts of DNA (Fig. 12). Thus DNA measurements of epithelial cells were useful as a parameter for the determination of the malignant potency, even in the individual case.

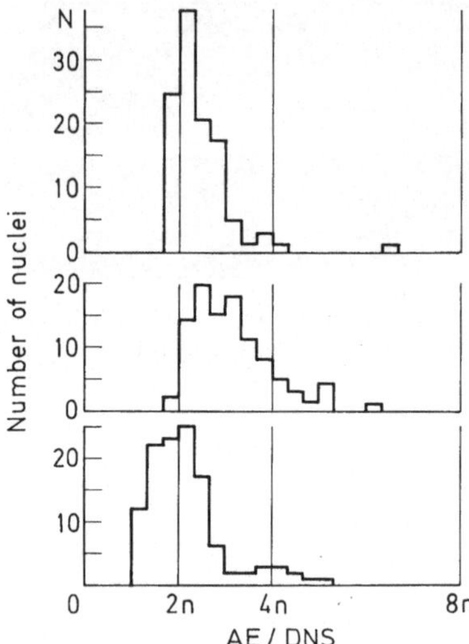

Fig. 9. Cytophotometric DNA determination of borderline ovarian tumors with mild proliferation of the surface epithelium. Distinct diploid maximum of the values

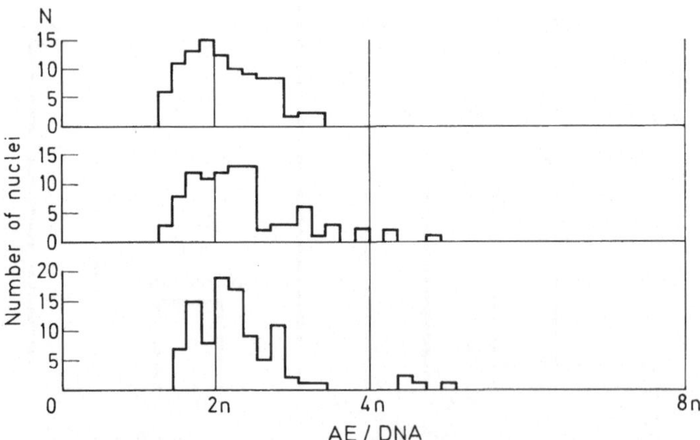

Fig. 10. Cytophotometric DNA determination of borderline ovarian tumors with distinct proliferation of the surface epithelium. Broader distribution of the DNA values around the diploid region compared to Fig. 9

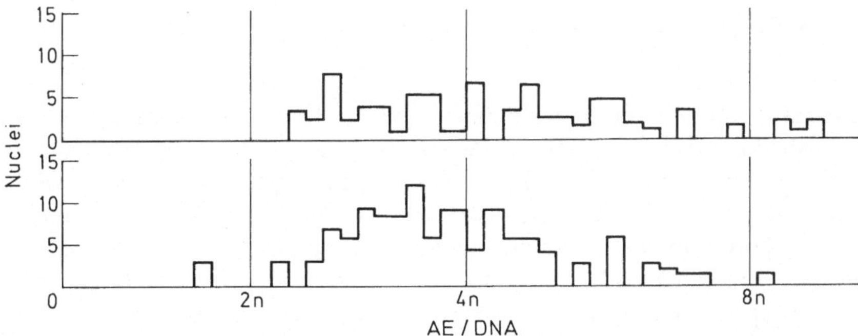

Fig. 11. Cytophotometric DNA determination of ovarian tumor with an irregular distribution of the values in the hyperploid region

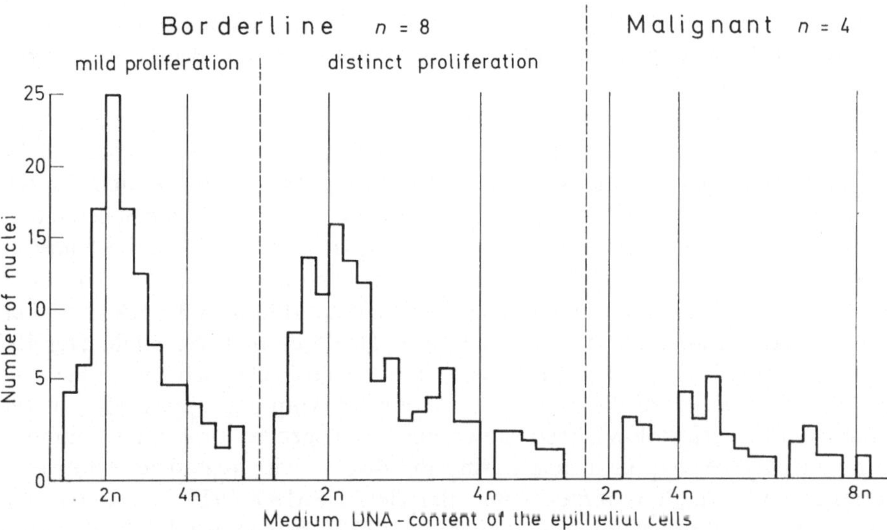

Fig. 12. Comparison of the average DNA values of ovarian tumor with mild or distinct proliferation, and of carcinomas

Electron Microscopy

Extensive ultrastructural examinations of borderline and malignant tumors revealed no characteristic criteria for discrimination. Neither the intracellular content nor the differentiation of organelles, i.e., microvilli, secretory granules, desmosomes or other, nor the morphology of the nuclei, show definite differences. Surface cells of borderline tumors with serous differentiation could not be distinguished from those in serous carcinomas. Mucinous carcinomas often consisted of highly differentiated epithelial cells, a fact which can lead to misdiagnosis at the ultrastructural level.

Conclusions

The statistical data on the incidence of ovarian tumors are in agreement with those published in other studies (Lingeman 1974; Hart 1977; Smith and Day 1979; Scully 1979). The peak incidence of BOTs was found to be 20 years earlier than that of the malignant lesion. This and the distinctly better prognosis of BOTs support the view that the borderline type of tumor represents an early stage of the malignant form. Of all borderline and malignant tumors of the ovary 8%–9% were diagnosed in young women up to the age of 30. A precise discrimination between the two forms is especially important in this group of patients, since a reserved therapy with conservation of fertility is possible in some cases. On the other hand, an insufficient treatment can result in a fast and extensive spreading of the tumor and in an adverse prognosis, which could have been prevented by a more radical therapy.

During the postmenopausal phase BOTs and MOTs appear at an equal rate. Whether certain hormonal constellations have any influence on the development of epithelial ovarian cancer is unknown. First clues on interactions between endocrine factors and the in vitro growth of epithelial tumor cells have been observed by Simon and Hölzel (1979).

The statistical data and the rather good 5-year survival rate of ovarian cancer diagnosed in stage I or II of the FIGO staging (Scully 1979; Dietel and Stegner 1981) emphasize strongly the necessity of an early diagnosis. In the search for tumor markers, a number of substances have been examined for ovarian specificity, i.e., placenta-like alkaline phosphatase (PLAP) (Malkin et al. 1978), alpha-fetoprotein, ABH antigens (Levin et al. 1976), Lewis antigen (Szulman 1977), human ovarian tumor associated antigen (OCA) (Knauf and Urbach 1980), and CEA (Levin et al. 1976; Malkin et al. 1978; Nagell et al. 1978; Heald et al. 1979; Stiglmayer 1978). The determination of OCA raises expectations since elevated levels have been found in early stages of the disease before clinical symptoms appear (Knauf 1980). Other tumor markers have been shown not to be specific for ovarian tumors and thus can only be helpful in monitoring the disease with regard to remission, recurrence, and formation of metastases (Barrelet and Mach 1975; Levin et al. 1976). As in the case of other organs (Wagner et al. 1967; Stiglmayer 1978; Wurster and Rapp 1979; Walker 1980), the immunohistochemically determined CEA positivity of epithelial ovarian tumors (Nagell et al. 1978; Heald et al. 1979) was correlated to staging, extent, and grading of the malignant potential of ovarian tumors. In our study, we paid special attention to the evaluation of the histochemical CEA determination in the diagnostic and prognostic assessment of the individual case. However, since there are always some carcinomas which are CEA-negative and a number of borderline tumors which are positive, the CEA determination is not very helpful in the discrimination between borderline and malignant forms of ovarian tumors and in the determination of the malignant capacity of the individual case.

The DNA determination of individual nuclei in tumor cells has often been used as a parameter for the assessment of the risk of dedifferentiation (Kother and Sandritter 1964; Wagner et al. 1967; Sachs 1971; Stegner et al. 1980). In tumorous lesions of the ovary this method can be of special use in the differentiation between benign, borderline, and malignant forms (Weiss et al. 1969; Sachs et al. 1974). In this investigation we demonstrated a correlation between the histologic appearance and the appropriate DNA histogram. A high amount of diploid nuclei of the surface epithelium corresponded to a well-differentiated light microscopic appearance with low tendency to proliferation. Spreading of DNA values in the hypo- and hyperploid region of the histogram found its expression in a higher degree of cellular and nuclear atypias with a stratification of the tumor cells. All examined cases of ovarian carcinomas showed an irregular distribution pattern of DNA, indicating severe heteroploidy with high malignant potency. Less than 10% of the MOTs cells contained diploid nuclei. Characteristic DNA distribution patterns could be obtained in all tumors investigated. There were no cases of benign tumors with a heteroploid DNA content and none of the carcinomas showed a diploid pattern. All BOTs contained nuclei with DNA values intermediate between benign and malignant DNA patterns. Thus DNA measurements of epithelial ovarian cells are useful as a parameter for the determination of the malignant potency even in the individual case. Similar results were reported by Schumann and Knörr-Gärtner (1975), using chromosome analysis for the assessment of the malignant potential of ovarian tumors.

In the literature, electron microscopic examinations of ovarian tumors are rare (Ferenczy and Richart 1974; Ferenczy 1976; Fenoglio et al. 1975), especially those dealing with borderline forms (Ferenczy 1974; Fenoglio 1975). Characteristic signs for the differentiation between borderline and malignant tumors have not been demonstrated (Ferenczy 1976). In ultrastructural observations we too were unable to find any specific criteria as diagnostic indicators. In borderline serous tumors the surface cells showed severe atypias at the electron microscopic level, whereas carcinomas consisted sometimes of rather highly differentiated cells. This observation is even more frequent in mucinous lesions, since mucinous carcinomas are often formed by highly differentiated signet-ring cells, which can be observed likewise in adenomas of mucinous character. Electron microscopy therefore does nothing to solve the differential diagnostic problems presented by epithelial ovarian tumors.

The two questions raised at the beginning of the investigation can be answered as follows:

1. The age distribution of the incidence of BOTs and MOTs, the light microscopic observations, and the measurements of the cellular contents of CEA and DNA support the possibility of a continuous conversion from benign to borderline and then to malignant epithelial tumors. Especially borderline tumors have a capacity for malignant change.
2. Among the methods examined, only DNA measurements proved to be a useful addition to conventional light microscopy in the diagnosis of the individual case. The difficult distinction between borderline and malignant tumors will therefore continue to be based mainly on light microscopy.

Acknowledgment. The excellent technical assistance of E. Lehmann and H. Meyer is gratefully acknowledged. For the DNA measurements I am indebted to my colleagues Dr. H. Sachs and Dr. K. Würthner. For help with the manuscript I would also like to thank Dr. F. Hölzel.

References

Aure JH, Høeg K, Kolstad P (1971) Clinical and histologic study of ovarian carcinoma. Am J Obstet Gynecol 37:1

Barrelet V, Mach JP (1974) Variations of the carcinoembryonic antigen level in the plasma of patients with gynecologic cancers during therapy. Am J Obstet Gynecol 121:164–168

Caselitz J, Seifert G, Jaup T (1981) Presence of carcinoembryonic antigen (CEA) in the normal and inflamed human parotid gland. J Cancer Res Clin Oncol 100:205

Dietel M, Dorn-Quint G (1980) By-pass secretion of human parathyroid adenomas. Lab Invest 43:116

Dietel M, Stegner HE (1981) Zur Klassifikation maligner Ovarialtumoren. Pathologie 2:226–232

Dietel M, Lehmann E, Kaspar M, Heitz P (1980) Distribution pattern of PTH in human parathyroid adenomas. An immunhistochemical study. Horm Metab Res 12:640

Fenoglio CM, Ferenczy A, Richart RM (1975) Mucinous tumors of the ovary. Ultrastructural features of mucinous cystadenomas with histogenetic considerations. Cancer 36:1709

Ferenczy A (1976) The ultrastructural morphology of gynecologic neoplasms. Cancer 38:463

Ferenczy A, Richart RM (1974) Female reproductive system. Dynamics of scan and transmission electron microscopy. Wiley & Sons, New York

Hart WR (1977) Ovarian epithelial tumors of borderline malignancy (carcinomas of low malignant potential). Hum Pathol 8:541

Heald J, Buckley CH, Fox H (1979) An immunohistochemical study of the distribution of carcinoembryonic antigen in epithelial tumours of the ovary. J Clin Pathol 32:918

Knauf S, Urbach GI (1980) A study of ovarian cancer patients using a radioimmunoassay for human ovarian tumor-associated antigen OCA. Am J Obstet Gynecol 138:1222

Kother L, Sandritter W (1964) Über den DNS-Gehalt des Carcinoma in situ. Gynaecologica 157:9

Levin L, McHardy JE, Poulton TA, Curling OM, Kitau MJ, Neville AM, Hudson CN (1976) Tumour-associated immune responses and isolated carcinoembryonic antigen and alpha feto-protein levels related to survival in ovarian cancer patients. Br J Cancer 33:363

Lingeman CH (1974) Etiology of cancer of the human ovary: A review. J Natl Cancer Inst 53:1603

Malkin A, Kellen JA, Lickrish GM, Bush RS (1978) Carcinoembryonic antigen (CEA) and other tumor markers in ovarian and cervical cancer. Cancer 42:1452

Munnell EW (1969) Is conservative therapy ever justified in stage I (IA) cancer of the ovary? Am J Obstet Gynecol 103:641

Nagell JR, Donaldson ES, Gay EC, Sharkey RM, Rayburn P, Goldenberg DM (1978) Carcinoembryonic antigen in ovarian epithelial cystadenocarcinomas. Cancer 41:2335

Sachs H (1971) Zytophotometrische Untersuchungen bei Präkanzerosen der Mamma. Beitr Pathol 143:360

Sachs H, Stegner HE, Würthner K (1974) Zytophotometrische Untersuchungen an papillomatösen Ovarialzystomen. Grenzfälle zur Malignität. Beitr Pathol 151:42

Samaan NA, Smith JP, Rutledge FN, Schultz PN (1976) The significance of measurement of human placental lactogen, human chorionic gonadotropin, and carcinoembryonic antigen in patients with ovarian carcinoma. Am J Obstet Gynecol 126:186

Schuhmann R, Knörr-Gärtner H (1975) Maligne Entartung von Ovarialtumoren (Zytogenetische und histologische Untersuchungen.) Arch Gynecol 219:179

Scully RE (1970) Recent progress in ovarian cancer. Hum Pathol 1:73

Scully RE (1979) Tumors of the ovary and maldeveloped gonads. In: Atlas of tumor pathology. Armed Forces Institute of Pathology, Washington D.C., pp 1–412

Serov SF, Scully RE, Sobin LH (1973) Histological typing of ovarian tumours. Internat. Histol Class of Tumours Nr 9, WHO 1–56

Simon WE, Hölzel F (1979) Hormone sensitivity of gynecological tumor cells in tissue culture. J Cancer Res Clin Oncol 94:307

Smith JP, Day TG (1979) Review of ovarian cancer at the university of texas systems cancer center, M.D. Anderson Hospital and tumor institute. Am J Obstet Gynecol 135:984

Sommers SC, Long ME (1972) Ovarian carcinoma: Pathology, staging, grading, and prognosis. Bull NY Acad Med 49:858

Stegner HE, Bahnsen J, Hinz B (1980) Cytophotometric analysis of nuclear DNA-content in So-called obliteraiting mastopathy with epithelial hyperproliferation. Pathol Res Pract 170:146

Sternberger LA (1979) Immunocytochemistry. Wiley & Sons, New York, p 104

Stiglmayer R (1978) Carcinoembryonales Antigen in der gynäkologischen Onkologie. Fortschr Med 96:1843

Swift H, Rasch E (1956) Microphotometry with visible light. In: Oster G, Pollister AW (eds) Cells and Tissues. Academic Press, New York (Physical Technics in Biol Res vol III)

Szulman AE (1977) The ABH and lewis antigens of human tissues during prenatal and postnatal life. 5th Int Convoc Immunol Buffalo, NY Karger, Basel, pp 426

Tobias JS, Griffiths CT (1976) Management of ovarian carcinoma. Current concepts and future prospects (first of two parts). N Engl J Med 294:818

Wagner E, Richart RM, Turner JY (1967) Deoxribonucleic acid content of presumed precursors of endometrial carcinoma. Cancer 20:2067

Walker RA (1980) Demonstration of carcinoembryonic antigen in human breast carcinomas by the immunperoxidase technique. J Clin Pathol 33:356

Wegener C, Csaszar H, Totovic V, Breuer H (1978) A highly sensitive method for the demonstration of carcinoembryonic antigen in normal and neoplastic colonic tissue. Histochemistry 58:1

Würthner K, Sachs H, Bahnsen J (1972) Zum Problem der Kernanschnitte bei der Zytophotometrie an histologischen Präparaten. Histochemie 32:261

Wurster K, Rapp W (1979) Histological and immunohistological studies on gastric mucosa. I. The presence of CEA in dysplastic surface epithelium. Pathol Res Pract 164:270

Yaker A, Benirschke K (1975) A ten year study of ovarian tumors. Virchows Arch [Pathol Anat] 366:275

Zur malignen Transformation mesothelialer Ovarialtumoren – Vergleichende histologisch-zytogenetische Untersuchungen

R. SCHUHMANN und H. KNÖRR-GÄRTNER[1]

Es darf heute als gesichert gelten, daß die maligne Entartung eines Gewebes, d.h. der Übergang vom regelrechten zum bösartigen Wachstum, schrittweise verläuft, sich über wechselnd lange Zeiträume erstreckt und mit komplexen Chromosomenveränderungen in Zahl und Struktur einhergeht. Über Chromosomenveränderungen des Ovarialkarzinoms liegen bereits zahlreiche Untersuchungen vor, wobei die Ergebnisse größtenteils an Tumorzellen von Malignomen fortgeschrittener Stadien und/oder Metastasen, Aszites oder Pleuraergüssen gewonnen wurden. Es werden hypo-, hyperdiploide, vornehmlich jedoch peritriploide Chromosomensätze beschrieben, die oft zusätzlich durch große Markerchromosomen als Zeichen grober Strukturveränderungen charakterisiert sind.

Diese Befunde vermögen jedoch keinen Hinweis auf einen stufenweisen Ablauf der malignen Transformation zu liefern, auch ist bislang unbekannt, zu welchem Zeitpunkt im Verlauf des Übergangs vom gutartigen zum bösartigen Wachstum *erstmals* Chromosomenveränderungen auftreten. Unbeantwortet ist weiterhin die Frage nach dem *histologischen* Äquivalent erster chromosomaler Aberrationen, da die frühen Vorstadien des Ovarialkarzinoms – anders als die frühen Vorstadien des Zervixkarzinoms – klinisch kaum erfaßbar sind.

Ansatzpunkte für die Abklärung dieser Fragen könnten diejenigen epithelialen Neoplasien des Ovars liefern, die vom histologischen Bild her hinsichtlich ihrer Dignität nach der Klassifizierung der FIGO als Tumoren mit „low potential malignancy“ eingeordnet werden.

Ausgehend von diesen Überlegungen wurden einige dieser Tumoren zytogenetisch und histologisch untersucht.

Methodisch wurde so vorgegangen, daß von den aus dem Tumor entnommenen und zur Kurzzeitkultivierung und zytogenetischen Untersuchung explantierten Gewebsstücken der Histologe jeweils ein Gewebsstück als sog. Referenzpräparat erhielt. Der Rest des Tumors wurde als sog. Routinehistologie in üblicher Weise histologisch aufgearbeitet.

Tabelle 1 zeigt die Zusammenstellung der untersuchten Borderline-Fälle. Im ersten Fall, einem einfachen serösen Zystom, ergab die Referenzhistologie eine beginnende maligne Entartung, während der Tumor in der Routinehistologie als gutartig beurteilt worden war. Zytogenetisch ließ sich eine abnorme Stammlinie mit 47 Chromosomen nachweisen, wobei das Extrachromosom morphologisch einem „D“-

1 Sektion Gynäkologische Zytologie und Histologie der Universitäts-Frauenklinik und Abteilung Klinische Genetik der Universität Ulm, D-7900 Ulm

Tabelle 1. Kombinierte histologische und zytogenetische Untersuchungen an mesothelialen Ovarialtumoren (Gruppe I b der FIGO-Klassifizierung - low potential malignancy)

Patient.	Fall Nr.	Routinehistologie	Ovar	Zytogenetische Analyse			Dignität	
				Normal	Abnorm	Abnorme Stammlinie	zytogenetisch	Referenzhistologie
B.M. 5. 6. 21	1	Cystoma serosum simplex	re.	+	+	47, XX, + „D“	Verdacht auf maligne Transformation	Beginnende maligne Entartung
Ö.B. 3. 8. 06	2	Cystoma serosum, papilliferum proliferans regional beginnend, maligne Transformation	re.	+	+	47, XX, +C	Verdacht auf maligne Transformation	Benigne Beginnende maligne Entartung
K.B. 25. 3. 44	3	Cystoma serosum papilliferum proliferans regional maligne	re. + li.	+	+	47, XX, +C	Verdacht auf maligne Transformation	Fehlt
K.A. 25. 6. 42	4	Cystoma serosum papilliferum proliferans	re. + li.	+	+	47, XX, +C	Verdacht auf maligne Transformation	Benigne Beginnende maligne Entartung
J.A. 21. 9. 14	5	Cystoma serosum papilliferum proliferans	re. + li.	+	+	47, XX, $+C_{10}$	Verdacht auf maligne Transformation	Örtlich beginnende maligne Entartung
J.V. 4. 4. 25	6	Cystoma serosum papilliferum proliferans	li.	+	+	47, XX, $+C_{10}$	Verdacht auf maligne Transformation	Beginnende maligne Entartung

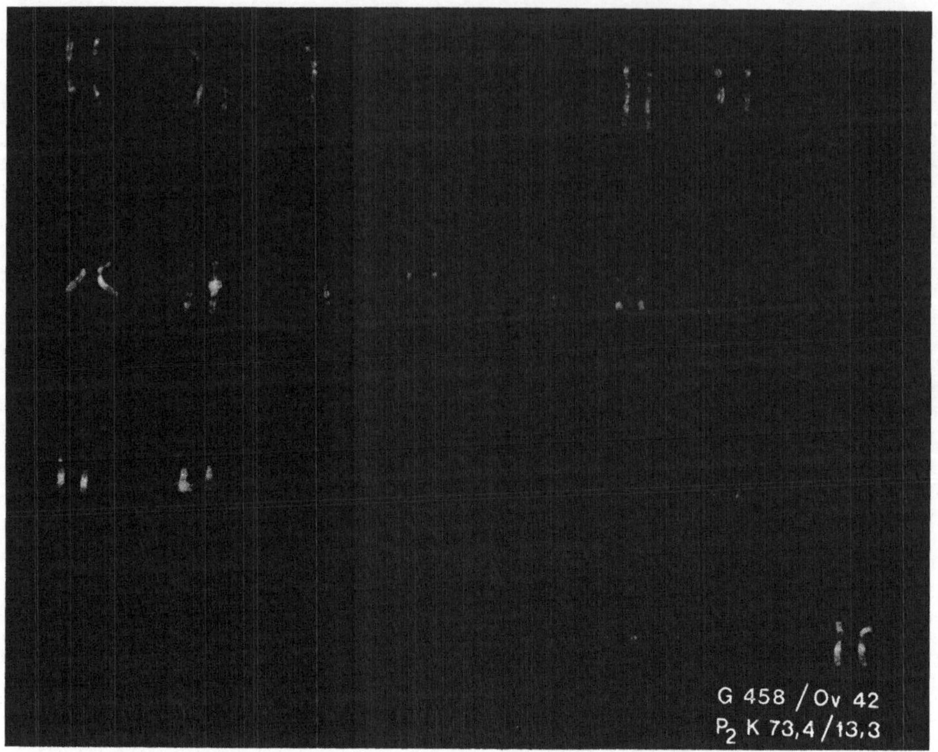

Abb. 1. Karyotypen eines Cystoma serosum papilliferum proliferans (Fall 6 der Tabelle 1), identifiziert mit Hilfe der Q-Banden-Technik. Karyotyp 47 XX + C_{10}

Chromosom entsprach. Besondere Aufmerksamkeit verdienen die nachfolgenden Beobachtungen 2–6, bei denen es sich histologisch um proliferierende Cystadenomata serosa papillifera handelte. In allen Fällen konnte eine Stammlinie mit 47 Chromosomen nachgewiesen werden. Das Extrachromosom entsprach bei konventioneller Färbetechnik morphologisch übereinstimmend einem der kleineren „C"-Chromosomen aus dem Bereich Nr. 10–12. In den letzten beiden Fällen kam zusätzlich die *Q-Banden-Technik* zur Anwendung. Mit ihrer Hilfe konnte das Extrachromosom jeweils eindeutig als Chromosom Nr. 10 identifiziert werden.

Abbildung 1 zeigt das trisom vorhandene Chromosom Nr. 10 – der Karyotyp entstammt dem letzten Tumor der Tabelle. Außerdem ließ sich zeigen, daß die abnorme Zellinie in die Polyploidisierung mit eingeht.

In Abb. 2 ist ein tetraploider – genauer gesagt pseudotetraploider – Chromosomensatz mit 94 Chromosomen dargestellt, wobei das Extrachromosom Nr. 10 ebenfalls verdoppelt ist.

Aus der Sicht des Zytogenetikers mußte in allen Fällen – je nach Ausprägung der Stammlinie und dem Grad der Polyploidie – der Verdacht auf eine beginnende oder bereits vollzogene maligne Transformation geäußert werden.

Am Beispiel des Falles 4 der Tabelle 1 sollen Einzelheiten der Ergebnisse erläutert werden:

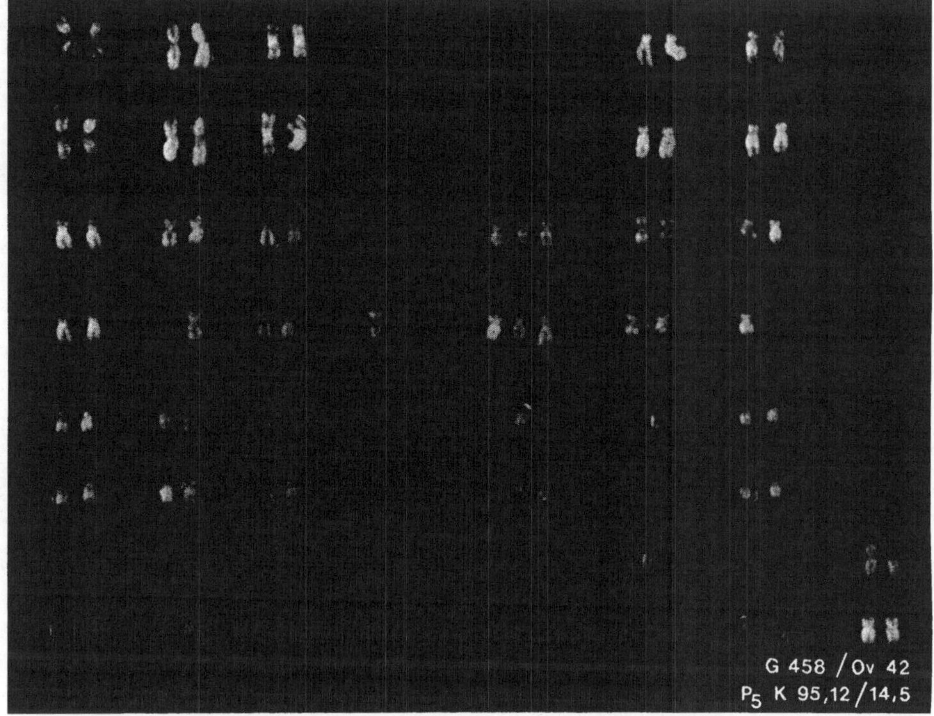

Abb. 2. Karyotyp eines Cystoma serosum papilliferum proliferans (Fall 6 der Tabelle 1), tetraploider bzw. pseudotetraploider Chromosomensatz. Karyotyp 94 XXXX+2 C_{10}. Das Extrachromosom Nr. 10 ist ebenfalls verdoppelt

Es handelte sich um eine 31jährige Patientin, die wegen doppelseitiger seröser Ovarialzysten mit papillärer Wandung operiert wurde. Von jeder Seite wurden zwei Gewebsproben untersucht.

In der ersten Probe der linken Seite ergab die Referenzhistologie einen gutartigen Befund (Abb. 3a). Bei der zytogenetischen Analyse (Abb. 3b) fanden sich zwei unterschiedliche Zellinien, unter denen die zahlenmäßig vorherrschende mit dem normalen Chromosomenkomplement 46 XX ausgestattet war; eine schwächere Zellinie – hier in 6% der karyotypierten Zellen vorhanden – enthielt dagegen 47 Chromosomen. Das Extrachromosom entsprach morphologisch einem der kleineren „C“-Chromosomen.

Im zweiten Präparat (Abb. 4a) fand sich ein gleichermaßen gutartiger histologischer Befund. Im Karyogramm ist die abnorme Zellinie mit 13% etwas deutlicher repräsentiert (Abb. 4b).

Die beiden Proben aus dem rechtsseitigen Tumor erbrachten unterschiedliche Ergebnisse. Während die erste Probe wiederum einen histologisch eindeutig gutartigen Befund und die Stammlinie 47 XX+C in einer Frequenz von 15% aufwies (Abb. 5a, b), zeigte die Histologie der zweiten Probe nunmehr eine Mehrschichtigkeit des Epithels mit zellulären Atypien und einer Polymorphie der Kerne und Zellen. Besonders fallen große helle Zellen mit teils bläschenförmigen Kernen auf, die

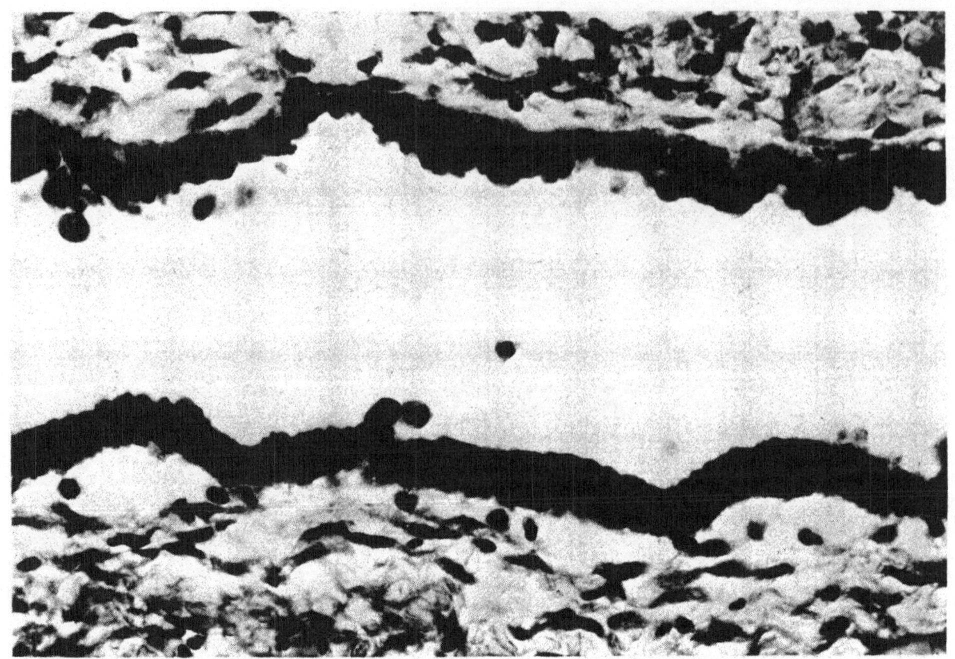

a

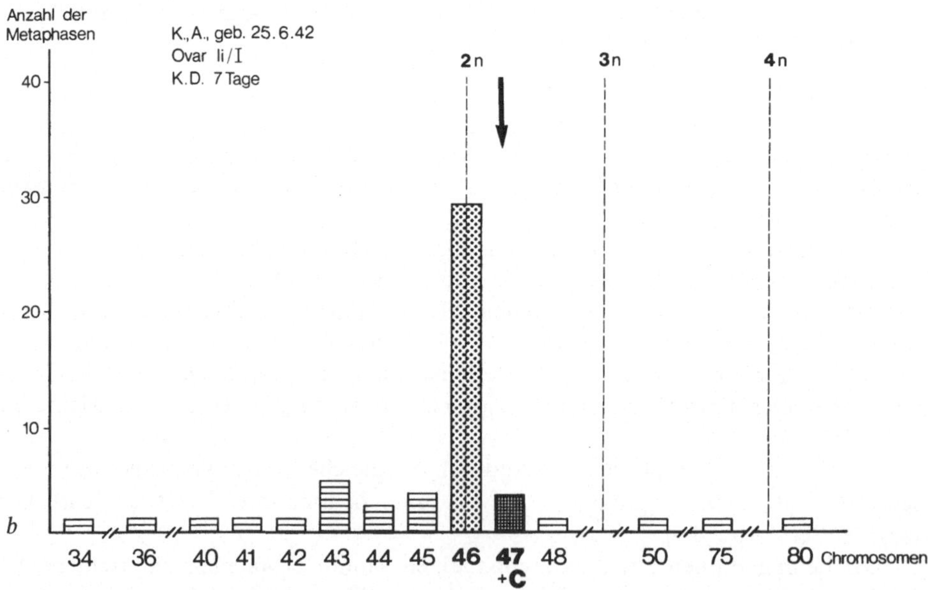

b

Abb. 3. *a* Histologisches Bild der Probe „links I" (Fall 4 der Tabelle 1). Gutartiges Cystoma serosum papilliferum, Eosin van Gieson, Originalvergr. ×100. *b* Häufigkeitsverteilung der Chromosomenzahlen

a

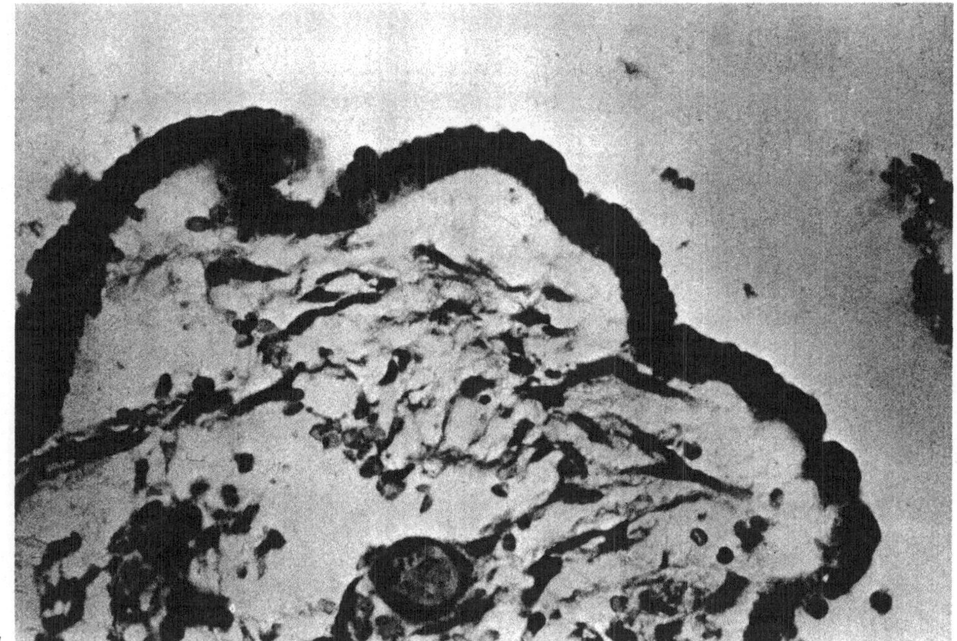

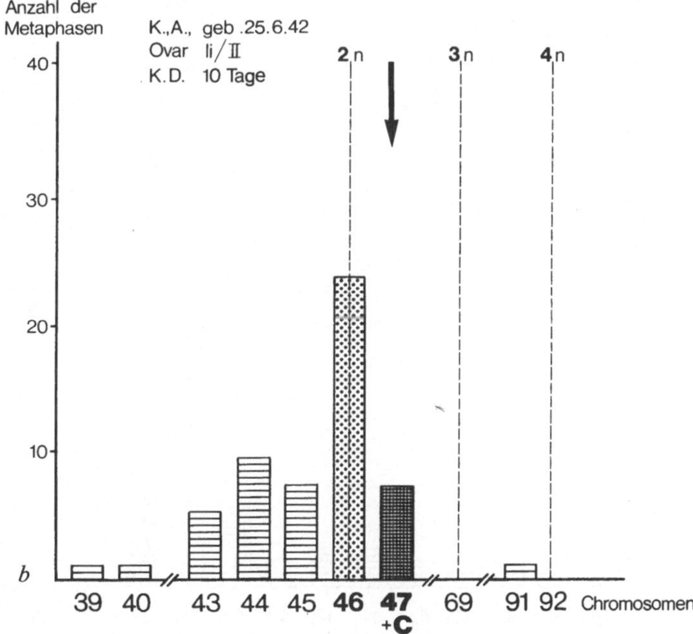

Abb. 4. *a* Histologisches Bild eines gutartigen Cystoma serosum papilliferum (Probe „links II", Fall 4 der Tabelle 1). Eosin van Gieson, Originalvergr. ×100. *b* Häufigkeitsverteilung der Chromosomenzahlen

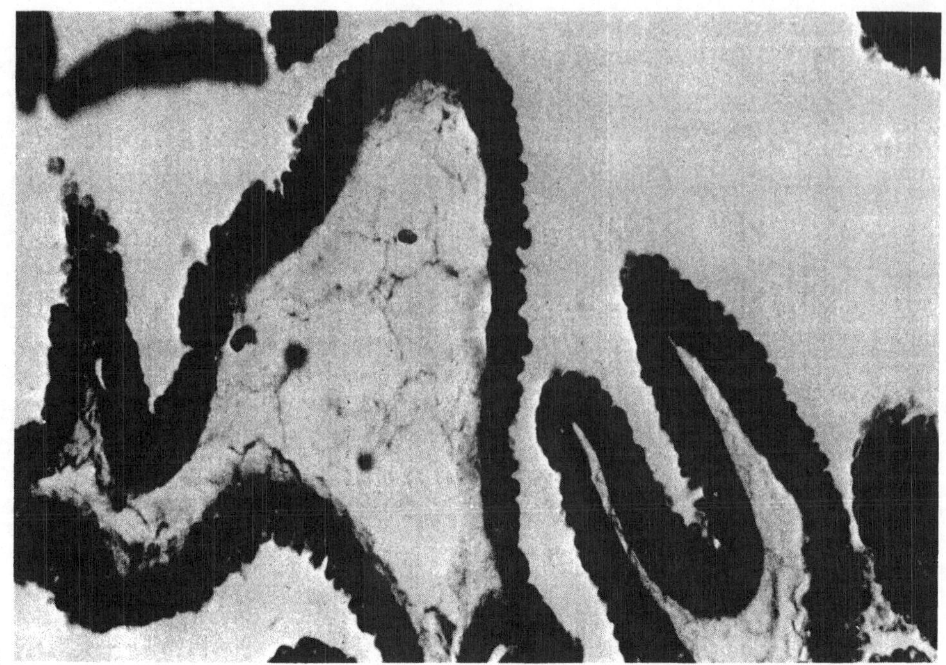

a

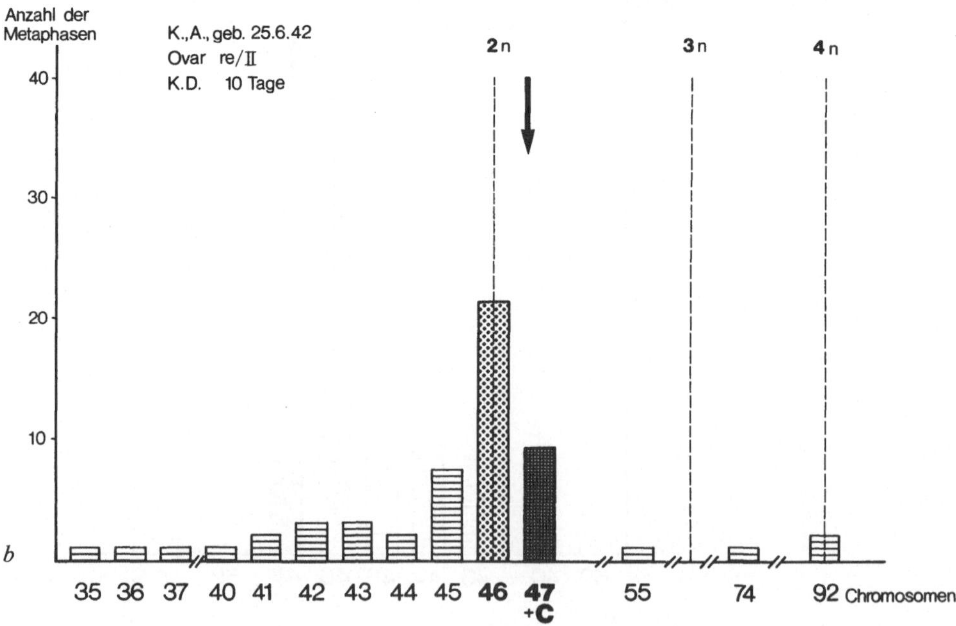

b

Abb. 5. a Histologisches Bild eines gutartigen Cystoma serosum papilliferum (Probe „rechts II", Fall 4 der Tabelle 1). Eosin van Gieson, Originalvergr. ×100. *b* Häufigkeitsverteilung der Chromosomenzahlen

a

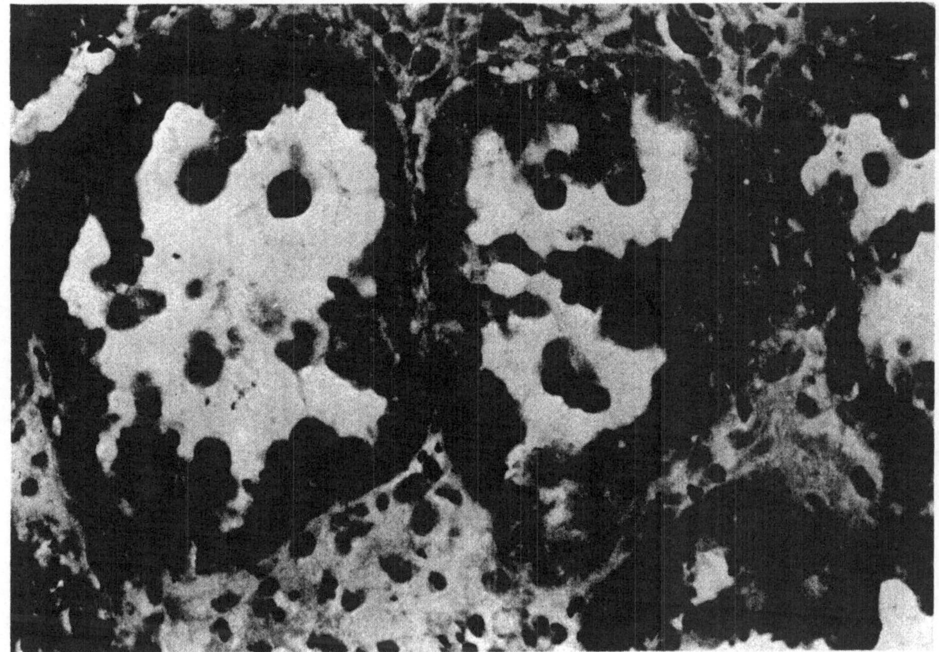

b

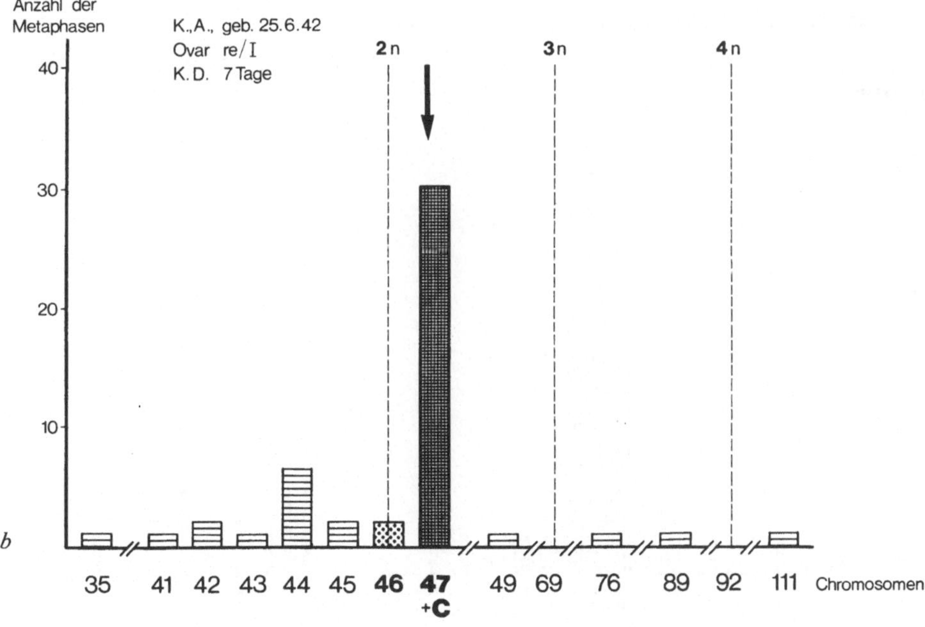

Abb. 6. a Histologisches Bild einer beginnenden malignen Transformation. Ausgeprägte zelluläre Proliferation, Mehrschichtigkeit, ausgeprägte zelluläre Atypie mit zahlreichen sog. hellen Zellen (Probe „rechts I", Fall 4 der Tabelle 1). Eosin van Gieson, Originalvergr. × 100. *b* Häufigkeitsverteilung der Chromosomenzahlen

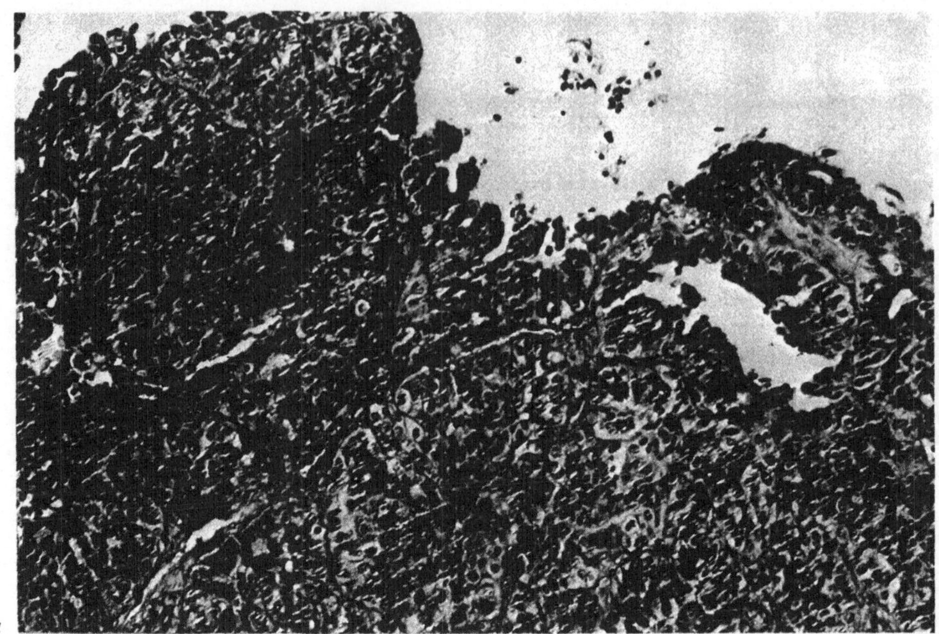

a

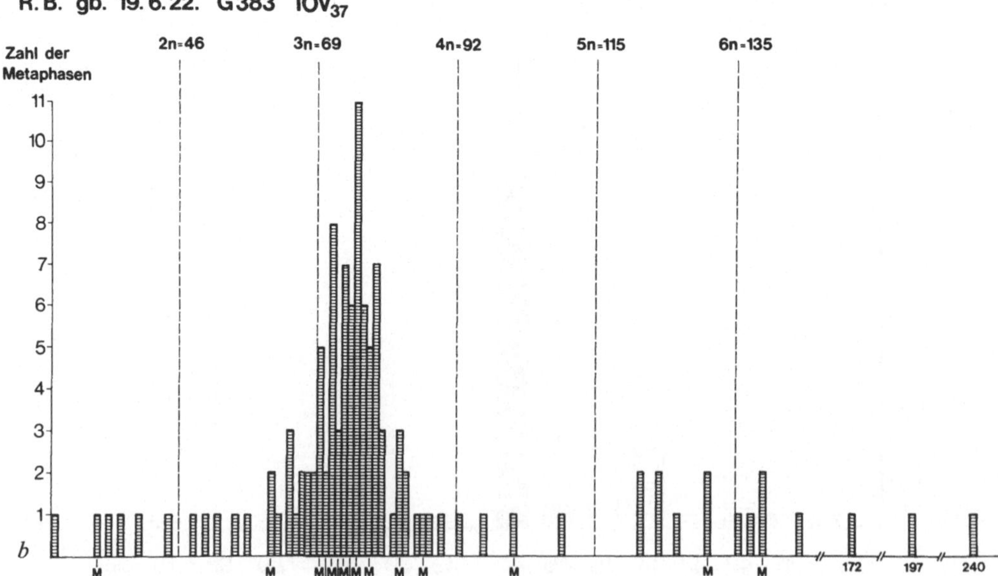

b

Abb. 7. *a* Entdifferenziertes Cystadenocarcinoma serosum; *b* Häufigkeitsverteilung der Chromosomenzahlen. Hochgradige Aneuploidie mit breitstreuenden Chromosomenzahlen vom hyperdiploiden bis zum hochgradig polyploiden Bereichen. Das mit „M" markierte B-ähnliche Markerchromosom findet sich in allen Ploidiebereichen

deutliche Nukleolen enthalten (Abb. 6a). Insgesamt wurde der Befund als beginnende maligne Entartung gedeutet.

Die zytogenetische Analyse (Abb. 6b) ergab, daß mehr als die Hälfte der Zellen, nämlich 61%, den pathologischen Karyotyp 47 XX+C aufwies. Die abnorme Zelllinie war etabliert, hatte also einen Selektionsvorteil gewonnen, wobei die zytogenetischen Kriterien der Malignität erfüllt waren. Zur Ergänzung seien die Befunde eines manifesten Karzinoms dargestellt.

In Abb. 7a ist ein entdifferenziertes Cystadenocarcinoma serosum dargestellt. Die zytogenetische Analyse ergab eine hochgradige Aneuploidie mit breitstreuenden Chromosomenzahlen von hyperdiploiden bis zu hochgradig polyploiden Bereichen (Abb. 7b). Das mit „M“ markierte „B“-ähnliche Markerchromosom findet sich in allen Ploidiebereichen. Bei dem beidseitigen Malignom fanden sich in allen Proben gleiche Chromosomensätze.

Bei der Interpretation der Befunde scheint bei aller gebotenen Vorsicht folgende Aussage möglich:

Die beginnende maligne Transformation kann sich *zytogenetisch* bereits durch eine abnorme Stammlinie anzeigen, wenn *histologisch* noch *keine Zeichen* der Entartung erkennbar sind. Im Fall der beschriebenen Cystomata serosa papillifera war der erste Schritt eine Stammlinie mit einer Trisomie Nr. 10. Es müssen weitere Untersuchungen an gleichen Tumoren vorgenommen werden, um eine Aussage darüber machen zu können, ob es sich hierbei um eine für diese Tumorgruppe *spezifische* abnorme Zellinie handelt. Weiter muß offen bleiben, ob dieser Prozeß *reversibel* ist, d.h., ob die abnorme Zellinie zumindest zeitweilig wieder von Zellen mit normalem Chromosomenkomplement überwuchert werden kann.

Hat aber die abnorme Stammlinie einen Selektionsvorteil gewonnen, wie es in den beschriebenen Gewebsproben evident wurde, dann werden auch *histologisch* Zeichen der malignen Transformation sichtbar. Schreitet der Malignisierungsprozeß fort, dann kommt es im Zuge der gesteigerten Proliferation zunehmend zu irregulär aneuploiden und polyploiden Chromosomensätzen, begleitet von gravierenden Umstrukturierungen der Chromosomen mit dem Auftreten von – meist großen – Markerchromosomen.

Der Histologe kann aus den vorgelegten Befunden entnehmen, daß es sich bei den Veränderungen, die bislang als vermehrte Proliferation mit zellulären Atypien und – je nach Ausprägung – noch als „gutartig“ oder schon als „Borderline-Befunde“ bezeichnet werden, tatsächlich um Präkanzerosen handelt, da auf der Ebene der Zytogenetik die maligne Transformation schon vollzogen ist.

Metastatic Tumors

B. CZERNOBILSKY [1]

Introduction

The ovary is a common site for metastases, which may be clinically silent, of microscopic size, or present as large bilateral masses. Direct spread of malignancy is common when the primary tumor is located in adjacent organs. Remote primaries reach the ovary more often through the blood vessels than through the lymphatics. As is the case with primary ovarian neoplasms, metastatic tumors in the ovary often tend to be cystic and sometimes papillary, which adds to the difficulty in distinguishing primary from metastatic tumors. Another feature which may occur in ovarian metastatic disease is luteinization of the surrounding stroma resulting in hormone production.

Metastases from Other Genital Organs

Ovary

About 30%–50% of all ovarian cancers are bilateral. However, the figure for bilateral involvement when there is no extraovarian spread, and which can therefore be assumed to represent multicentric bilateral ovarian neoplasms rather than metastases from one ovary to the other, is about 25%. Furthermore, since lymphatic pathways between ovaries are of minor importance, even in the presence of extraovarian tumors [6] one can only be reasonably sure that one is dealing with metastases to the opposite ovary. In other words, it is actually very difficult to be certain which cases of bilateral ovarian cancer constitute multicentricity and which constitute true metastases.

Fallopian Tube

Tumors of the fallopian tube are rare, but involve the ovary by direct extension in about 13% of cases [11]. When both tube and ovary are involved by massive tumor it

1 Medical School of the Hebrew University and Hadassah, Jerusalem, Department of Pathology, Kaplan Hospital, Rehovot, Israel

becomes almost impossible to determine which of these organs harbors the primary neoplasm. For these cases the term "tubo-ovarian carcinoma" has been coined. Microscopic examination does not always resolve the question of the primary site, since tubal and ovarian cancers may be histologically similar.

Uterus

Endometrium

The endometrium is a common source of ovarian metastases, being identifiable as such in about 40% of autopsies and in 5%–10% of surgical specimens. However, since ovarian endometrioid carcinoma with its frequent association of corpus carcinoma emerged as an entity, the problem whether these are both primary concomitant tumors, or whether one is metastatic to the other, if often difficult to resolve. This association was present in 15% of cases of ovarian endometrioid carcinoma in our series [1]. In most instances the endometrial tumor in these patients is focal, with or without minimal invasion, and with adjacent precancerous changes. These patients are doing much better than could be expected for metastatic disease. All this is in favor of two independent neoplasms in these instances.

Cervix

Carcinoma of the cervix only metastasizes to the ovary in less than 1% of cases. It is of interest that two of the three cases of ovarian primary squamous cell carcinoma described by Scully [7] also had cervical squamous cell carcinoma in situ.

Choriocarcinoma

According to data given in the Armed Forces Institute of Pathology (AFIP) fascicle on tumors of the placenta, out of 263 cases of uterine choriocarcinomas, 16 (6%) metastasized to the ovaries [2]. It should be emphasized, however, that not all instances of choriocarcinoma in the ovary are metastatic, since rare pure primary ovarian choriocarcinomas presenting both cyto- and syncytiotrophoblast do exist. The presence of syncytiotrophoblastic cells alone does not justify the diagnosis of choriocarcinoma.

Metastases from the Breast

Metastases to the ovary from carcinom of the breast are common and often bilateral. In patients with known metastatic carcinoma of the breast whose ovaries were removed to decrease estrogen production, there was ovarian involvement without ovarian enlargement in 20%–30% of cases. On the other hand, in patients without extraovarian metastases the frequency of metastatic breast cancer in prophylactically removed ovaries was 2%–11% [3]. Obviously the frequency of ovarian involvement discovered in autopsies on patients dying from carcinoma of the breast is much higher and can reach 40% [5].

Grossly the ovaries may be of normal size or enlarged and nodular. They can also be cystic. On microscopic examination the tumor infiltration may be discreet and can even be missed on low magnification when the cancer deposits are located in the walls of follicles or within a corpus luteum. They can also simulate stromal hyperplasia. Differential diagnosis includes ovarian lymphomas and granulosa cell tumor. In other instances the metastatic foci may be clearly identifiable and sharply demarcated from the normal stroma. In most cases the tumor cells are similar to the primary tumor in the breast. Mucin-filled signet-ring cells of the Krukenberg type can also be encountered.

Metastases from the Stomach

Most gastric carcinomas which metastasize to the ovary appear as typical Krukenberg tumors. However, the Krukenberg tumor, which is characterized by mucin-filled signet-ring tumor cells, is not exclusively derived from the stomach and some metastatic carcinomas from the large intestine and breast may present a similar histology. There also exist rare so-called primary ovarian Krukenberg tumors in patients in whom no other malignancy can be found [4]. At the Massachusetts General Hospital, Krukenberg tumors of gastric origin comprised about 30% of all ovarian metastases [10].

Typically the ovaries appear as enlarged, rounded, firm, lobulated masses. Occasionally cysts may be present. In most cases the tumors are bilateral. On microscopic examination the tumor cells are of the signet-ring type, filled with mucin. They can be individually scattered or arranged in small glandular patterns. Cysts lined by mucinous epithelium have sometimes been described in addition to the characteristic cells scattered around them. A prominent tubular pattern can simulate a Sertoli-Leydig cell tumor. Occasionally sclerosal stromal tumors and clear cell carcinomas may also constitute problems in differential diagnosis.

Metastases from the Intestinal Tract

The most common primary neoplasm of the intestinal tract which metastasizes to the ovary is the colonic adenocarcinoma. As with other ovarian metastases the tumor may be solid, or predominantly cystic simulating primary carcinoma of the ovary. On microscopic examination the tumor is usually similar to the primary cancer of the intestines showing glands and goblet cells. Rarely signet-ring cells may be present.

Differential diagnosis with primary ovarian mucinous carcinoma may be difficult. The presence of benign-appearing areas favors a primary mucinous tumor. When mucus-containing cells are lacking it may also become difficult to rule out a primary endometrioid carcinoma. However the presence of squamous or squamoid elements helps to establish the diagnosis of a primary endometrioid carcinoma.

Tumors which have metastasized from the appendix to the ovary are, of course, much more infrequent than those from the colon, but present special problems. In cases of mucinous carcinomas of the appendix with ovarian involvement and pseudomyxoma peritonei it is often difficult if not impossible to determine whether the tumor in the appendix or that in the ovary constituted the primary neoplasm [12].

Another tumor which is relatively rare, accounting for no more than 2% of metastases to the ovary [8], is the metastatic carcinoid. Although the primary intestinal carcinoid may be small, the ovarian metastases, which are usually solid, may be large. In contrast to primary ovarian carcinoids, the metastatic tumor is almost always bilateral.

Histologically these are insular or trabecular carcinoids. The insular pattern is characteristic of the midgut while the trabecular appearance is of the foregut and hindgut types.

Differential diagnosis includes Brenner tumor, granulosa cell tumor, adenofibroma, and adenocarcinoma. Staining for agentaffin granules and their ultrastructural identification is, of course, helpful. The carcinoid syndrome in patients with metastatic ovarian carcinoid tumor is a frequent occurrence. Most of these patients also had metastatic carcinoid elsewhere.

Luteinization of the Ovarian Stroma in the Presence of Ovarian Metastases

It is a well-known fact that many primary benign and malignant, as well as metastatic, ovarian tumors have a stroma that secretes steroid hormones as a result of the appearance of luteinized cells within it. The endocrine effect may be estrogenic, androgenic, progestogenic or mixed.

The stroma of these neoplasms differentiates into large theca externa, theca interna, or Leydig cells. These cells contain lipid and exhibit oxidative enzymes and alkaline phosphatase activity characteristic of steroid-hormone-producing cells. The term "enzymatically active stromal cells" (EASC) has been coined to describe the latter [9]. Among metastatic ovarian tumors with this type of stroma, the gastrointestinal neoplasms are the most common.

The endocrine manifestations present in some but by no means all the metastatic tumors with functioning stroma, together with the histologic picture of epithelial structures surrounded by luteinized cells, may mislead the pathologist to diagnose a sex cord stromal tumor.

Lymphoma and Leukemia

With very few exceptions, such as the primary ovarian Burkitt's lymphoma, these entities are always secondary to the ovary. The ovaries in these cases are enlarged, forming, smooth, nodular masses. The tissue is characteristically rubbery and white to tan, except for chloromas (granulocytic sarcoma), which are greenish. Here too, as in other ovarian tumors, cysts may be prominent. In most instances there is bilateral involvement.

The difficulties for the pathologist arise because the tumor cells may be grouped as islands or appear in rows simulating carcinoma especially from the breast. Lymphoma can also be confused with dysgerminoma and granulosa cell tumors. Of the different types of lymphomas and leukemias, ovarian involvement is most common in lymphocytic and histiocytic lymphoma, and in acute myelogenous leukemia.

References

1. Czernobilsky B, Silverman BB, Mikuta JJ (1970) Endometrioid carcinoma of the ovary. A clinicopathologic study of 75 cases. Cancer 26:1141–1152
2. Hertig AT, Mansell H (1956) Tumors of the female sex organs, Part 1. Hydatidiform male and choriocarcinoma. Armed Forces Institute of Pathology, Washington, D.C., p 23
3. Johansson H (1960) Clinical aspects of metastatic ovarian cancer of extragenital origin. Acta Obstet Gynecol Scand 39:681–697
4. Joshi VV (1968) Primary Krukenberg tumor of ovary. Review of literature and case report. Cancer 22:1199–1207
5. Luisi A (1968) Metastatic ovarian tumors. In: Gentil F, Junqueira AC (eds) Ovarian cancer. Springer-Verlag, Berlin Heidelberg New York (UICC Monograph Series, vol 11), pp 87–104
6. Scully RE (1978) Atlas of tumor pathology, 2nd ser, fasc 16. Tumors of the ovary and maldeveloped gonads. Armed Forces Institute of Pathology, Washington D.C., pp 38–39
7. Scully RE (1978) Atlas of tumor pathology, 2nd ser, fasc 16. Tumors of the ovary and maldeveloped gonads. Armed Forces Institute of Pathology, Washington D.C., pp 143–144
8. Scully RE (1978) Atlas of tumor pathology, 2nd ser, fasc 16. Tumors of the ovary and maldeveloped gonads. Armed Forces Institute of Pathology, Washington D.C., p 340
9. Scully RE, Cohen RB (1964) Oxidative-enzyme activity in normal and pathologic human ovaries. Obstet Gynecol 24:667–681
10. Scully RE, Richardson GS (1961) Luteinization of the stroma of metastatic cancer involving the ovary and its endocrine significance. Cancer 14:827–840
11. Sedlis A (1961) Primary carcinoma of the fallopian tube. Obstet Gynecol Surv 16:209–226
12. Shanks HGI (1961) Pseudomyxoma peritonei. J Obstet Gynecol Br Commonw 68:212–224

Tumor-like Conditions

B. CZERNOBILSKY [1]

Introduction

Tumor-like conditions can be defined as conditions which macroscopically and/or microscopically may appear as neoplasms but are not truly neoplastic. The World Health Organization (WHO) classification includes such a category [24], which is enlarged upon in this presentation as follows:

1. Solitary follicle cysts and corpus luteum cysts
2. Solitary luteinized follicle cysts of pregnancy and puerperium *
3. Multiple luteinized follicle cysts and/or corpora lutea
4. Pregnancy luteoma
5. Stromal hyperplasia and hyperthecosis
6. Polycystic ovaries
7. Surface-epithelial inclusions and cysts
8. Unusual mesothelial inclusions *
9. Surface papillary structures *
10. Endometriosis
11. Massive edema
12. Simple cysts
13. Inflammatory lesions
14. Hilus cell hyperplasia *
15. Splenic-gonadal fusion *
16. Ovarian pregnancy *
17. Torsion of the normal ovary and tube *
18. Parovarian inclusions and cysts
19. Hyperplasia of tubal epithelium *
20. Two further types of epithelial inclusions *
    a) In the pelvic lymph nodes
    b) In the peritoneum

1. Solitary Follicle Cysts and Corpus Luteum Cysts

In various textbooks the sizes of normal follicles or corpura lutea vary. I adhere to the definition given in Anderson's textbook of pathology [15], in which 3 cm is the

---

* Not discussed in the "Tumour-like Conditions" of the WHO International Histological Classification of Tumours.

1 Medical School of the Hebrew University and Hadassah, Jerusalem, Department of Pathology, Kaplan Hospital, Rehovot, Israel

limit of normal. These cysts, which are not always truly solitary, rarely exceed 8 cm in diameter. Many of the follicle cysts are actually atretic follicles which have become cystic. Histologically, follicle cysts do not differ from the smaller follicles, but because of the intraluminal pressure their granulosa layer may become thinned or completely obliterated. Thus, a good number of the so-called simple cysts are probably follicle cysts in which the lining can no longer be identified. Bleeding into the cavity of these cysts can occur, and in these cases, especially when the lining is no longer identifiable, it may become difficult to rule out endometriosis. The importance of these innocuous cysts is that they can lead to unnecessary surgical exploration. Occasionally they may also be subject to torsion. Follicle cysts can be a source of excessive estrogen secretion and sexual precocity in children [25]. A corpus luteum cyst may occasionally cause menstrual irregularities [19], or rupture. The luteinic character of the corpus luteum cyst is not always obvious. Some of these are actually corpus albicans cysts. In most instances solitary follicle cysts and corpus luteum cysts regress spontaneously.

2. Solitary Luteinized Follicle Cysts of Pregnancy and Puerperium

Clement and Scully [3] have recently described solitary follicle cysts of 8–26 cm in diameter with marked nuclear atypicality of the luteinized granulosa cell layer during pregnancy or 6–7 weeks postpartum. These patients had no endocrine changes. The cysts are most likely luteinized follicle cysts related to high gonadotropin levels of pregnancy.

3. Multiple Luteinized Follicle Cysts and/or Corpora Lutea

In this condition the ovaries can become very large, exceeding 20 cm in diameter with numerous cysts, undergoing hemorrhage, infarction, and rupture with ascites and hydrothorax, and thus obviously simulate neoplasms. This type of ovarian enlargement is often due to the presence of hydatidiform mole or choriocarcinoma [6]. However, this condition can also occur in cases of erythroblastosis fetalis, twin pregnancies, and occasionally even in a normal single pregnancy. In general the basis for hyperreactio luteinalis, which is another term for this condition, is an increase in chorionic gonadotropin titers. Lately this ovarian picture has also been described in patients who have received clomiphene or gonadotropin to stimulate ovulation, especially when the underlying disorder was the Stein-Leventhal syndrome [20]. Histologically there is prominent luteinization of theca and sometimes granulosa cells. These cysts retrogress and eventually disappear after removal of the primary cause.

4. Pregnancy Luteoma

Luteomas occurring in pregnancy are nodular, solid, or hemorrhagic large masses within the ovary, are orange-brown, and may be single or multiple, unilateral or bilateral. Histologically they are composed of large, luteinized stromal cells intermediate in size between luteinized granulosa and theca cells. Mitoses may be numerous and even atypical. The cells are lipid poor or lipid free. There may be focal ballooning degeneration and hyaline necrosis. Nucleoli are prominent. The reticulum stain surrounds groups of cells rather than individual cells. These lesions are usually discovered during caesarian section in multiparous women, particularly black women [10]. Occasionally they may be virilizing [17], but they always regress when pregnancy terminates since they are dependent on chorionic gonadotropin stimulation. For unknown reasons pregnancy luteomas do not usually occur with choriocarcinoma, in which HCG levels are high. In contrast to the solid pregnancy luteoma, the corpus luteum of pregnancy has a festooned margin and contains both granulosa and theca lutein cells, colloid droplets, and small calcifications. Histologically it may be impossible to differentiate pregnancy luteoma from lipid cell tumors, but the association of pregnancy, the multiplicity of the pregnancy luteomas, the absence of lipid within the cells, and the abundance of mitoses are helpful differentiating features. Luteinized thecomas have more spindle cells than pregnancy luteomas.

5. Stromal Hyperplasia and Hyperthecosis

In stromal hyperplasia there is bilateral enlargement of the ovaries, often in a nodular fashion. The hyperplasia of the stroma is primarily medullary but may also involve the cortex. The presence of single or clusters of lutein cells within this hyperplastic stroma warrants the diagnosis of hyperthecosis, which has also been called thecosis, thecomatosis, and diffuse luteinization of the ovarian stroma. The luteinized stromal cells usually contain lipids and oxidative enzymes. This entity is more common in perimenopausal women but may also be seen at a younger age, when it is often accompanied by follicle cysts with luteinization of the theca. Thus, in these patients it becomes difficult to separate hyperthecosis from the syndrome of polycystic ovaries [11]. It is not too difficult to differentiate stromal hyperplasia and hyperthecosis from thecoma and other stromal neoplasms since the former are bilateral while the tumors are almost always unilateral.

The clinical picture can be that of the classic Stein-Leventhal syndrome, namely infrequent anovulatory bleeding, sterility, and obesity, but can also show virilism, hypertension, and a disturbance of glucose metabolism resembling Cushing's syndrome. As is the case with polycystic ovaries, stromal hyperplasia can also cause endometrial hyperplasia or carcinoma, and the question of an estrogen-secreting tumor has to be ruled out in these cases.

In patients with virilism hyperthecosis is usually present, and then the condition has to be differentiated from androgen-secreting ovarian tumors. Wedge resection is generally not effective in the treatment of hyperthecosis with severe endocrine disturbances.

6. Polycystic Ovaries

As mentioned above, it is often almost impossible to separate stromal hyperplasia with polycystic changes from polycystic ovaries with stromal hyperplasia. The ovaries are enlarged, pale, and grossly cystic. On microscopic examination the outermost portion of the cortex (and not the capsule) is thickened and collagenized. The follicle cysts show proliferation and luteinization of the theca interna and there is usually a variable amount of medullary stromal hyperplasia, sometimes with some hyperthecosis.

The syndrome begins in the early reproductive years and occasionally follows a pregnancy or the withdrawal of oral contraceptive therapy [1]. There is infrequent anovulatory bleeding and sterility with hirsutism, and rarely virilism. Wedge resection of the ovaries and ovulation-inducing drugs can reverse this condition. Endometrial hyperplasia or low-grade endometrial adenocarcinoma is not unusual in these patients.

7. Surface-Epithelial Inclusions and Cysts

These are extremely common structures. The importance of these inclusions, which may become cystic, is their metaplastic and neoplastic potential. As a matter of fact, the epithelial lining of these structures is rarely that of the surface epithelium but usually shows a spectrum of müllerian type epithelia which can all be found in the various "common epithelial tumors" of the ovary. Sometimes one can also see psammoma bodies or larger calcifications within the structures, as well as hyperplastic or papillary areas, which makes them appear as microscopic versions of some of the common epithelial tumors. As a matter of fact sometimes the only difference between such structures and true tumors is their size. The origin of these inclusions in the surface epithelium has been proven by their occasional continuity with this epithelium. The previously used term "germinal inclusion cysts" is of course a misnomer, since the germ cells do not derive from the surface epithelium.

8. Unusual Mesothelial Inclusions

These inclusions, which we described [14] in 6 out of 57 patients with endometriosis, are of the same origin as the previously described surface epithelium inclusions but of different histologic appearance. Unusual inclusions do not show the various types of metaplastic epithelia which are so characteristic of the ordinary inclusions. The epithelium of these unusual inclusions is actually similar to the surface epithelium. While the ordinary inclusions are not crowded together and are often cystically dilated with much stroma between them, the unusual inclusions are small, irregular, often crowded, noncystic, and can create a pseudoinvasive pattern, and thus may actually simulate malignancy. Similar inclusions have been reported in other sites, such as hernial sacs, pleura, and hydrocele, in association with chronic inflammation and fibrosis, as well as in ovaries in which they were present within inflammatory areas or in close association with fibrosis. In our cases there were no inflammatory changes and no fibrosis, but in all the patients there was ovarian or pelvic endometriosis, which was always situated in areas other than the inclusions. We favored the theory that a common stimulus is responsible for the development of both the endometriosis and the unusual inclusions from the pelvic mesothelium. The nature of this stimulus is unknown but the known hormonal relationship to endometriosis, and the experimental work of McClure and Graham [9, 16], who produced a spectrum of mesothelial lesions on the uterine serosa of squirrel monkeys following prolonged diethylstilbestrol administration, points to the possibility of a hormonal histogenetic mechanism in these patients.

9. Surface Papillary Structures

Other structures which originate in the surface epithelium of the ovary are small papillary excrescences. These are extremely common, especially in older women, and should not be confused with papillary neoplasms. They have a fibrous core and are lined by cuboidal serous type cells, thus resembling small papillary cystadenofibromas. It is for this reason that we somewhat arbitrarily made 1 cm the dividing line between tumor-like and true neoplastic papillary surface lesions [5].

10. Endometriosis

Endometriosis is listed in the WHO classification [24] both as one of the common epithelial tumors and as a tumor-like condition. In our opinion the distinction between these two types of endometriosis is not always possible. In this presentation, however, I shall adhere to the WHO classification and to the opinions expressed in the Armed Forces Institute of Pathology (AFIP) fascicle on ovarian tumors [21]. According to these views, true benign endometrioid neoplasms include polyploid adenoma, adenofibroma, and adenoacanthofibroma – all of course with glands of endometrioid type. All other forms of endometriosis are tumor-like conditions. Thus, non-neoplastic endometriosis may range from microscopic to large so-called chocolate cysts. Most investigators believe that in the ovary the multipotential surface epithelium and the inclusion cysts which derive from it may give rise to endometriosis by a metaplastic process. Although it is obvious that in order to make an unequivocal diagnosis of endometriosis both endometrial type glands and endometrial type stroma should be present, this is not always the case. In the absence of these elements, which can be destroyed by repeated bleeding, a presumptive diagnosis of endometriosis can often be made in a cyst in which the stroma contains the so-called pseudoxanthoma cells with hemosiderin and abundant scarring with collagen and spindle-shaped fibroblasts.

In a study of 194 cases of ovarian endometriosis we found severe epithelial atypism, characterized by nuclear pleomorphism, eosinophilic cytoplasm, occasional squamoid features, tufting, and stratification, in 7 (3.6%) cases [4]. When one carefully examines the epithelium in endometriosis adjacent to endometrioid carcinoma, one occasionally finds similar atypical changes. It is still to be determined whether this atypism is of reactive nature only, or may occasionally signify a premalignant change.

11. Massive Edema

Since massive edema was first described in 1969 [12], a total of about 16 cases have been reported. The lesion is clinically characterized by the onset of sudden abdominal pain or the appearance of a mass in young women. In most cases only the right ovary was involved. Grossly the ovary is markedly enlarged, but the outer cortex is not involved in the process. The rest of the parenchyma is extremely edematous and swollen.

On microscopic examination there is diffuse interstitial edema of the stroma with dilation of vascular channels but preservation of the follicles. Follicles are not seen within fibromas or thecomas, with which this lesion can sometimes be confused. Clusters of luteinized stromal cells in massive stromal edema may possibly be related to the occasional virilization which has been reported. An impairment of the venous and lymphatic drainage of the ovary due to torsion of the mesovarium has been implicated. Another theory is that the basic process is stromal hyperplasia or hyperthecosis, and that the edema is a secondary phenomenon due to torsion of an already enlarged organ [2]. The recognition of this entity is extremely important in order to avoid unnecessary radical operation for a completely benign condition.

12. Simple Cysts

Simple cysts are cysts without identifiable lining cells and may be either tumor-like conditions such as follicle cysts or endometriosis, or neoplastic cysts usually belonging to the common epithelial tumors, which cannot be diagnosed because of the lack of lining elements. Rarely a cystic granulosa cell tumor may present at least in part as a simple cyst. Sometimes cystic teratomas are converted into simple cysts but multiple sections may reveal in the wall large vacuoles of fatty material surrounded by foreign body giant cells, which are the clue to the true origin of such a cyst. In general, whenever a so-called simple cyst is present within the ovary, numerous sections should be made in an attempt to reach a more specific diagnosis.

13. Inflammatory Lesions

Inflammatory lesions of the ovary can cause enlargement and distortions which simulate neoplasms. Most ovarian inflammations are secondary to inflammatory diseases of the fallopian tubes. Sometimes inflammation spreads to the ovary from the adjacent bowel, as in colonic diverticulitis or acute appendicitis. Severe pelvic inflammatory disease can result in acute oophoritis characterized by large, edematous, hyperemic ovaries or abscesses binding together the ovary and fallopian tube. The resulting granulation tissue may be rich in foamy histiocytes which may be mistaken for luteinized cells. Fibrosis and adhesions resulting from oophoritis may stimulate serosal proliferation and cause inclusions of the surface epithelium.

14. Hilus Cell Hyperplasia

This as well as the next three items are not listed in the WHO classification of tumor-like conditions, but appear in the new fascicle of ovarian tumors by Scully [22]. This hyperplasia may appear during pregnancy, but a form of hyperplasia with bizarre shapes of cells and nuclei in postmenopausal women can be particularly worrisome and should not be confused with foci of metastatic carcinoma.

15. Splenic-Gonadal Fusion

This is a rare condition in which a mass of splenic tissue is adherent to the ovary as a result of fusion of the anlage of both organs during intrauterine development.

16. Ovarian Pregnancy

In the past this was a very rare condition, but has become more frequent since the introduction of the intrauterine device [8]. Since ectopic pregnancy in the fallopian tube is much more common, a diagnosis of ovarian pregnancy should only be made if the fallopian tube is intact and clearly separated from the ovary, and if the gestational sac is definitely situated within the ovary.

17. Torsion of the Normal Ovary and Tube

This can produce a palpable mass and thus simulate a tumor. It is particularly apt to occur in children. Autoamputation of the mass can result in calcification.

18. Parovarian Inclusions and Cysts

The common microscopic tubules which one finds in the parovarian region arise from the remnants of the wolffian duct. These are lined by a single layer of cuboidal epithelium surrounded by well-demarcated muscular tissue in which one can sometimes distinguish an inner circular and an outer longitudinal layer.

These wolffian remnants can enlarge and become cystic. The inner lining of the cysts is similar to that of the microscopic inclusions. Sometimes papillary projections may be present. The muscular layer, which is very prominent in the microscopic tubules, disappears in most instances from the wall of these cysts, probably as a result of the intraluminal pressure. Actually the absence of muscle, the presence of papillary infoldings and the proximity of the cysts to the ovary frequently make it difficult to distinguish these tumor-like parovarian cysts from true cystic neoplasms of the ovary. They may also undergo torsion with hemorrhagic infarction.

19. Hyperplasia of Tubal Epithelium

This has classically been described in cases of tuberculosis of the fallopian tubes [18], but can also occur in nonspecific salpingitis. In such cases the epithelial structure of the tube becomes extremely complex and crowded, but absence of invasion and lack of epithelial atypia distinguish this from neoplastic disease.

20. Two Further Types of Epithelial Inclusion

a) Epithelial Inclusions in Pelvic Lymph Nodes

Similar in structure to the surface epithelial inclusion cysts of the ovary, epithelial inclusions in the pelvic lymph nodes in females are quite common. In our series we found them in 14% of routine autopsies [13]. Their origin is in the surface mesothelium and they should not be confused with endometriosis or with metastatic disease.

b) Epithelial Inclusions and Papillary Structures in the Peritoneum

These too are of the same origin as the ovarian and pelvic lymph node inclusions described above. Occasionally they can also show psammoma bodies. When found in the presence of ovarian epithelial neoplasms, they can easily be confused with metastatic disease. A careful histologic study will, however, show that these foci have no malignant characteristics [7, 23].

References

1. Beaconsfield P, Dick R, Ginsburg J, Lewis P (1974) Amenorrhea and infertility after the use of oral contraceptives. Surg Gynecol Obstet 138:571–575
2. Case records of the Massachusetts General Hospital (1971) Case 24–1971. Ovarian hyperthecosis with massive edema. N Engl J Med 284:1369–1375
3. Clement PB, Scully RE (1980) Large solitary luteinized follicle cyst of pregnancy and puerperium. A clinico-pathological analysis of 8 cases. Am J Surg Pathol 4:431–438
4. Czernobilsky B, Morris WJ (1979) A histologic study of ovarian endometriosis with emphasis on hyperplastic and atypical changes. Obstet Gynecol 53:318–323
5. Czernobilsky B, Borenstein R, Lancet M (1974) Cystadenofibroma of the ovary. A clinicopathologic study of 34 cases and comparison with serous cystadenoma. Cancer 34:1971–1981
6. Girouard DP, Barclay DL, Collins CG (1964) Hyperreactio Luteinalis. Review of the literature and report of 2 cases. Obstet Gynecol 23:513–525
7. Goepel JR (1981) Benign papillary mesothelioma of peritoneum: A histological, histochemical and ultrastructural study of six cases. Histopathology 5:21–30
8. Graff G, Lancet M, Czernobilsky B (1972) Ovarian pregnancy with intrauterine device in situ. Obstet Gynecol 40:535–538
9. Graham CE, McClure HM, Collins DC (1980) Uterine tumors in nonhuman primates after estrogen exposure. In: Dallenbach-Hellweg G (ed) Functional morphologic changes in female sex organs induced by exogenous hormones. Springer, Berlin Heidelberg New York, pp 29–38

10. Greene RR, Holzwarth D, Roddick JW (1964) "Luteomas" of pregnancy. Am J Obstet Gynecol 88:1001–1011
11. Judd HL, Scully RE, Herbst AL, Yen SSC, Ingersol FM, Kliman B (1973) Familial hyperthecosis. Comparison of endocrinologic and histologic findings with polycystic ovarian disease. Am J Obstet Gynecol 117:976–982
12. Kalstone CE, Jaffe RB, Abell MR (1969) Massive edema of the ovary simulating fibroma. Obstet Gynecol 34:564–571
13. Karp LA, Czernobilsky B (1969) Glandular inclusions in pelvic and abdominal para-aortic lymph nodes. A study of autopsy and surgical material in males and females. Am J Clin Pathol 52:212–218
14. Kerner H, Gaton E, Czernobilsky B (1981) Unusual ovarian, tubal and pelvic mesothelial inclusions in patients with endometriosis. Histopathology 5:277–283
15. Kraus FT (1977) Female genitalia. In: Anderson WAD, Kissane JM (eds) Pathology, 7th edn. Mosby, St. Louis, p 1731
16. McClure HM, Graham CE (1973) Malignant uterine mesotheliomas in squirrel monkeys following diethylstilbestrol administration. Lab Anim Sci 23:493–498
17. Norris HJ, Taylor JB (1967) Nodular theca lutein hyperplasia of pregnancy (so-called "pregnancy luteoma"). A clinical and pathologic study of 15 cases. Am J Clin Pathol 47:557–566
18. Pauerstein CJ, Woodruff JD (1966) Cellular patterns in proliferative and anaplastic disease of the fallopian tube. Am J Obstet Gynecol 96:486–492
19. Piver MS, Williams LJ, Marcuse PM (1970) Influence of luteal cysts on menstrual function. Obstet Gynecol 35:740–751
20. Schenker JG, Polishuk WZ (1975) Ovarian hyperstimulation syndrome. Obstet Gynecol 46:23–28
21. Scully RE (1979) Tumors of the ovary and maldeveloped gonads. Atlas of tumor pathology, 2nd ser, fasc 16. The Armed Forces Institute of Pathology, Washington D.C., pp 92–110
22. Scully RE (1979) Tumors of the ovary and maldeveloped gonads. Atlas of tumor, pathology, 2nd ser, fasc 16. The Armed Forces Institute of Pathology, Washington D.C., pp 387–388
23. Scully RE (1979) Tumors of the ovary and maldeveloped gonads. Atlas of tumor pathology, 2nd ser, fasc 16. The Armed Forces Institute of Pathology, Washington D.C., pp 392–393
24. Serov SF, Scully RE, Sobin LH (1973) International histological classification of tumours, No 9: Histological typing of ovarian tumors. WHO, Geneva, pp 17–21
25. Steiner MM, Hadawi SA (1964) Sexual precocity. Association with follicular cysts of ovary. Ann J Dis Child 102:28–36

Ovarian Tumors of Childhood

H.-E. STEGNER[1]

Introduction

Ovarian tumors comprise about 1% of all tumors in children under 15 years old. The relative frequencies of childhood solid tumor types are shown in Table 1. Since Wilms' tumor appears to occur with constant frequency throughout the world, a number of investigators have suggested using it as an index to show the relative frequencies of other tumors. In the series of Young et al. (1978) there are for each case of Wilms' tumor 3.2 cases of brain tumors, and about 0.4 cases of gonadal tumors.

Table 1. Relative frequency of solid tumors in childhood. (Young et al. 1978)

Tumor type	% of all tumors	Frequency relative to Wilms tumor
Central nervous system	33.1	3.22
Neuroblastoma	14.2	1.37
Wilms' tumor	10.3	1.00
Other soft tissue tumors	5.7	0.55
Rhabdomyosarcoma	5.5	0.54
Osteosarcoma	4.6	0.45
Retinoblastoma	4.5	0.43
Gonadal/germ cell	3.7	0.36
Ewing's sarcoma	3.2	0.31
Liver	2.4	0.23
Miscellaneous	13.1	1.28

Among the patients of the Department of Gynecology and Obstetrics at the University of Hamburg, 35 cases in children and women under 21 were found among 712 ovarian blastomas from 1971 to 1979 (Fig. 1). Eight of these were malignant. The ratio of malignant to benign tumors is accordingly 1 : 4.

1 Universitäts-Frauenklinik, Martinistr. 52, D-2000 Hamburg 20

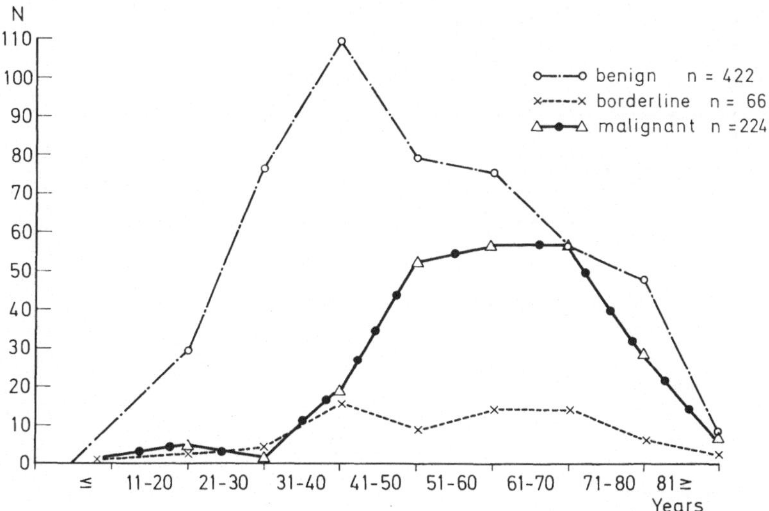

Fig. 1. Age distribution of 712 ovarian tumors. Department of Gynecology and Obstetrics, University of Hamburg 1971–1979. The line of *black circles* indicates benign ($n=422$); the line of *crosses*, borderline ($n=66$); and the line of *diamonds*, malignant tumors ($n=224$)

Histologic Types

The histologic classification of ovarian tumors in childhood shows a broad spectrum of types. In the series of Groeber (1963) and that of the Armed Forces Institute of Pathology (Norris and Jensen 1972), germ cell tumors predominate (Fig. 2). They make up roughly 50% of all ovarian tumors and are to be regarded as age-specific malignancies (Cangir et al. 1978). The dysgerminoma is the classic representative, 80% occurring before the 30th year of life and 5% before the 10th year of life. On the other hand, the seminoma (the homologous testicular tumor) is manifested very much later. Thus the age peak for the occurrence of the classic seminoma is the 40th year of life, and that of the polymorphic spermatocytic seminoma actually the 50th year of life (Hedinger 1980).

This observation permits interesting conclusions with regard to the etiology of these tumors. The cell of origin is for both tumors the germ cell. It is a prerequisite for tumor development that the stimulus for neoplastic transformation falls upon a cell compartment which is able to divide. The mitotic proliferation of the oocytes is already completed in the sixth fetal month, however. Afterwards the oocytes are in an arrested (resting) stage of meiotic prophase which is only resumed after ovulation. In contrast the germ cells of the testis regenerate mitotically over the entire period of male sexual maturity. They thus remain susceptible to carcinogenic noxae up to the end of life.

The diversity of childhood germ cell tumors is shown by Fig. 3. The pluripotency of germ cells is such that they can give rise to all conceivable somatic differentiation products. Phenotypically, then, they are capable of the diversity of all organizational elements of the body, including monstrous aberrations. Nevertheless, the diversity

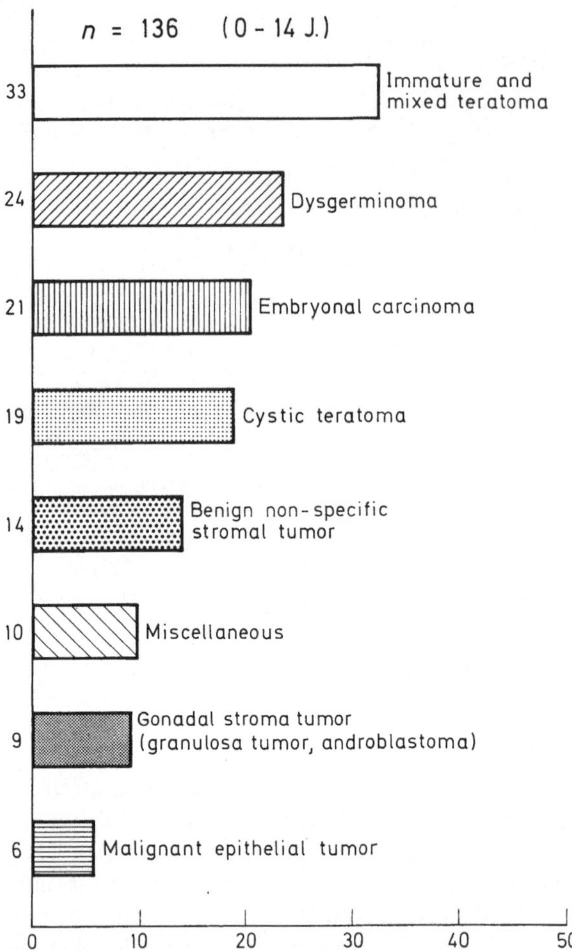

Fig. 2. Ovarian tumors in children up to 14 years old. Distribution of histologic types ($n = 136$). (Norris and Jensen 1972)

of manifestations can be reduced in practical diagnostics to a few clearly defined types, although overlapping due to combination forms is very frequent.

Clinical Significance of the Type Diagnosis

A differentiated histologic diagnosis in childhood cancers is of primary clinical importance, since there are extreme differences in the biologic behavior of the tumors and their sensitivity to radiologic or cytostatic therapy. Thus sarcomas and neuroblastomas in general show a good response to radiation therapy. The dysgerminoma in its pure form is one of the most radiosensitive tumors. Complete tumor sterilization can be achieved by a dosage which does not necessarily destroy the func-

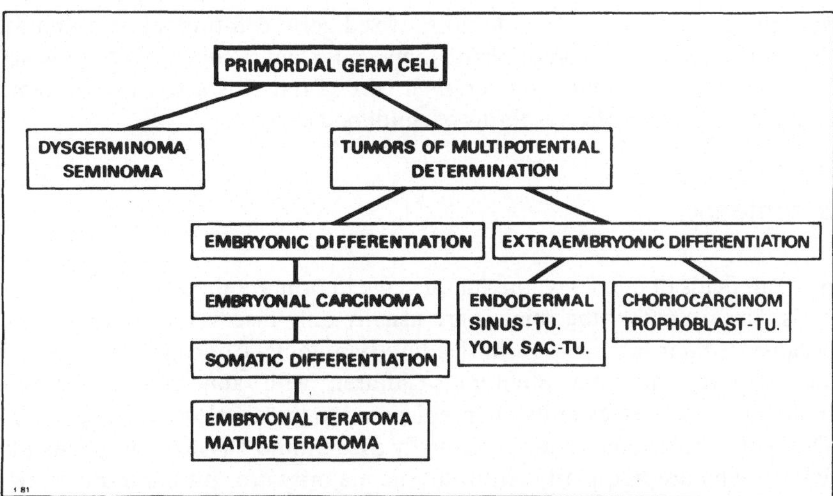

Fig. 3. Classification of germ cell tumors. [Adapted from Teilum G (1976) Special tumors of ovary and testis. Lippincott, Philadelphia Toronto]

Table 2. Recommendation for adequate treatment for various forms of childhood cancer

Tumor	Treatment
Granulosa stromal cell tumor Sertoli-Leydig cell tumor Mature teratoma	Unilateral adnexectomy
Dysgerminoma Sarcoma Neuroblastoma	Postoperative irradiation
Embryonal and extra-embryonal carcinoma Immature teratoma Adenocarcinoma	Additive polychemotherapy

tional structures of the normal gonads. I have seen patients who experienced more than one pregnancy following postoperative pelvic irradiation for dysgerminoma, and who gave birth to healthy offspring.

The experience reported in various papers demonstrates, however, that except in the case of dysgerminomas irradiation is not indicated in most ovarian germ cell tumors. In the case of a 12-year-old girl who was admitted because of abdominal pain extending into the right leg, laparotomy revealed a right ovarian tumor 20 cm in diameter. Microscopic diagnosis was endodermal sinus tumor. Irradiation was ineffective. The patient died 6 months later with widespread bone and lymph node metastases.

In various germ cell tumors of poor prognosis, however, substantial advances have been achieved during the last 10 years by polychemotherapy. Administration of certain chemotherapeutic agents has significantly improved the survival rates, especially in endodermal sinus tumors, mixed germ cell tumors, and immature teratomas (Cangir 1978). In choriocarcinoma consistent treatment with folic acid antagonists enables long remissions or even cure. Table 2 is a tentative schema for adequate treatment of various forms of childhood cancers.

Symptoms

As in all fields of oncology, the tumor stage in primary therapy determines the prognosis. Unfortunately the tumors are usually only discovered in an advanced stage because of their late or even misleading symptoms. Concomitant symptoms therefore require particular attention. Children with abnormal chromosome constellations and intersexuality are predisposed to the development of gonadal tumors. Thus gonadoblastomas and occasionally dysgerminomas occur in young phenotypic females who are frequently virilized. The majority are chromatin-negative and possess a Y chromosome (Scully 1970; Talerman 1980). Disturbances of sexual maturation may be a secondary manifestation of an ovarian tumor. Symptoms of a pubertas praecox are found in about 20% of malignant ovarian tumors (Moore et al. 1967). Primary amenorrhea or virilism may be the leading symptom of an ovarian tumor, especially in the case of androgen-secreting gonadal stromal tumors.

In the undifferentiated and sarcomatous forms of androblastoma the histologic diagnosis may be difficult. The basic structure of these tumors is formed by a highly cellular blastema consisting of irregularly arranged elongated or roundish tumor cells. A hint of fascicular, trabecular or even a rosette-like arrangement can be discerned. The blastema is rich in capillaries or even cavernous spaces (Fig. 4). The

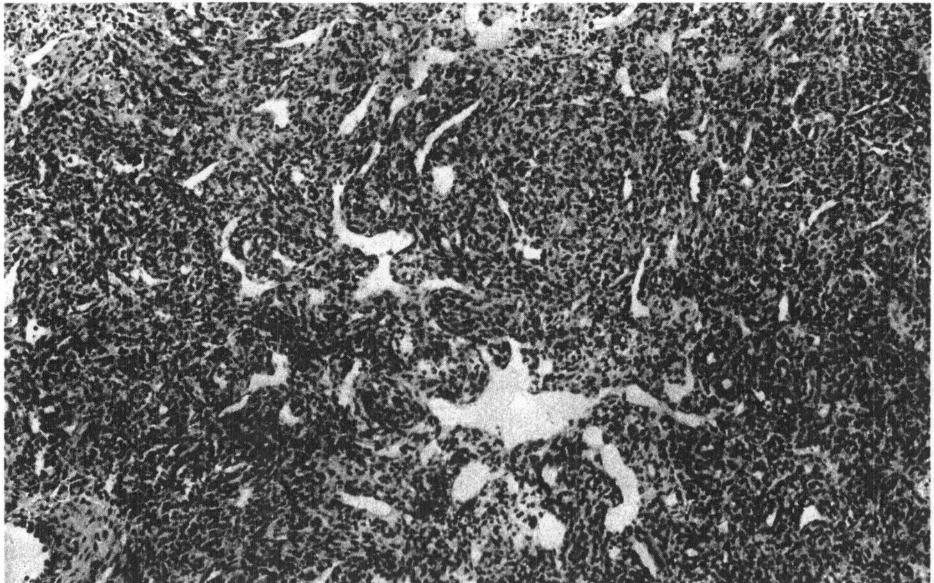

Fig. 4. Sarcomatous type of androblastoma

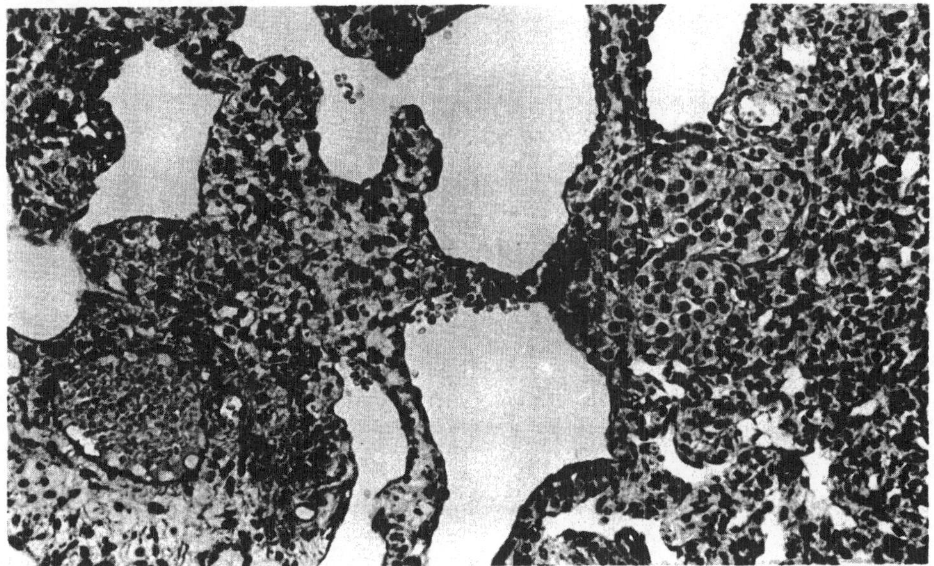

Fig. 5. Sarcomatous type of androblastoma. Clusters of Leydig cell elements adjacent to cavernous spaces

demonstration of Leydig cells is decisive for the diagnosis: these are chiefly to be found in the periphery of the blastema or in the interstitium near to the capillaries (Fig. 5).

We observed four cases of sarcomatoid androblastoma which could be followed for up to 7 years (Table 3). These tumors are in general semimalignant. Prognosis is not always favorable, however. In case 4496/77, peritoneal metastasis was manifested 6 months after the operation and resulted in death within 2 years. This case differed histologically from the three further cases listed in the table in its intense nuclear pleomorphism and higher mitotic activity (Fig. 6a, b). In our experience a prognostically relevant prediction of malignancy seems possible within the same tumor type by nuclear grading.

The examples described make it evident that in ovarian tumors of childhood and adolescence a prominent endocrinopathy frequently masks the underlying neoplastic condition. Abdominal symptoms directly deriving from the tumor often show a rapid development over a few weeks or even hours, namely when an acute complication such as torsion or tumor perforation necessitates immediate laparotomy and then confronts the surgeon with an unexpected situation. The gross morphology does not permit any reliable distinction between benign and malignant tumors. The frozen section does not enable any definitive clarification. This applies especially to mixed germ cell tumors and immature (embryonic) teratomas. The nature and proportion of undifferentiated components determine the prognosis. The biopsy taken for the frozen section is not representative for the often complex structure of the overall tumor. Not every cystic teratoma is fundamentally benign and nor do peritoneal metastases render the case hopeless from the beginning. Thus in mature teratomas, peritoneal inoculation metastases (glial implants) may be found which can

Table 3. Casuistics of four sarcomatous androblastomas observed at the Department of Gynecology and Obstetrics, University of Hamburg 1974 – 1981

Name	Code	Age	Diagnosis	Symptoms	Therapy	Follow-up
S. A.	4496/77	16	Sarcomatous androblastoma	Primary amenorrhea Virilism Hypertrophy of clitoris Testosterone: > 2000 pg/ml	Unilateral Adnexectomy	Recurrence 1977 Radiation therapy Exitus 1978
T. J.	2487/74	16	Sarcomatous androblastoma	Primary amenorrhea Virilism Hypertrophy of clitoris	Unilateral adnexectomy	Alive No recurrence
R. H.	73/81	18	Sarcomatous androblastoma	Secondary amenorrhea Hirsutism Testosterone: 185 pg/ml	Unilateral adnexectomy	Alive No recurrence
C. A.	5722/79	17	Sarcomatous androblastoma	Menometrorrhagia Virilism Hypertrophy of clitoris	Unilateral adnexectomy postop. radiation therapy	Alive No recurrence

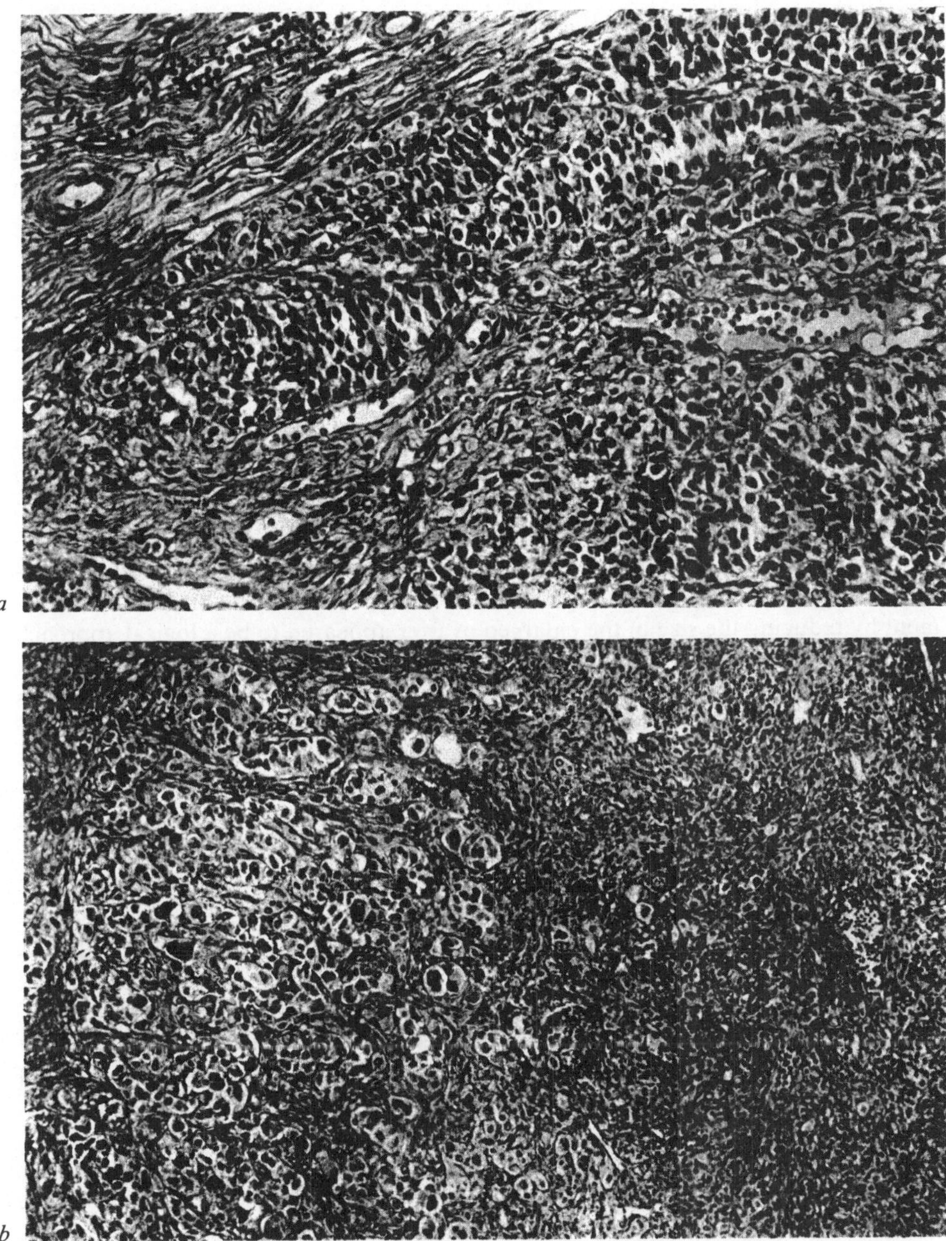

Fig. 6a, b. Ovarian androblastoma in a 16-year-old girl. *a* typical trabecular arrangement of the neoplastic cells; *b* areas of marked cellular pleomorphy

regress spontaneously after removal of the primary tumor (Robboy and Scully 1970).

There is another potential source of error in treating ovarian tumors in children: the so-called tumor-like conditions which may easily render an indication for unnecessary radical treatment. Follicle cysts and polycystic ovaries have been encountered not only in adolescents, but even in infants and prepuberal children, in whom they may produce sexual precocity. Although they rarely exceed 8 cm in diameter they are not seldom considered neoplastic, and the ovaries completely removed.

In a 6-year-old girl with sexual precocity pelvic examinatio revealed cystic enlargement of both ovaries. Estrogen excretion was ranging from 3 to 6 μg/day. Prolactin and plasma gonadotrophines were not increased, showing low infantile profiles. LH-RH stimulation test was negative.

At operation both ovaries were found to be enlarged to 8 cm in diameter with numerous small follicles visible just below the surface. Microscopic examination of frozen sections revealed typical basic structures of ovarian cortex with numerous primordial germ cells and cystic follicles. There was no thecal stimulation or luteinization as frequently found in gonadotrophic hyperstimulation. Corpora lutea, corpora albicantia, and interstitial cells could not be demonstrated. Conservative treatment by reducing the size of the enlarged ovaries appeared to be a logical approach to therapy.

The pathogenesis of those simple or multiple follicle cysts in infantile ovaries without demonstrable gonadotrophic stimulation remains to be clarified.

Therapy

In summary the following conclusions may be drawn. The ovarian tumors of childhood are almost paradigmatic for individual tumor therapy based on a subtile histopathologic diagnosis. There are few areas of cancer therapy which can present such substantial advances as pediatric oncology. The nephroblastoma (Wilms' tumor) is an example of this. In the 1930s survival rates of 8%–10% were achieved by surgical treatment. The combination of surgery and irradiation which predominated in the 1950s gave rise to an improvement of 17%–47%. With the application of highly effective polychemotherapy, survival rates of 45%–90% are attained today (Landbeck 1978; Exelby 1980). Similarly good results are to be recorded in cases of juvenile rhabdomyosarcoma, osteosarcoma, and in the highly malignant teratoid and extraembryonic germ cell tumors. These are all tumors in which the prognosis was to be regarded as poor even a few years ago. The results are due to effective combinations of chemotherapeutic agents. The child's body has an enormous capacity for regeneration, so that oncocidal chemotherapeutics can be applied in a higher dosage and with a lower risk of severe complications than in adults. The choice of adequate therapy requires close cooperation between clinical oncologists and pathologists.

Malignancies in childhood are rare but tragic events. There is no reason for defeatism, however. Most of the young patients are primarily managed by general surgeons in association with a preoperative diagnosis of acute appendicitis or other acute abdominal condition. At laparotomy the surgeon is confronted with an unexpected situation. In all questionable cases it seems preferable to carry out a conservative resection and then refer the patient to a specialized treatment center which alone can guarantee optimal therapy.

Literature

1. Cangir A, Smith J, Eys J van (1978) Improved prognosis in children with ovarian cancers following modified VAC (Vincristine sulfate, Actinomycin, and Cyclophosphamide) Chemotherapy. Cancer 42:1234–1238
2. Exelby PR (1980) Improved curability and changing concepts in pediatric cancer surgery. In: Status of the curability of childhood cancers. Raven, New York
3. Gröber WR (1963) Ovarian tumors during infancy and childhood. Am J Obstet Gynecol 86:1027–1035
4. Hedinger C (1980) Pathologie der Hodentumoren. Pathologe 1:179–187
5. Landbeck G (1978) Tumoren im Kindesalter. Verh Dtsch Krebs Ges 1:265–273
6. Moore JG, Schifrin BS, Erez S (1967) Ovarian tumors in infancy, childhood, and adolescence. Am J Obstet Gynecol 99:913–922
7. Norris HJ, Jensen RD (1972) Relative frequency of ovarian neoplasms in children and adolescents. Cancer 30:713–719
8. Robboy SJ, Scully RE (1970) Ovarian teratoma with glial implants on the peritoneum. Hum Pathol 1:643–653
9. Scully RE (1970) Gonadoblastoma. A review of 74 cases. Cancer 25:340–356
10. Talermann A (1980) The pathology of gonadal neoplasms composed of germ cells and sex cord stroma derivatives. Pathol Res Pract 170:24–38
11. Van Eys J, Sullivan MP (1980) In: Status of the curability of childhood cancers. Raven, New York
12. Young JL Jr, Heise HW, Silverberg E, Myers MH (1978) Cancer incidence, survival and mortality for children under 15 years of age. American Cancer Society, New York

Die Ovarialtumoren im Eingangsmaterial eines Pathologischen Institutes 1966–1976

G. Zieger und W. Hirsch[1]

Kein anderes Organ zeigt eine derartige Vielfalt an benignen und malignen Neubildungen wie das Ovar. Die Klassifikation der Ovarialtumoren hat daher schon immer Schwierigkeiten bereitet. Die derzeitige allgemein gebräuchliche Einteilung ist die der WHO, die auch von uns verwendet wurde.

Unter 200 000 Eingängen der Jahre 1966–1976 fanden sich an unserem Institut 640 Ovarialgeschwülste (Abb. 1). Sie wurden nachmikroskopiert und reklassifiziert sowie die Krankheitsverläufe bei malignen und semimalignen Tumoren mit Hilfe der behandelnden Fach- oder Hausärzte oder durch direkte Befragung der Patientin ermittelt.

Knapp ein Drittel aller Geschwülste war maligne, 8% davon waren Metastasen im Ovar.

Mehr als 50% aller Ovarialtumoren gehörten zur Gruppe der vom Oberflächenepithel abstammenden Geschwülste. Von 148 serösen Tumoren waren 11 semimaligne, 21 maligne, von 137 muzinösen Tumoren 7 semimaligne und nur 6 maligne. Das Entartungsrisiko scheint bei serösen Geschwülsten höher als bei den muzinösen zu sein. Etwas häufiger wurden endometrioide Karzinome gefunden; es waren 27 Fälle. Die gemischten Karzinome lagen mit 14 Fällen höher als die undifferenzierten Karzinome mit 6. Einzelfälle unter den malignen Tumoren waren ein Mesonephroma ovarii, ein mesodermaler Mischtumor und ein maligner Brenner-Tumor.

Die Zahl der vom spezifischen Ovarialstroma ausgehenden Tumoren war geringer als die der unspezifischen Stromatumoren (Abb. 1). Sie bestanden aus 15 Granulosazelltumoren (Abb. 2), gefolgt von 12 Thekazelltumoren sowie von 3 mäßig bis gut differenzierten Androblastomen (Abb. 3). Es bestand keine Korrelation zwischen der hormonalen Aktivität und dem Differenzierungsgrad des Tumorgewebes. Unter 6 zusammen mit den Granulosazelltumoren übersandten Uteri wurde dreimal eine glandulär-zystische Schleimhauthyperplasie, unter 12 Thekazelltumoren dreimal ein Adenokarzinom des Corpus uteri und zweimal eine glandulär-zystische Schleimhauthyperplasie beobachtet. Die Androblastome zeigten keine hormonale Aktivität.

Unter den Keimzellgeschwülsten lagen die der zystischen Teratome mit 156 Tumoren weit an der Spitze, gefolgt von 4 Dysgerminomen und 4 unreifen soliden Teratomen. Eine Dermoidzyste mit maligner Transformation – nämlich mit einem verhornenden Plattenepithelkarzinom – kam einmal vor. Histogenetisch besonders interessant waren die monodermalen, hochspezialisierten Teratome: Von diesen hatten wir zweimal eine Struma ovarii (Abb. 4) und einmal ein Karzinoid. Differen-

1 Pathologisches Institut der Universität des Saarlandes, D-6650 Homburg/Saar

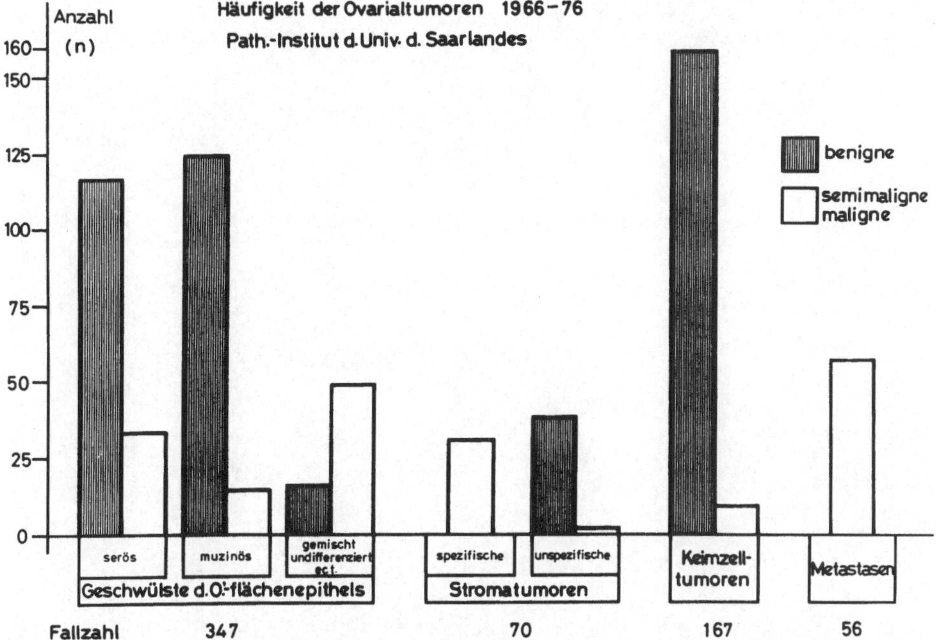

Abb. 1. Maligne und benigne Tumoren des Ovars, der Klassifikation der WHO entsprechend aufgeschlüsselt. Fast jeder 3. Tumor ist maligne und jeder 12. Tumor metastatisch

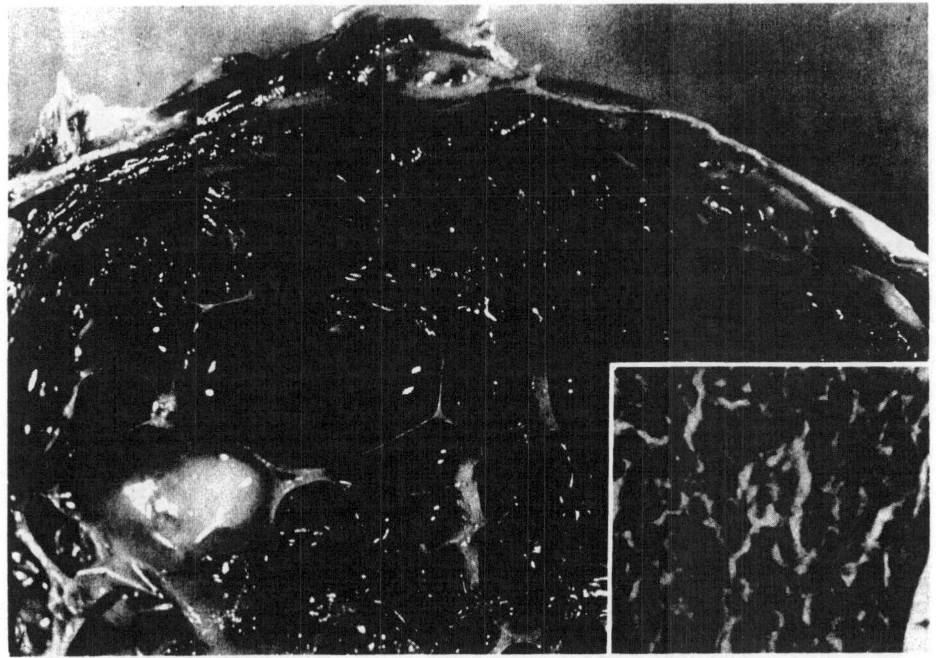

Abb. 2. Ausschnitt aus einem seltenen zystischen Granulosazelltumor, die Hohlräume mit blutiger Flüssigkeit gefüllt. (Dazugehöriges histologisches Bild mit angedeutet follikuloiden Strukturen *rechts unten.*) HE, ×256

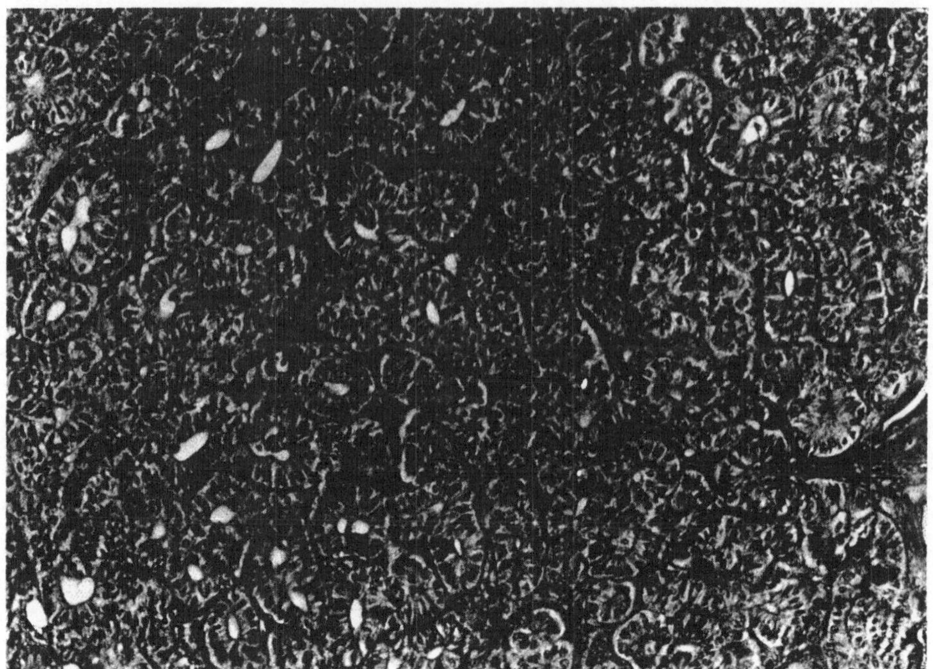

Abb. 3. Hochdifferenziertes Androblastom: Dicht liegende tubuläre Drüsenschläuche vom Typ der Sertoli-Zellen (tubuläres Adenom). Masson-Goldner, ×160

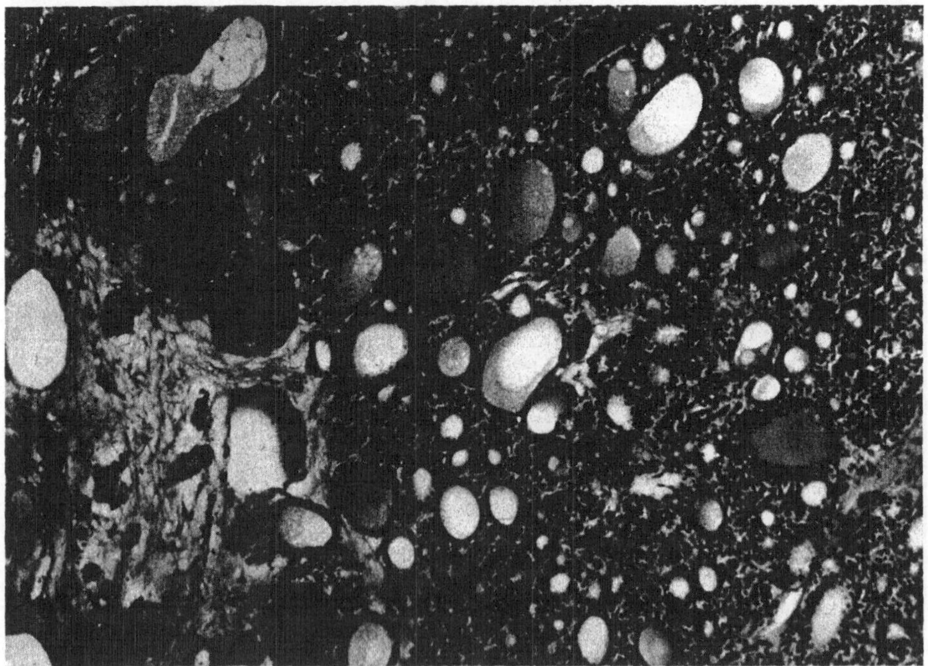

Abb. 4. Struma ovarii: Monodermal differenzierte Keimzellgeschwulst mit typischen kolloidgefüllten Follikeln. HE ×160

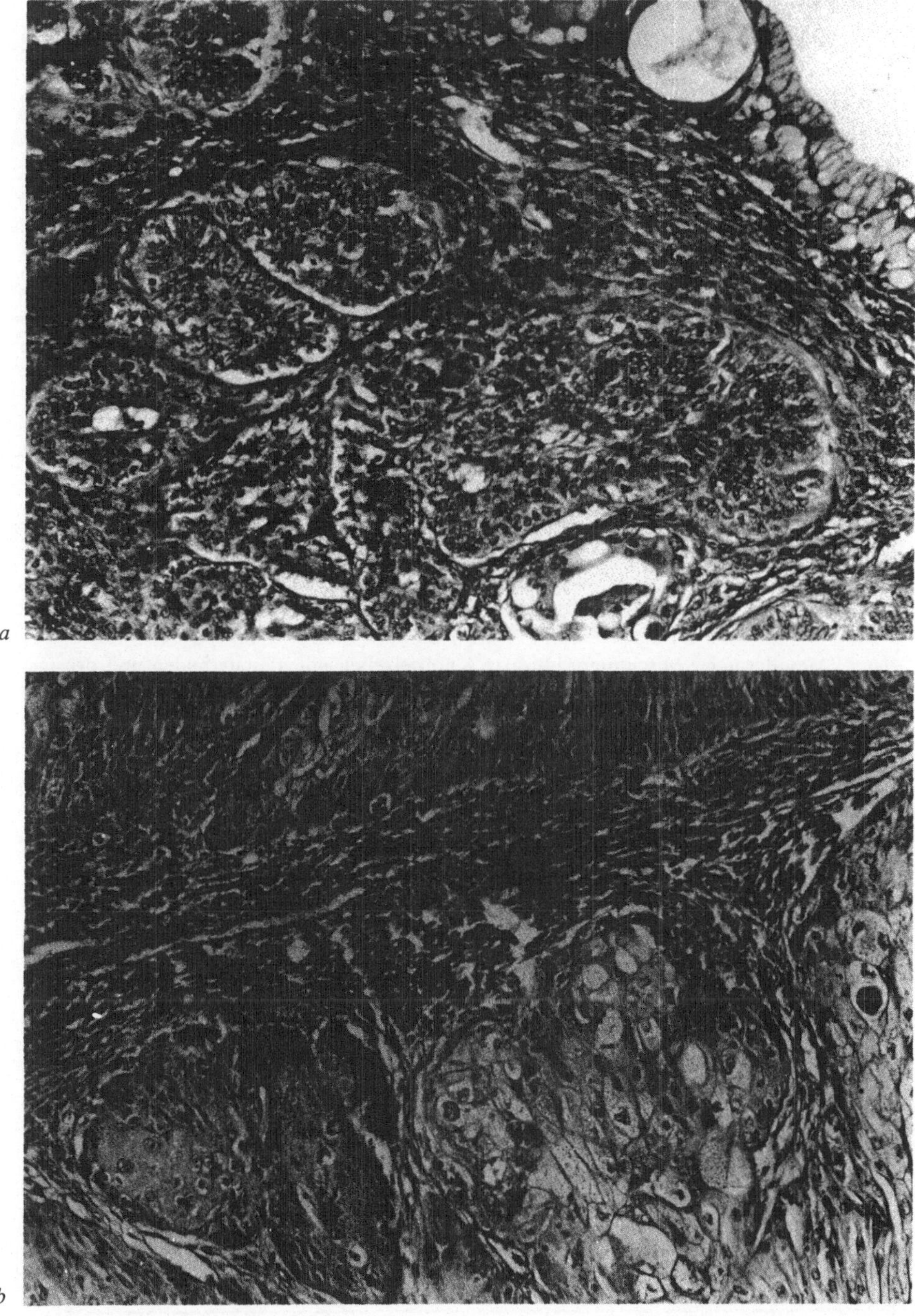

Abb. 5a, b. Maligne entarteter Brenner-Tumor; *a* an Urothel erinnernde proliferierende solide Zellkomplexe und muzinöse Zystenwandanteile; *b* plattenepithelial differenzierte Bezirke, z. T. an ein hochdifferenziertes Plattenepithelkarzinom erinnernd. HE ×160

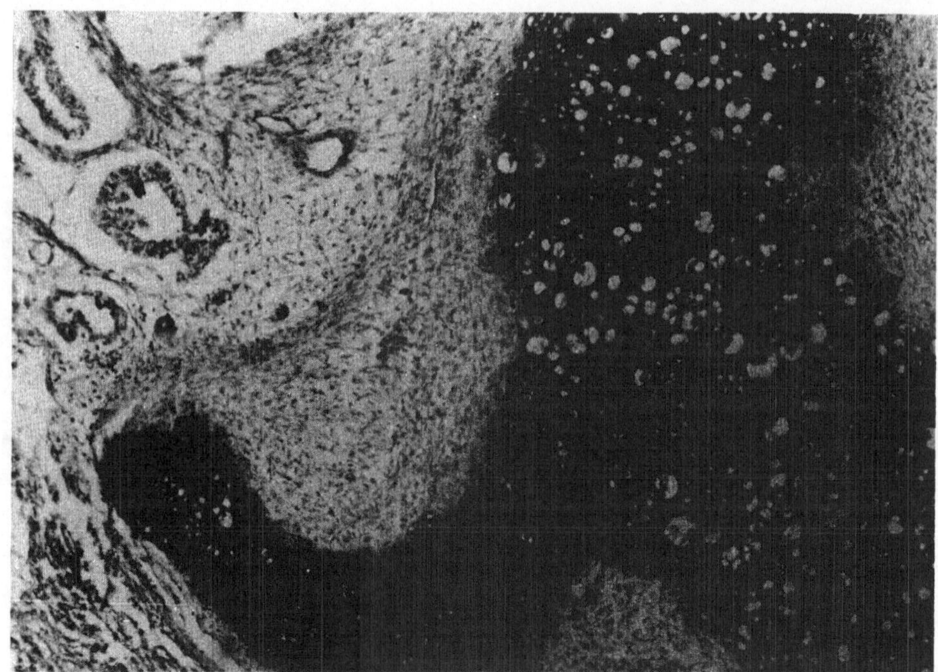

Abb. 6. Mesodermaler Mischtumor: Bizarre Knorpelzellen mit mesodermalen und drüsigen, z. T. drüsig-papillären Strukturen des ektodermalen Anteils zwischen wechselnd zellreichen, lockeren Faserstrukturen. Giemsa, × 160

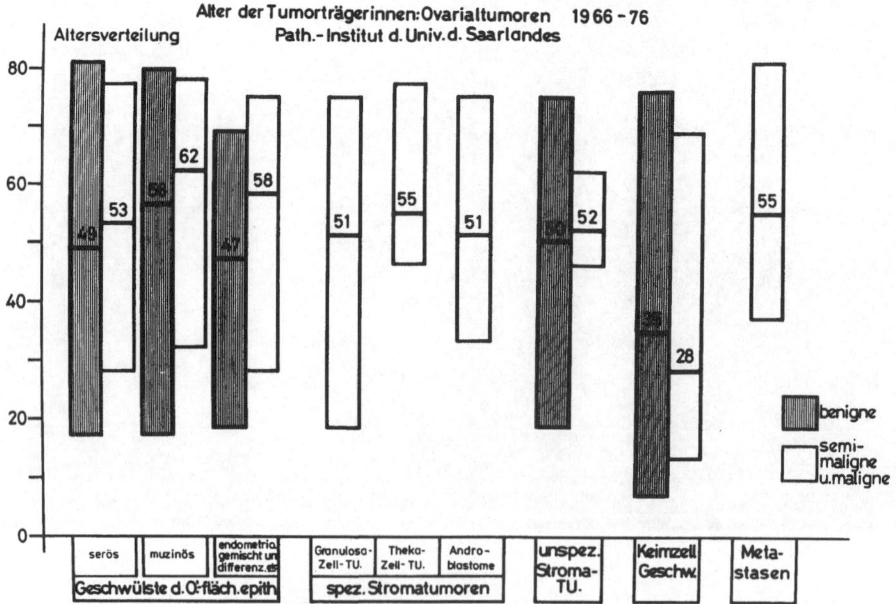

Abb. 7. Ovarialtumoren kommen in jedem Alter vor. Das mittlere Erkrankungsalter liegt bei Keimzelltumoren im jugendlichen Erwachsenenalter

tialdiagnostische Schwierigkeiten hatten wir, abgesehen von den undifferenzierten Tumoren, bei 2 Geschwülsten: Ein maligne entarteter Brenner-Tumor war gegen ein zystisches Teratom abzugrenzen. Für den Brenner-Tumor sprach a) die Kombination mit einem muzinösen Cystadenom, b) ein umschriebenes Areal mit fibrösem Stroma und typischen epithelartigen Zellnestern, c) der Wechsel zwischen muzinösem, Übergangs- und Plattenepithel, und d) das Fehlen von Hautanhangsgebilden (Abb. 5).

Bei der zweiten Geschwulst handelte es sich um einen mesodermalen Mischtumor bei einer 56jährigen Patientin. Differentialdiagnostisch hatten wir zunächst auch an ein unreifes solides Teratom gedacht. Für den mesodermalen Mischtumor sprachen die bizarren Knorpelzellen des mesodermalen und die drüsig-papillären Elemente des epithelialen Anteils (Abb. 6), das Fehlen von ektodermalen und neuroektodermalen Strukturen sowie das Alter der Patientin.

Ovarialtumoren kommen in jedem Alter vor (Abb. 7). Das Durchschnittsalter der Dysgerminompatientinnen betrug 22 Jahre. Dieser Gruppe folgten die Teratomträgerinnen mit 35 Jahren. Das Maximum der maligne entarteten serös-papillären Cystadenome lag zwischen 50–55 Jahren, das der muzinös-papillären etwa 10 Jahre später. Die Granulosazelltumoren traten zwischen dem 18. und 75. Lebensjahr auf, mit einem Maximum zwischen 46 und 55 Jahren. Die jüngste Frau mit Metastasen im Ovar war 37 Jahre alt. Am häufigsten wurden diese bei Frauen um 55 Jahre gefunden. Nehmen wir alle benignen und malignen Ovarialgeschwülste zusammen, so werden sie am häufigsten zwischen dem 50. und 60. Lebensjahr beobachtet.

Die schlechteste Prognose hatten die Patientinnen mit Metastasen im Ovar und unreifen Teratomen, gefolgt von den Patientinnen mit undifferenzierten Karzinomen. Von den Patientinnen mit serös-papillären Cystadenokarzinomen, endometrioiden und gemischten Karzinomen starben 50%. Von 10 Fällen mit muzinös-papillären Cystadenomen, die wir aufklären konnten, sind 3 Patientinnen gestorben, die übrigen befanden sich in einem mäßigen Allgemeinzustand. Unter den „Borderline“-Fällen ist keine Patientin ihrem Geschwulstleiden erlegen. Die Prognose der vom spezifischen Ovarialstroma stammenden Geschwülste hängt vom Differenzierungsgrad ab. Drei Patientinnen mit undifferenzierten Granulosazelltumoren, z.T. schon mit Metastasen in der Umgebung, starben kurz nach der Operation. Die übrigen Patientinnen sind beschwerdefrei. Die Patientinnen mit Thekazelltumoren und Androblastomen haben ebenfalls überlebt. Von den Dysgerminomträgerinnen ist die Hälfte verstorben.

So vielfältig und bedeutungsvoll zweifellos die Gruppe der primären Ovarialkarzinome ist, so muß das Ovar doch als Sitz von Metastasen besonders in Betracht gezogen werden. Jedes 4. Ovarialmalignom war eine Metastase. Wir haben die Erfahrung gemacht, daß solche metastatischen Wucherungen öfters verkannt werden. Wie so oft in der pathohistologischen Diagnostik, kommt es daher darauf an, überhaupt an die Möglichkeit eines metastatischen Prozesses zu denken. Der häufigste Sitz des Primärtumors war das Corpus uteri und das Kolon, an zweiter und dritter Stelle lagen Mamma und Magen.

Ovarialtumoren machen nur einen kleinen, aber wichtigen Anteil im Einsendegut eines pathologischen Instituts aus. Sie sind wichtig deshalb, weil ein Drittel aller Tumoren maligne ist und maligne Geschwülste in jedem Alter auftreten können.

Experimentelle Erzeugung

Zur experimentellen Erzeugung von Ovarialtumoren

B. VON SCHILLING [1] und A. LLOMBART BOSCH [2]

Wenig Modelle für das Karzinom des Ovars

Die Bemühungen um die experimentelle Erzeugung von Ovarialtumoren im Versuchstier erbrachten seit Zondek's Entdeckung (zitiert nach Biskind u. Biskind 1944) des Östrogenabbaus in der Leber (1934) zahlreiche Modelle für die funktionellen Granulosazelltumoren des Eierstocks. Für das bei der Frau wesentlich häufigere und bedeutungsvollere Karzinom in seinen verschiedenen Formen fanden sich dagegen bisher nur vereinzelte Modelle, die meist unreproduziert blieben und für die Prüfung neuer Wege in der Therapie oder die Aufdeckung pathogenetischer Prinzipien in größerem Maß nicht genutzt werden.

Dontenwill u. Squartini revidieren 1966 das einschlägige Schrifttum und ermittelten 96 Abhandlungen über experimentell erzeugte Granulosazelltumoren, deren Ursprung eine vorangehende Zerstörung der Oozyten durch Röntgenbestrahlung oder mechanische Beschädigung voraussetzte und deren Wachstum von der ungehemmten Sekretion oder exogenen Zufuhr gonadotroper Hormone aus dem Hypophysenvorderlappen abhing. Über epitheliale Malignome im Sinne der Ovarialkarzinome der Frau findet sich dagegen nichts in diesem ausführlichen Kapitel des *Handbuches über die Erzeugung von Krankheitszuständen durch das Experiment.*

An diesem Zustand der Dinge hat sich auch bis in die jüngste Zeit nichts wesentliches geändert. Wenn man von den heute vielfach geübten Versuchen einer peroperativen Einpflanzung von menschlichen Ovarialtumorproben in „nude mice" absieht, die dem behandelnden Arzt Auskunft über vorhandene Hormonrezeptoren, Radiosensibilität oder chemotherapeutische Beeinflußbarkeit des individuellen Tumors geben sollen, finden sich in der Literatur nur drei Arbeiten, denen karzinomatöse Neubildungen im Versuchstier zugrundeliegen.

Die experimentellen Karzinome des Ovars

1969 erzeugte Ivankovic nach einmaliger Gabe von 10–80 mg/kg Äthylnitrosoharnstoff bei trächtigen Ratten trabekuläre hellzellige Ovarialkarzinome bei 31 von 124 Tieren nach ca. 550 Tagen. Die knotigen Tumoren erreichten beachtliche Dimen-

1 Bio-Investigación MERCK, E-Barcelona
2 Pathologisches Institut, Universität Valencia, E-Valencia

sionen (in der Abbildung entspricht der Durchmesser des Tumors der doppelten Länge eines Uterushorns). An nichtträchtigen Tieren auch anderer Spezies gelang es dagegen nicht, mit diesem potenten Karzinogen Eierstockgeschwülste zu erzeugen. Ivankovic führt sein positives Ergebnis auf die Sondersituation der Gravidität der Versuchstiere zurück.

Ozols et al. (1978) beschreiben ein dem menschlichen Ovarialkarzinom ähnliches spontanes Karzinom in der Maus, das sie weiterverpflanzten und zur Wirkungsprüfung von Zytostatika verwendeten. 1979 führten Sekiya et al. mit Dimethylbenzanthracen (DMBA) getränkte Seidenfäden durch das Rattenovar und erhielten nach 5 Wochen bei 39% der Tiere Adenokarzinome. Folgearbeiten, die auf den genannten Beobachtungen beruhten, fanden sich nicht.

Die experimentellen Granulosazelltumoren

Die Erzeugung nichtepithelialer Geschwülste, die sich von der Membrana granulosa herleiten, war dagegen viel erfolgreicher. Die Bemühungen gehen hier fast so

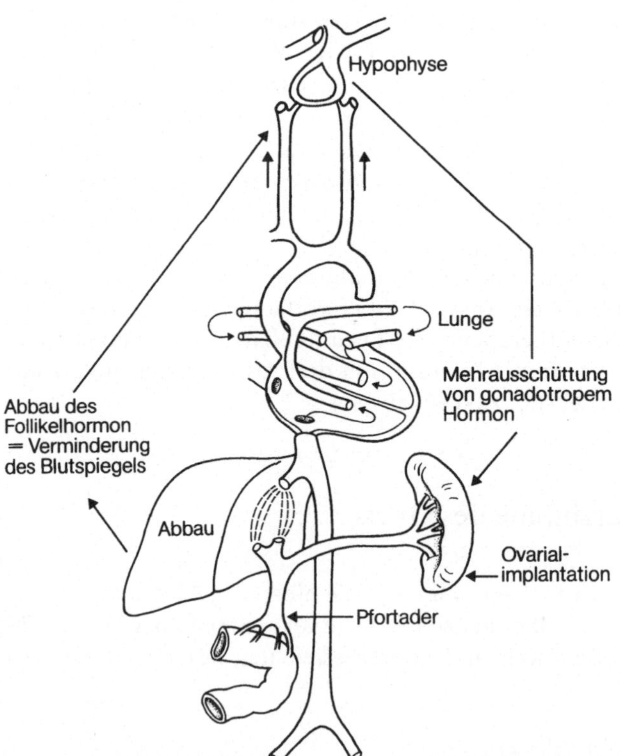

Abb. 1. Schematische Darstellung der Versuchsanordnung nach Biskind u. Biskind (1944) und der Hormonsekretion des in die Milz transplantierten Ovarialgewebes (aus Dontenwill u. Squartini 1966)

weit zurück wie die historische Aufklärung erster Zusammenhänge zwischen Struktur und Wirkung der steroiden Geschlechtshormone. Wir überschauen heute die Veröffentlichungen von praktisch fünf Jahrzehnten und können die eingangs erwähnte Entdeckung des Östrogenabbaus durch die Leber (Zondek 1934) an den Anfang stellen. Sie führte zu der von Biskind u. Biskind (1944) beschriebenen Versuchsanordnung mit Einpflanzung eines Eierstocks in den exklusiven Abflußbereich des lebergängigen Pfortaderkreislaufs wie z. B. der Milz der Ratte nach gleichzeitiger Entfernung des anderen Ovars (Abb. 1).

Das Biskind-Modell

Durch die Hemikastration wird die Rückmeldung zirkulierenden Östrogens an die Hypophyse unterbrochen und eine reaktive Mehrausschüttung der Gonadotropine FSH und LH veranlaßt, die im Laufe von 12 Monaten das Milzovar in einen geschwulstartigen hyperplastischen Knoten von 1–1,5 cm Durchmesser umwandelt, vorausgesetzt, daß die exklusive venöse Leberdrainage des Implantats nicht durch Verwachsungsbrücken mit dem Zwerchfell oder der Bauchwand umgangen worden war.

Biskind u. Biskind (1944) hatten die Eierstöcke nicht in der Erwartung verpflanzt, diese „hyperplasiogenen Anpassungsgeschwülste" zu entdecken, wie sie Büngeler u. Dontenwill (1959) in ihrer kritischen Auseinandersetzung mit diesen Tumoren benannt haben, sondern nur, um den Östrogenabbau durch die Leber auf seine Dauer auch unter einer Mangeldiät zu überprüfen. Dazu kontrollierten sie den sich fortsetzenden Steroidabbau anhand des konstanten Anöstrus im Scheidenabstrich der Ratten. Die unerwartete Tumorbildung bezeichneten sie als eine ausgezeichnete Gelegenheit, die enthemmte Stimulation der von den Fesseln zirkulierenden Follikelhormons befreiten Hypophyse am Ovar zu beobachten.

Biskind u. Biskind (1944) stellten eine weitgehende morphologische Ähnlichkeit zwischen den Milzovartumoren ihrer Ratten und den Geschwülsten ortsständig verbliebener Eierstöcke fest, die Furth u. Butterworth (1936) und Brambell et al. (1927) durch Röntgenbestrahlung hervorgerufen hatten. Damit wird hier zum ersten Mal eine exogene Schädigung des Eierstocks angesprochen, die zur Unterbrechung seiner Steroidsekretion und zur reaktiven Überstimulierung des Hypophysenvorderlappens führt, die das verbliebene funktionelle Stroma des Ovars nun zur Proliferation anregt.

Zunächst finden sich luteinisierte Zellelemente, die sich bis zur Bildung von Luteomen vermehren können. Im Laufe der Zeit verschwinden diese Luteinisierungszeichen jedoch wieder, und nun wird das Gesichtsfeld mehr und mehr von Granulosazellen mit Mitosen eingenommen, die sich in follikuloiden oder strangförmigen Verbänden anordnen. Diese Morphologie wurde bei dem Biskind-Versuchsmodell immer wieder beschrieben und wird auch von den Verfassern der vorliegenden Abhandlung an Ratte und Hamster bestätigt.

Das Biskind-Milzovar diente ab 1944 zahlreichen Forschern zur Beantwortung onkologischer und endokrinologischer Fragestellungen, von denen die aus heutiger Sicht belangvollsten herausgegriffen seien:

Untersuchungen am Biskind-Milzovar der Ratte und Maus

Altersabhängigkeit

Ausgehend von der Feststellung, daß alte Mäuse nur selten spontane Ovarialtumoren entwickeln, untersuchte Klein (1952) die Frage nach der Tumorbildung in einem senil in die Milz transplantierten Ovar. Er verpflanzte Ovarien aus drei Altersklassen: Aus abgesetzten Jungmäusen (28 Tage), jungen erwachsenen Mäusen (100–140 Tage) und senilen Mäusen (690–855 Tage). Als Empfänger dienten die Milzen kastrierter Männchen und Weibchen. Die senilen Ovarien wurden 68–169 Tage alten Männchen implantiert. Die Eierstöcke abgesetzter Jungmäuse gingen an kastrierte Männchen zwischen 100 und 140 Tagen. Die Ovarien erwachsener Mäuse (100–140 Tage) wurden auf Männchen und Weibchen gleichen Alters übertragen. Tumoren fanden sich in allen Gruppen. Die meisten (91%) fanden sich in den kastrierten männlichen Empfängern von Ovarien 28 Tage alter abgesetzter Mäuse, die wenigsten (immerhin 67%) bei den Männchen, die senile Implantate erhalten hatten. Die mittlere Beobachtungszeit betrug 210 Tage. Die Hauptfrage Klein's nach der Rezeptivität auch des alten Ovars der Maus für eine Tumorbildung war für ihn damit im positiven Sinne beantwortet. Zweifellos wird hier das hyperplastische Wachstum des stimulierten Ovarialstromas mit einem neoplastischen Geschehen identifiziert.

Wirkung zusätzlichen Gonadotropins

Nachdem subkutane Implantate von Hypophysenvorderlappen (HVL) bei Mäusen die Zahl spontaner Mammakarzinome steigerte und auch bei kastrierten, ovarimplantierten Männchen die zusätzliche Einpflanzung von HVL die Häufigkeit spontaner Brustdrüsenkarzinome anhob, untersuchten Silberberg et al. (1951) den Effekt von vier zusätzlich eingepflanzten HVL auf das Biskind-Milzovarmodell, dessen hormoneller Wachstumsanstoß ohnehin von dem eigenen enthemmten HVL ausgeht.

Als Ergebnis fand er Wachstumsförderung und schnellere Alterung der Milzovarien; epitheliale Tubuli und im Vergleich älteres luteinisiertes Gewebe traten verfrüht auf oder waren gegenüber den Kontrollen vermehrt. Intralienäre Tumoren traten auch früher auf, und das Verhältnis zwischen Granulosazelltumoren und Luteomen verschob sich zugunsten der letzteren. Diese Wirkungen wurden den follikelstimulierenden und luteinisierenden Hormonen aus dem implantierten HVL zugeschrieben.

Geschwulstmorphologie

1955 erzielte Gardner in einer umfangreichen Untersuchung über die Entwicklung und das Wachstum von Eierstockstumoren eines in die Milz transplantierten Ovars kastrierter Mäuse 42 Geschwülste aus 74 Implantaten. Sie hatten sich nach durchaus uneinheitlichen Induktionszeiten entwickelt. Gemäß Perioden der Ruhe und der Wucherung unterschied er 5 Wachstumstypen. Desgleichen beschrieb er 5 verschiedene histologische Muster, die mit den Wachstumstypen jedoch nicht korrelieren:

I. Groß- und blaßzelliger Typ mit Aufbau aus groben Zellsträngen (10 Beispiele)
II. Tubulär-adenomatöser Typ, z.T. zystisch, einmal teratomatöse (12 Beispiele)
III. Follikuloider Typ mit unregelmäßiger Anordnung der Granulosazellen und zahlreichen Mitosen (6 Beispiele)
IV. Massierte Zellanordnung mit wenig Stroma ohne bestimmte Struktur (8 Beispiele)
V. Schmalleistige Granulosazelltumoren (4 Beispiele).

Cortisonwirkung

1956 befaßte sich Mardones u. Lipschutz mit der damals aktuellen Wirkungsaufklärung des Cortisons (Cortisonacetat) auf Wachstum und Metastasierung maligner Tumoren. Beide Phänomene waren nach früheren Untersuchern in konträrer Weise beeinflußt worden, d.h. Cortison hemmte das lokale Wachstum und förderte die Tumoraussaat. Auch gingen die Verfasser von der Beobachtung von Li (1948) aus, der bei einer Maus mit Milzovar nach Biskind (unter zusätzlicher Progesteronbehandlung) nach 220 Tagen neben dem Hauptknoten in der Milz satellitäre Granulosazelltumoren fand, die er als Metastasen ansah.

Der Tumor war außerdem auf andere Mäuse verpflanzbar, so daß sowohl für Li wie auch für die andere Verfassergruppe die Kriterien der Malignität erfüllt waren. So wollte Mardones den Cortisoneinfluß auf das Wachstum und die Streuung der unter einem hormonellen Ungleichgewicht entstandenen Milzovartumoren nach Biskind bei der Maus untersuchen. Cortisonacetat wurde ohne Angabe der Gesamtdosis als 40%iger Anteil mit 60% Cholesterol in einem Preßling subkutan eingepflanzt (tägliche Absorption 30–90 μg). Als Ergebnis bei 37 Mäusen fand sich eine Verlangsamung des Wachstums der Milztumoren und kein Fall von Metastasierung. Gegenüber den Granulosazelltumoren überwogen Luteome.

Sequenzumkehr des Zellbildes

Besondere Aufmerksamkeit fand die Umkehrung der gewohnten orthologen Reihenfolge des zellulären Aspekts: In den Geschwülsten folgten in der Regel einer anfänglichen Luteinisierung und Luteombildung als Endstadium paradoxerweise die Granulosazellen, und zwar nunmehr ohne lichtmikroskopische Zeichen einer Gelbkörperreaktion. Myhre versuchte 1964, diesen Widerspruch durch autoradiographische Untersuchungen zu klären. Anhand nachgewiesener mitotischer Teilungen der luteinisierten Tumorzellen bezeichnet er die im Spätstadium nachfolgenden und verbleibenden Granulosazellen als deren Tochterzellen.

Nachweis der Steroidhormonsynthese

Deane u. Fawcett (1956) verpflanzten Ovarien kastrierter Ratten nicht nur in die Milz, sondern auch in die Niere und Leber, um eine histochemische Hormonaktivitätsbestimmung am Implantat durchzuführen gemäß der von Deane (1952) angegebenen Methode zur Identifikation der physiologischen Aktivität der verschiedenen Gewebskomponenten des Ovars. Nach geeigneter Fixierung wurden hierbei die histochemischen Parameter Zellbasophilie (Granulosa-Lutein-Zellen), Lipide, Carbonylgruppen, Cholesterin, Glykoproteine und alkalische Phosphatase färberisch nachgewiesen. Im normal funktionierenden Ovar enthalten die Steroidhormonvorläufer in der inneren Theka, dem Zwischengewebe und den Gelbkörpern Lipidtröpfchen, die bei aktiver Sekretion klein, cholesterinarm und carbonylreich sind. Bei schwacher Sekretion vergrößern sich die Lipidtropfen unter Cholesterinzunahme und Carbonylabnahme. Die alkalische Phosphatase ist in den Blutgefäßwänden reichlich nachweisbar, die sezernierende Parenchymzellen umgeben.

Bei den in die *Nieren* verpflanzten Ovarien der Kastraten fand sich kein histochemischer Unterschied von normalen Ovarien. Sie bewirkten normale Östruszyklen. Auch die in die *Leber* eingepflanzten Eierstöcke führten nicht zum Anöstrus. Die dem eingepflanzten Ovar nachgeschaltete Leberparenchymstrecke schien nicht auszureichen, um das Östrogen voll abzubauen. In 37 *Milzovarien* bestand dagegen Anöstrus bis auf neun Ratten, bei denen nach einigen Monaten die Verhornung des Scheidenepithels (Östrus) auf einen von der Leber nicht mehr zu bewältigenden Überschuß von Östrogen aus dem Milzovar hinzuweisen schien. Mühlbock et al. (1952, 1958) vermutet auch eine allmählich nachlassende Kapazität der Leber zum Östrogenabbau. Histologisch beobachteten die Verfasser wieder das beschriebene Mischbild aus lutealen und Granulosazellelementen, wobei im ersten Drittel der neunmonatigen Beobachtungsphase die Luteinisierung überwog, im zweiten Drittel das Bild granulosazellreicher wurde und im letzten Drittel bei 9/14 Ratten erneut die luteale Phase in den Vordergrund trat.

Histochemisch zeigten die Milzovarien nach 6 Monaten Steroidaufbereitung mit stark positiver Glykoproteinreaktion des Follikelsekretes und carbonyl- und lipidtropfenhaltige Thekazellen mit positivem Cholesterinnachweis. In ihrer Umgebung waren die Blutgefäße reich an alkalischer Phosphatase. Von Interesse ist die Feststellung, daß es nicht die Granulosazellen waren, die Steroidbildung anzeigten, sondern die sie umgebenden und sich dazwischen schiebenden Thekazellverbände.

Morphologie, Sekretion und Verpflanzbarkeit

1957 beschrieb Green Morphologie, Sekretion und Verpflanzbarkeit von 10 Milzovartumoren der Maus. Die Steroidsekretion maß er histologisch an den Erfolgsorganen: *Progesteron* bewirkt am Mäuseendometrium eine vesikuläre Umwandlung der Stromazellkerne mit deutlichem Nukleolus und feinem Chromatinmuster. *Östrogen* geht mit Stromaödem, Drüsenentwicklung und Epithelerhöhung einher. *Androgen*sekretion erkennt man am Ausbleiben einer Samenblaseninvolution und an der Größe der Azinuszellen der Unterkieferspeicheldrüsen.

Von den 10 Primärtumoren zeigten *4* eine gesicherte Östrogensekretion, davon *1* in Kombination mit Progesteronsekretion. Eine fünfte Maus zeigte Progesteron und Androgensekretion. Auch in den ersten Passagen im Zweitwirt fand sich erneut Östrogenbildung.

Beim Vergleich zwischen Zellbild und ermitteltem Hormontyp fand sich nur eine sehr ungefähre Übereinstimmung zwischen Granulosazellaufbau und Östrogensekretion, bzw. Luteomaufbau und Progesteronsekretion, so daß nach Green für die Beurteilung des Sekrettyps die Tumormorphologie keinen sicheren Hinweis gibt.

Milzovar in Parabiose

Mühlbock beschrieb 1952 die experimentelle Genese von Ovarialtumoren bei der Maus 1,5–2 Jahre nach Röntgenganzkörperbestrahlung oder Einzelbestrahlung der freigelegten Eierstöcke. Im Milzovar erreichte er eine schnellere Tumorbildung durch folgende Abänderung:

Die mit Implantat versehene, kastrierte Maus wurde auf einer Seite parabiotisch mit einem weiteren kastrierten Weibchen und dies wiederum mit einem dritten anastomosiert. Nachdem die Hormone des HVL leicht von einem Parabiosepartner zum anderen überkreuzten, kombinierte sich im Milzovar die dreifache gonadotrope Stimulation. Da Östrogen dagegen schlecht diffundiert und über den mittleren Partner nicht hinauskommt, entfiel mit dieser Versuchsanordnung in Parabiot II und besonders in Parabiot III jegliches Östrogen aus dem Milzovar, das dem Leberabbau evtl. entgangen sein und die Hypophyse hemmen könnte.

Unter den Fernwirkungen der Milzovartumoren erwähnt Mühlbock die mitunter zu beobachtende schwammartige Erweiterung der Lebersinusoide mit Hypervolämie, einem Äquivalent zur „Peliosis hepatis", die beim Menschen nach Anwendung androgener Anabolika beschrieben wird (Bartok 1969; McGiven 1970; Rübner 1970; Ross 1972; Bagheri 1974; Nadell 1977; Shapiro 1977; Chopra 1978). Eine Spekulation am Ende jener Abhandlung erscheint belangreich: „Wenn eine relative Überproduktion des gonadotropen Hormons der verursachende Faktor für das Entstehen von Ovarialtumoren ist, dann ist es auffallend, daß nicht mehr Granulosazelltumoren bei Frauen nach der Menopause gesehen werden ... Die lange Induktionszeit scheint hierfür ein Faktor von Bedeutung zu sein." Auch erwartet Mühlbock im Jahre 1952 für die kommenden Dezennien die Möglichkeit einer signifikanten Ovarialtumorzunahme bei den Japanerinnen, die der Strahlenexposition der Atombomben in Hiroshima und Nagasaki 1945 ausgesetzt waren.

Malignität

Die Frage der *Malignität* der besprochenen experimentellen Granulosazelltumoren des Ovars ist umstritten. Büngeler u. Dontenwill (1959) weisen mit Letterer auf den grundsätzlichen Unterschied zwischen dem Verhalten dieser Neubildungen und dem invasiv-destruktiven und metastasierenden Wachstum echter Malignome hin, das keinem erkennbaren Regulationsmechanismus unterworfen ist. Die Entstehung und anfängliche Entwicklung der hier diskutierten Neubildungen ist dagegen bis zum Moment eines autonomen Wachstums von einer hormonellen Steuerung abhängig, und der morphologische Aspekt dieser Tumoren ist i. allg. von sarkomatösen oder anaplastischen Bildern weit entfernt.

Das autonome Wachstum in der Spätphase und die Verpflanzbarkeit auf kastrierte und intakte Zweitwirte beiderlei Geschlechts mit weiteren Tumorpassagen wird aber dennoch von verschiedenen Untersuchern als Kriterium für eine echte Malignität angesehen (Li 1947; Gardner 1955; Green 1957) und die gelegentlich beobachteten hämatogenen Absiedlungen in Leber und Lunge unterstützten diese Auffassung.

Trotzdem führte die Suche nach malignen Ovarialtumoren mit aggressiverem Verhalten sowohl am orthotopen wie am Milzovar zum zusätzlichen Einsatz von anderen karzinogenetischen Agenzien.

Tumormodelle am orthotopen Ovar

9,10-Dimethyl-1,2-benzanthracen (DMBA) am orthotopen Ovar

Die Entstehung von Ovarialtumoren bei der Maus durch kutane Applikation des oben genannten Kohlenwasserstoffes (Abb. 2) wurde bei Mammakarzinogeneseversuchen von Howell zufällig entdeckt. Die Nachprüfung (Howell et al. 1954) an 88 Mäusen ergab nach 14tägig einmaliger Aufbringung von 16 Tropfen (1,25 mg) DMBA auf die Haut der 4 Seiten der Tiere bei 52 Mäusen unilaterale, und bei 1 Maus bilaterale Granulosazelltumoren. Histologisch wurde nachgewiesen, daß der Tumorentstehung die Zerstörung der Eizellen vorangegangen war.

Das Vaginalzellbild zeigte 3 Varianten: Entweder verschwand die Östrusphase völlig nach immer länger werdenden Diöstrusperioden oder sie trat nach ca. 7 Monaten plötzlich und dann aber permanent wieder auf, oder – als dritte Variante – sie wurde schon von Anfang an immer länger, um schließlich zur Dauerphase zu werden. Dieses letztere Verhalten bei 7 Mäusen mit Granulosazelltumoren war mit der bisherigen Anschauung einer obligaten hypophysären Gonadotropinmehrausschüttung aufgrund fehlender Östrogenrückmeldung nicht verständlich und blieb auch für die Verfasser eine offene Frage.

Tumorverhinderung bei Anwesenheit normaler Ovarien

Um so mehr ging es einer der Mitautoren Howell's, Marchant (1960), nun darum, nachzuweisen, daß selbst unter DMBA in der Maus keine Eierstocktumoren entstehen, wenn normales Ovarialgewebe vorhanden ist, das eine Überstimulierung der adenohypophysären Gonadotropinbildung verhindert (Tabelle 1).

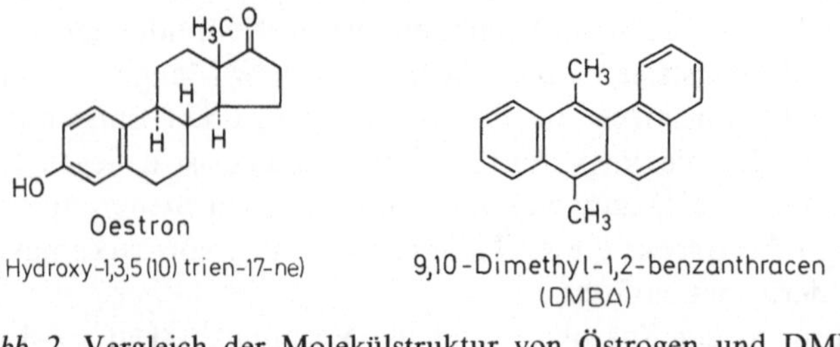

Abb. 2. Vergleich der Molekülstruktur von Östrogen und DMBA. (Merck Index, 9th edn. Merck, Rahway)

Tabelle 1 Versuchsanordnung nach Marchant (1960) (*) Ovarium aus DMBA-behandelter Maus; (O) Ovarium aus unbehandelter Maus

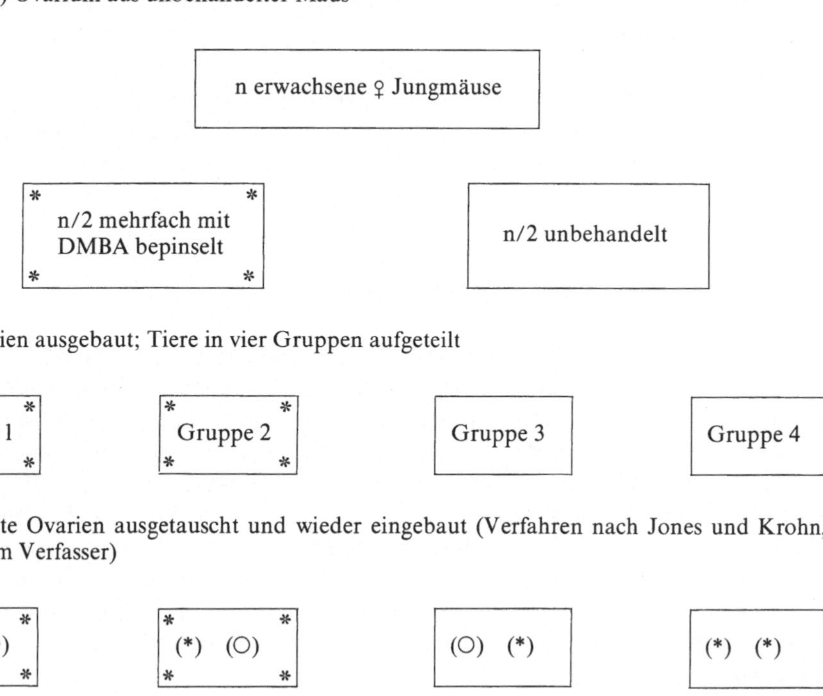

Sektionsergebnis: 13 Granulosazelltumoren entstanden nur in Gruppe 4 (unbehandelte Mäuse mit Ovarien aus DMBA-behandelten Tieren). Rest tumorfrei. Die Gegenwart eines normalen Ovariums verhinderte damit die Tumorbildung in den Gruppen 1, 2 und 3. Zur Onkogenese am Ovar der Maus bedarf es der „kokarzinogenen“ Wirkung von DMBA und Gonadotropin. Östruszeichen traten bei diesem Versuch in der Tumorgruppe 4 nur in der Spätphase auf, zum Zeitpunkt einer vermutlichen Tumorautonomie.

DMBA nur kokarzinogen

Den endgültigen Beweis für die *nur kokarzinogene Wirkung des DMBA* lieferte Jull (1969) ebenfalls durch Ein- und Ausbau von Eierstöcken, wobei er die Information aus den Marchant-Versuchen noch ergänzen konnte.

Links ovariektomierten Mäusen setzte Jull subkutan ein DMBA-bepinseltes Ovar ein. Die Frage ging um die Anzahl zu erwartender Tumoren am Implantat nach Entfernung des verbliebenen rechten Ovars: Bei sofortiger Entfernung bildeten sich große Tumoren an 56% der Implantate. Bei Entfernung nach 6 Wochen entstanden nur noch mikroskopisch sichtbare Granulosazellgeschwülste an 25% und nach 12 Wochen an 17% der Implantate. Verblieb das rechte Ovar an Ort und Stelle, so atrophierte das DMBA-bepinselte subkutane Implantat.

An einer weiteren Gruppe von Mäusen ließ Jull nach der subkutanen Einpflanzung des DMBA-vorbehandelten Ovars zwei Trächtigkeiten mit Würfen ablaufen, um dann zu kastrieren. 33% der Implantate wurden neoplastisch. Wiederholte er diese Versuchsanordnung mit Einpflanzung vorher unbehandelter Eierstöcke, so entstanden nach dem zweiten Wurf und nachfolgender Kastration an 11% der Implantate auch Tumoren, also eine reine Gonadotropinwirkung. (Vermutlich war hier aus dem subkutan eingepflanzten normalen Ovar zu wenig Östrogen in den Kreislauf gelangt, um die Hypophyse zu hemmen.)

DMBA an anderen Spezies (außer der Maus)

Kuwahara versuchte 1976, durch DMBA orthotope Ovarialtumoren auch bei Ratte, Kaninchen, Hamster und Meerschweinchen zu erzeugen. Es gelang nur bei der Maus, und zwar sowohl durch Fütterung als nach i.p.- und nach i.v.-Applikation mit Tumorausbeuten von 59, 36 und 57%. Mit Ausnahme eines papillären Adenokarzinoms entstanden nur Granulosazelltumoren, so daß der Verfasser die deutliche Affinität des DMBA zu hormonbildenden oder hormonreaktiven Zellen wie die der Mamma oder Hypophyse auf die stereochemische Ähnlichkeit zwischen DMBA und den Steroidhormonen zurückführen möchte (Abb. 2). Der nach DMBA-Applikation beobachtete Schwund der follikulären Strukturen und der Oozyten veranlaßte Kuwahara, von einer strahlenmimetischen Wirkung dieses Kohlenwasserstoffs zu sprechen.

Oozytenzerstörung

Die durch DMBA bewirkte Zerstörung der Oozyten als erste Stufe der nachfolgenden Onkogenese wies Krarup (1969a) durch Zählung der verbleibenden Eizellen 22 Tage, 9 Wochen und 12 Monate nach ein- oder mehrfacher Bepinselung der freigelegten Gonaden der Maus nach. Zu den genannten Fristen sank die Anzahl von 3400 auf 1700 und auf 250 Oozyten.

Seine morphologischen Befunde entsprechen denen anderer schon zitierter Autoren. Das Auftreten eines Granulosazelltumors an nur einem der beiden orthotopen Ovarien bei Atrophie des gegenseitigen betrachtet Krarup (1969b) als Folge eines kompetitiven Geschehens: Das erste der beiden von Oozyten entledigte, teils luteinisierte und neoplastisch proliferierende Ovar, das Autonomie erlangt und Östrogene zu produzieren beginnt, wird die bis dahin erfolgte Gonadotropinausschüttung aus dem HVL eindämmen und damit dem etwas später nachfolgenden zweiten Ovar, welches bis dahin analoge Umwandlungen mitgemacht hat, die weitere Wachstumsmöglichkeit entziehen und es zur Atrophie freigeben.

Versuche aus den Jahren 1969–1979. Malignisierung

Zunächst seien Hilfrichs erfolgreiche Bemühungen erwähnt (1972, 1973), die Tumoren im Milzovar der Ratte durch einmal wöchentliche subkutane DMBA-Injektionen (2 mg/kg) bis zum Spontantod der Tiere in 5–6 cm große metastasierende invasive maligne Geschwülste umzuwandeln, die meist durch zentrale Autolyse und intraabdominale Blutungen zum Verenden der Tiere führten.

Histologisch handelte es sich hier um maligne Thekome und Granulosazelltumoren. Begann diese Medikation zugleich mit der Ovarialeinpflanzung in die Milz, so erzielte Hilfrich 30% Malignome, setzte sie erst 25 Wochen später ein, erhielt er 65%.

Weitere chemische Karzinogene

Vol'fson erzielte 1976 Granulosazelltumoren an der Maus durch intravaginale Applikation vom Synestrol, Polyurethan, DMBA und 8-Hydroxychinolin.

Überprüfung der experimentellen Ergebnisse aus 30 Jahren

Armuth u. Berenblum überprüften schließlich 1979 alle die bis dahin berichteten Erfahrungen noch einmal in einem Kombinationsversuch an der Maus unter Beobachtung der orthotopen und der in die Milz eingepflanzten Ovarien mit und ohne DMBA.

Folgende Versuchsanordnungen wurden gewählt:

Gruppe 1: Kastration. Milzovar. Ergebnis: 50% Milzovargeschwülste. Dies entsprach bisherigen Erfahrungen eines gonadotropen Promotionseffekts.

Gruppe 2: Hemikastration. Milzovar. Ergebnis: Kein orthotoper und kein Milzovartumor.
Dies entsprach bisherigen Erfahrungen einer verhinderten Gonadotropinpromotion dank des verbliebenen normalen Ovar.

Gruppe 3: Kastration. Milzovar. Einmal DMBA oral. Ergebnis: 43% Milzovargeschwülste.
Entsprach bisherigen Erfahrungen, daß zusätzliche DMBA-Gaben den gonadotropen Wachstumsimpuls im Milzovar der Maus nicht verstärken.

Gruppe 4: Hemikastration. Milzovar. Einmal DMBA oral. Ergebnis: Nur 1 lokaler Ovarialtumor, aber 47% Milzovargeschwülste. Keine Vergleiche in der Literatur, da neuartige Versuchsanordnung. Theoretisch erstaunt die geringe neoplastische Wirkung des DMBA + Gonadotropin am verbliebenen Einzelovar. Die Verfasser begründen dies mit dem von Krarup (s. o.) diskutierten kompetitiven Mechanismus zwischen den beiden stimulierten Ovarien, wobei das in der Milz befindliche offenbar schneller „autonom" wird.

Gruppe 5: Beide Ovarien in situ. DMBA oral, einmal. Ergebnis: Keine Tumoren.
Dies entsprach nicht bisherigen Erfahrungen, da Tumoren zu erwarten gewesen wären. Seitens der Verfasser keine Diskussion.

Gruppe 6: Unbehandelte Kontrolltiere: Kein Tumor, kein Kommentar.

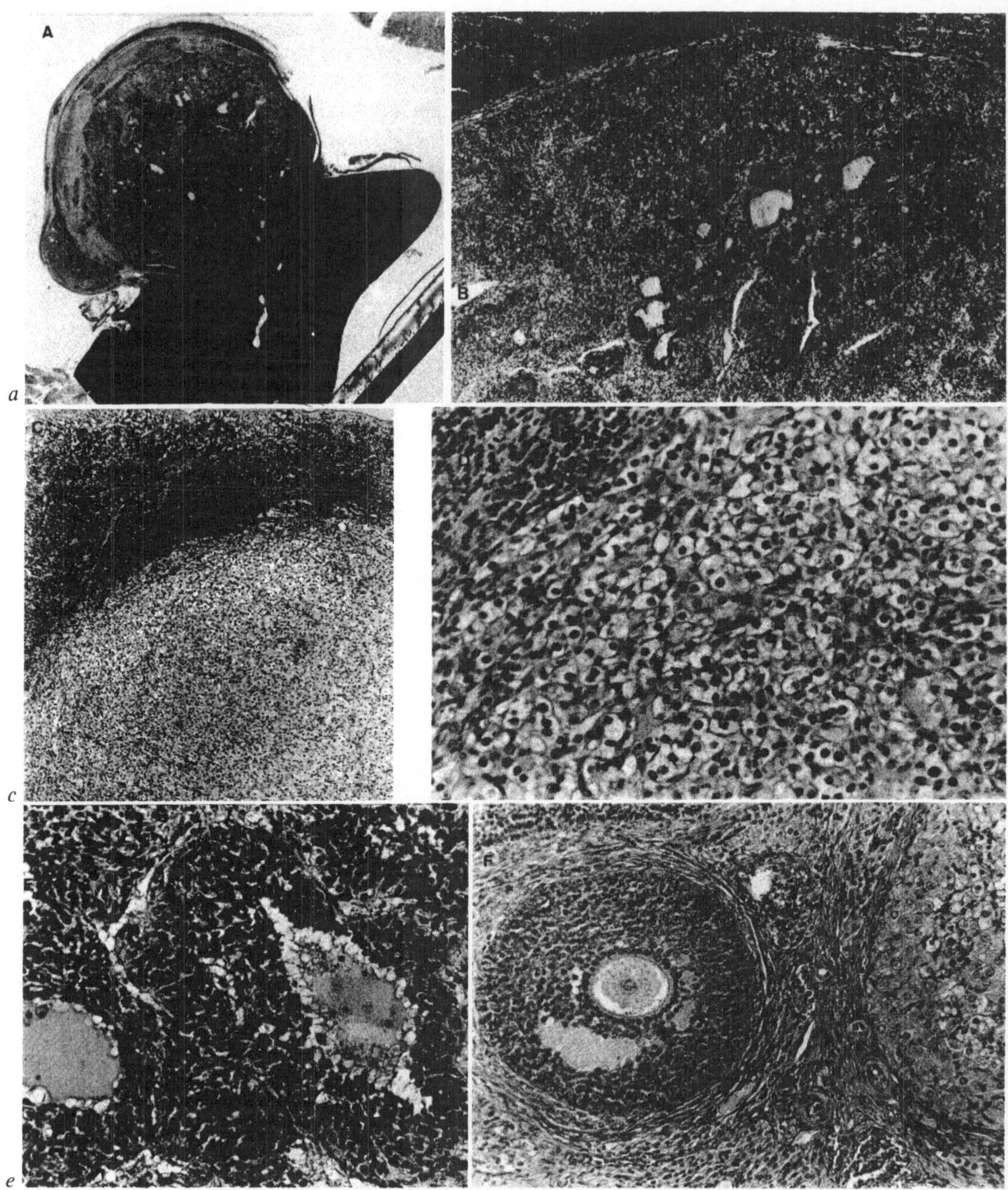

Abb. 3. *a* Milzovar, Ratte, Granulosazelltumor (GZT), ×2*; *b* Ausschnitt aus *a*, ×8; *c* Milzovar, luteinisiert, ×20; *d* Ausschnitt aus *c*, ×80; *e* GZT mit follikuloidem Aufbau, ×63; *f* normales Rattenovar, Follikel und Gelbkörper, ×50

---

* alle Maßstäbe mikroskopisch, nicht photographisch

Zur Ultrastruktur der experimentellen Ovarialgeschwülste

Durch Einpflanzung des Ovars in die Milz und einmal monatliche orale DMBA-Gaben an 17 Ratten erzeugten die Verfasser im Laufe eines Jahres 5 Granulosazelltumoren mit luteinisierten und thekomatösen Anteilen (Abb. 3). Daneben entstanden 11 weitere bösartige Tumoren an Haut, Darm, Brust, ZNS, Nieren und blutbildenden Geweben der Tiere.

Elektronenmikroskopisch fanden sich neben perivaskulär angeordneten, zytoplasmaarmen, spindelförmigen, myofibroblastenähnlichen Elementen des Stromas als Hauptkontingent zytoplasmareichere, epitheloide Granulosazellen ohne und mit lipiden Einschlußvakuolen. Glattes, endoplasmatisches Retikulum fand sich zwischen den Lipidvakuolen neben einem regelrecht gestalteten Golgi-Apparat. Eine intramitochondriale pigmentkörnige Steroidsynthese fand sich in einzelnen Zellen (Abb. 4).

Kuwahara versuchte 1976 beim Hamster vergeblich, durch DMBA orthotope Ovarialtumoren zu erzeugen. Nach monatlich einmaliger Gabe von 8 mg DMBA an weibliche Hamster erzielten die Verfasser innerhalb von 9 Monaten bei 8/32 Tieren Ovarialtumoren (35%). Histologisch fand sich wieder ein Aufbau aus follikuloiden Granulosazellverbänden, die elektronenmikroskopisch teilweise Zeichen der Luteinisierung und Steroidsynthese (Vakuolen) und dicht gelagerte Mitochondrien mit tubuloveskulären Leisten enthielten. Laminär konzentrisch gestaltete kristalloide Einschlüsse ließen darüber hinaus eine Paraproteinsynthese vermuten. Ferner fanden sich fingerabdruckartige, fädig geschichtete Eiweißkörper im Interstitium, die entfernt an Reinke-Kristalle erinnerten (Abb. 5).

Die von Laffargue u. Adechy-Benkoël (1972) aufgezählten ultrastrukturellen Merkmale der luteinisierten Granulosazellen stimmen hinsichtlich der Mitochondrien, dem an tubulovesikulären Schläuchen reichen endoplasmatischen Retikulum und den zahlreichen Fetttropfeninklusionen mit den Aspekten überein, die sich im DMBA-initiierten und gonadotrop promovierten Granulosazelltumor des Hamsters fanden. Die kristallinen Einschlüsse, die in Abb. 5 gezeigt werden, ähneln den von oben genannten Autoren gezeigten Korpuskeln in der Thekazelle des humanen Gelbkörpers.

Die Ultrastruktur des Gelbkörpers des unter die Haut verpflanzten Rattenovars zeigt nach Bagwell et al. (1976) ein regressives Bild, einen kleineren Golgi-Apparat und kleinere Mitochondrien als im orthotopen Rattenovar. Dagegen sind im Transplantat sowohl die Vakuolen wie auch die Lysosomen und kristallinen Einschlüsse häufiger als im orthotopen Rattenovar.

Zusammenfassung

Bisher hat die experimentelle Onkogenese noch kein leicht manipulierbares Modell des beim Menschen häufigsten bösartigen Ovarialtumors, des Karzinoms, geliefert. Sogenannte funktionelle Tumoren, z. B. Luteome, Granulosazelltumoren und Granulosathekome, sind dagegen in erheblicher Anzahl erzeugt worden seit dem im Jahre 1934 entdeckten Östrogenabbau in der Leber. Ein in die Milz eingepflanzter

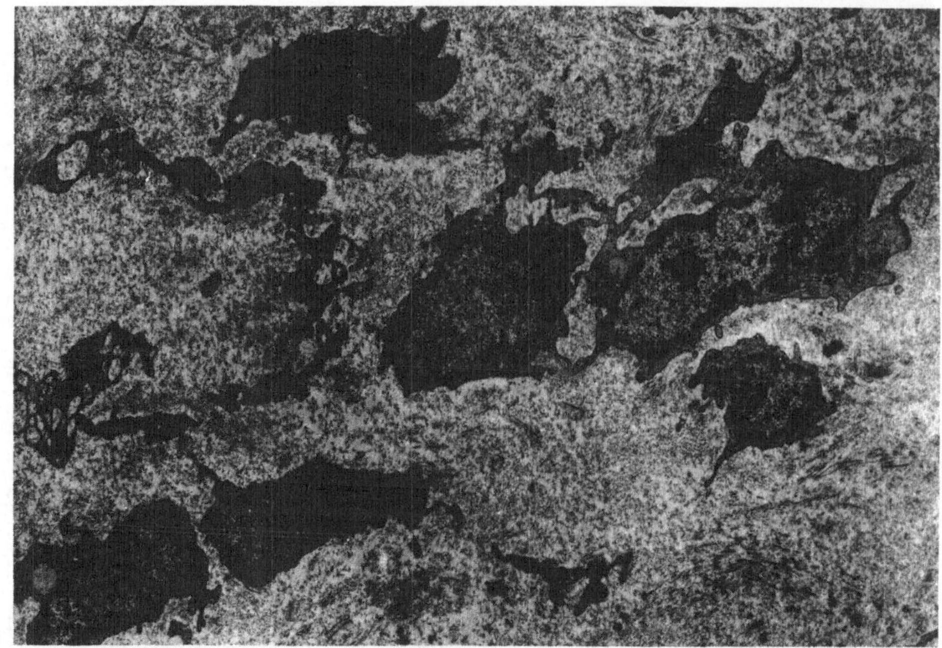

a

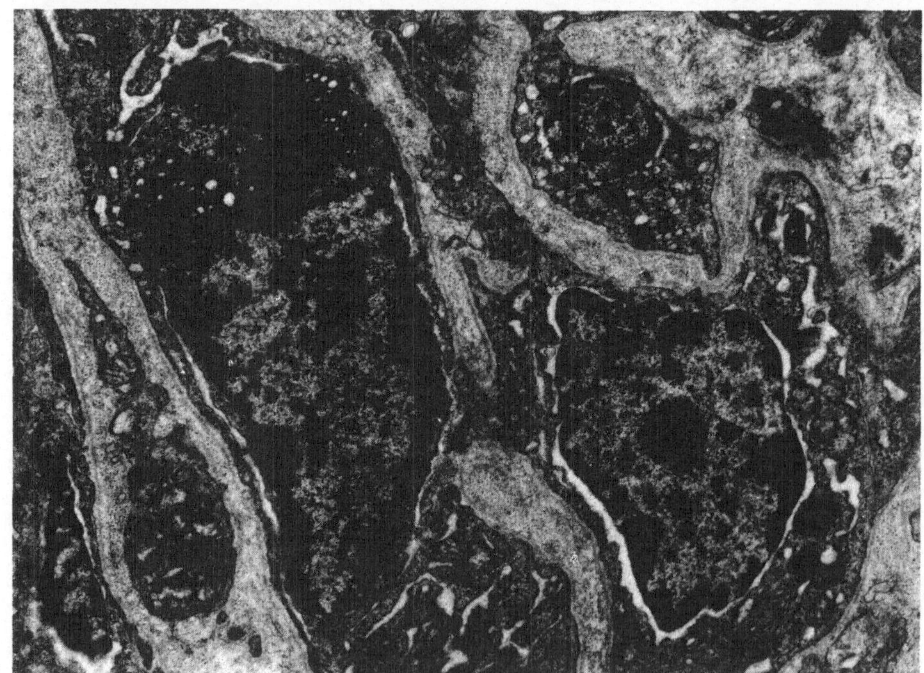

b

Abb. 4. a Fibromyoblastische Elemente mit wenig Organzellen im Zytoplasma. Milzovar Ratte (Llombart B.), ×2500; *b* enger Kontakt zwischen den Fibroblasten mit abgerundeten Kernen. Milzovar Ratte, ×3000; *c* Milzovar Ratte (Llombart B.). Luteinisierung mit aktiver Lipidvakuolenbildung, ×6000; *d* Lipidsynthese (Steroide). Aktivierung des Golgi-Apparates, ×10000; *e* intramitochondriale Proteinsynthese, ×12000

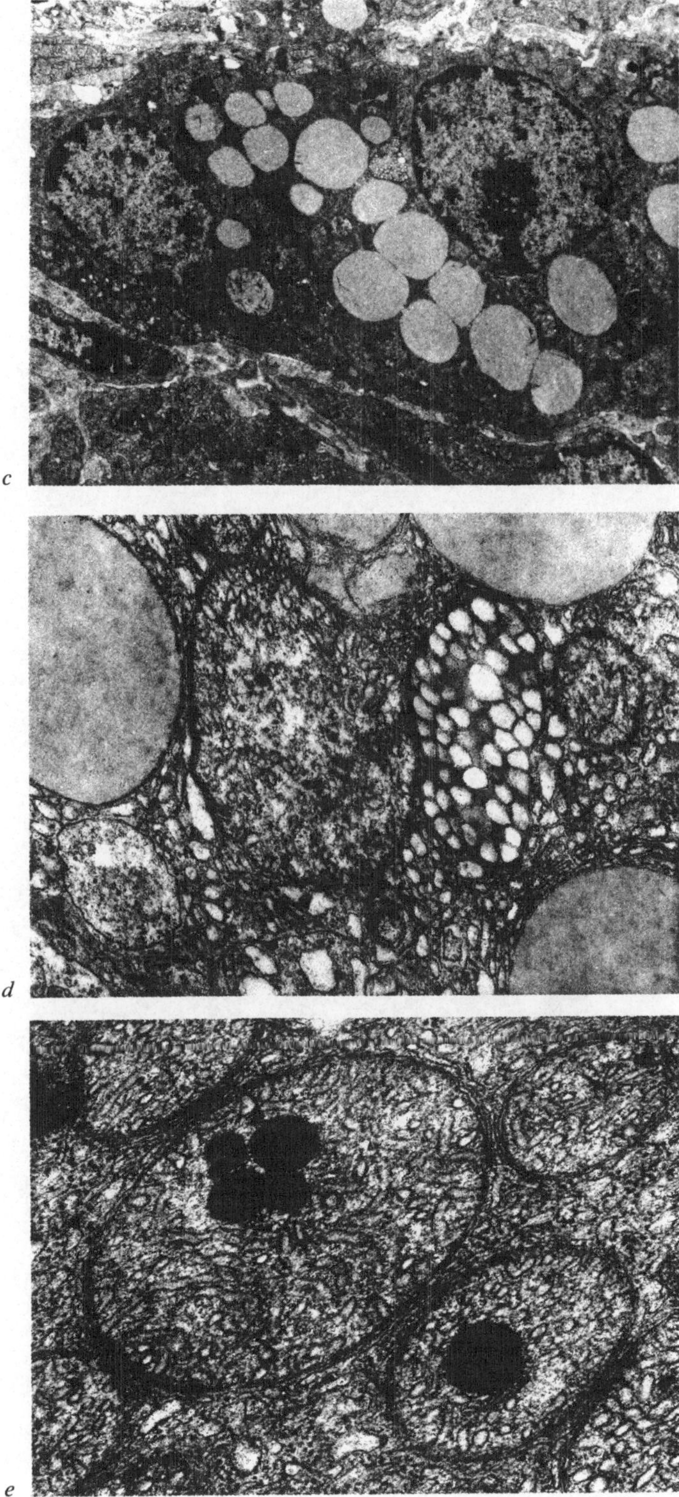
c
d
e

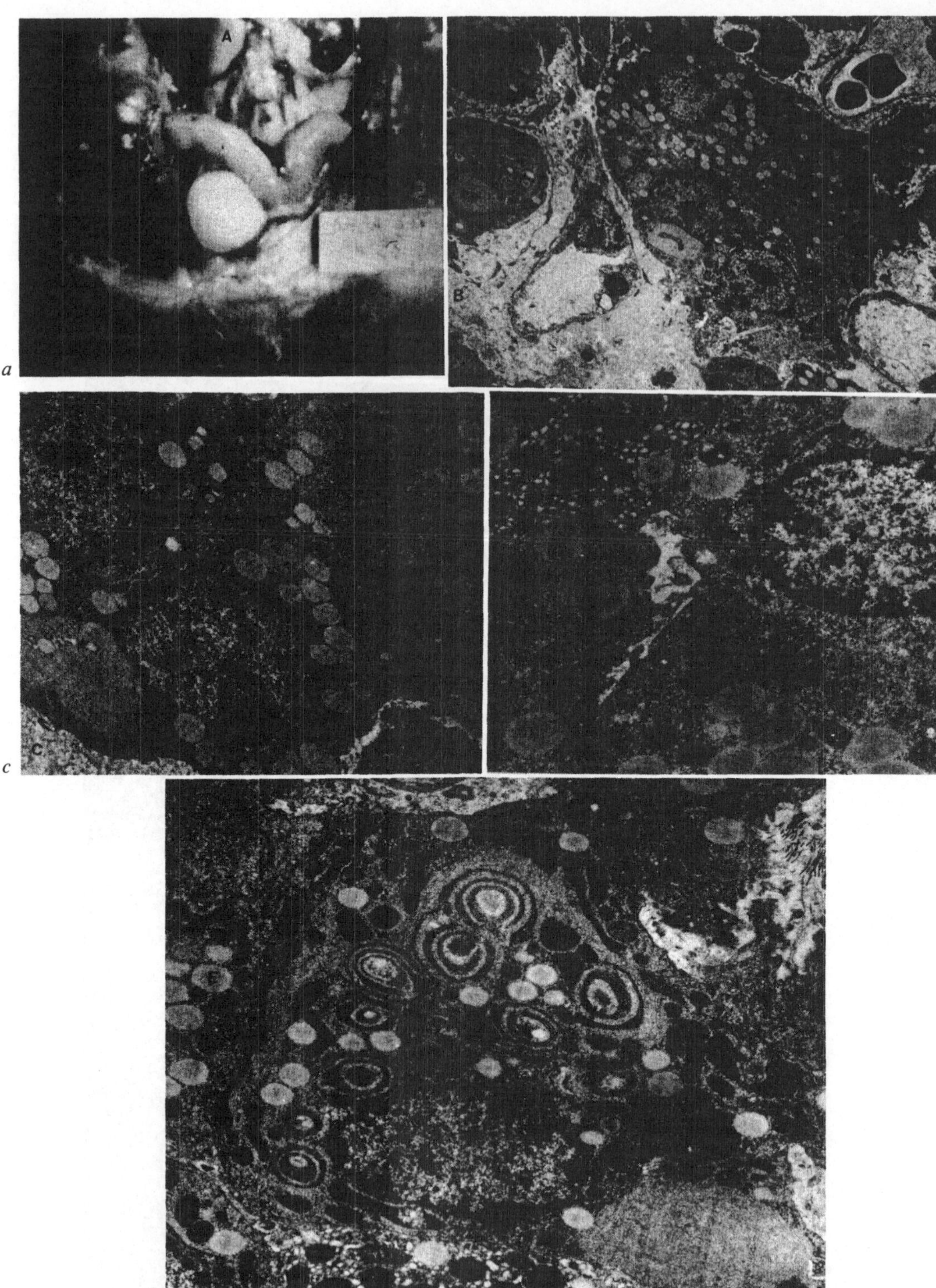

Abb. 5. *a* Unterbauchsitus, Hamster, G. Großer Granulosazelltumor, rechtes Ovar. *b* Granulosazelltumor, Hamster. Granulosazellen mit und ohne Luteinisierung (Vakuolen), enger Kontakt mit Kapillaren. ×3000; *c* vakuoläre Lipidsynthese. Dichte Mitochondrien. ×6000; *d* Ausschnitt aus *c*. Dichte Mitochondrien mit tubulovesikulären Leisten. ×8000; *e* Kristalloide Paraproteinsynthese, pseudolamellär. Rechts unten Reinke-Kristall-ähnliches Gebilde.

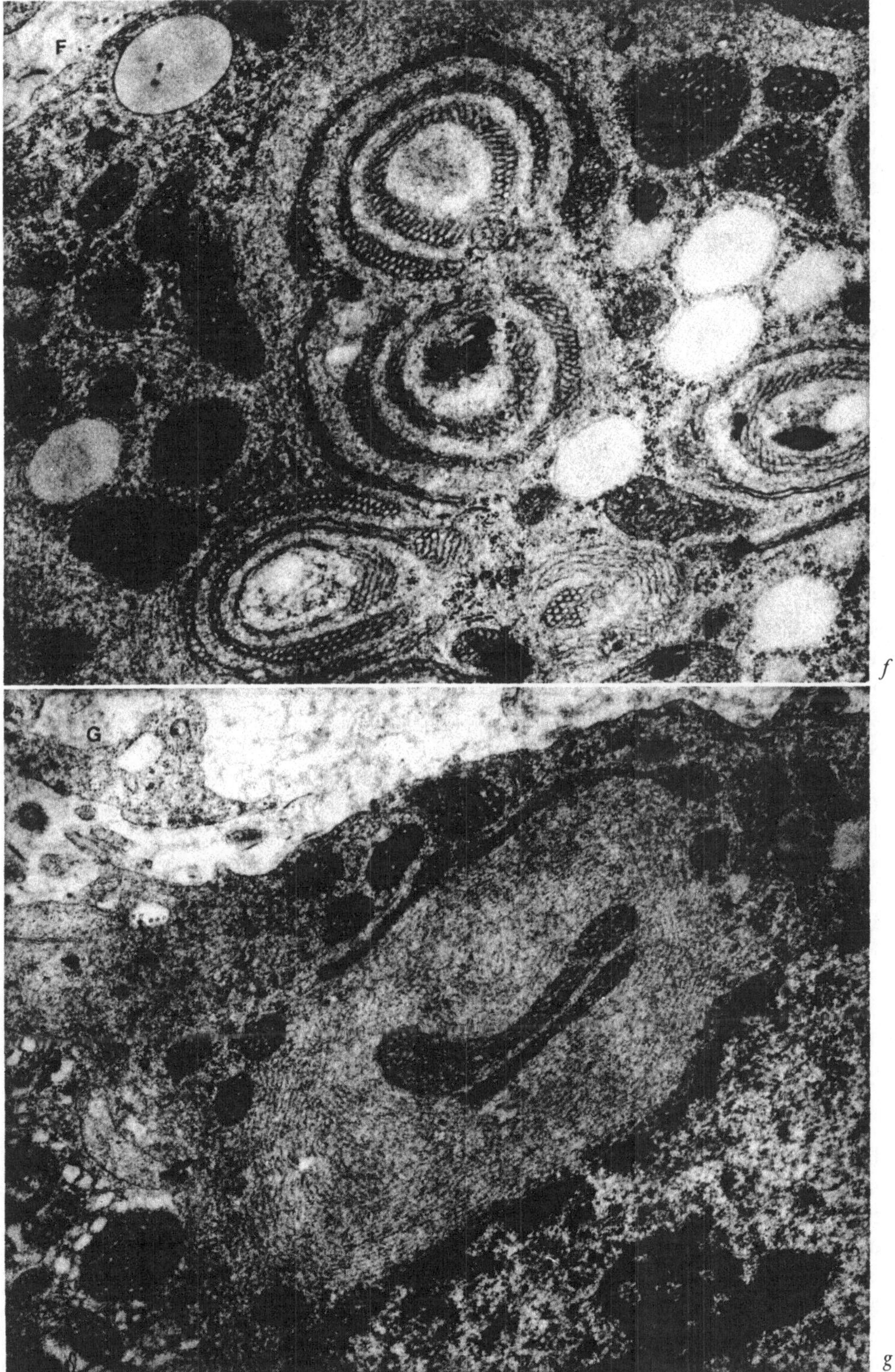

×10000; *f* Ausschnitt aus *e* zur Erkennung der in konzentrische Ringe umgewandelten Mitochondrien innerhalb der filamentös geschichteten kristalloiden Proteinsynthese; ×12000; *g* lamellär geschichtete Proteinsynthese in einer Zwischenzelle. Fingerabdruckähnliche Lagerung der Substanz. Darum Mitochondrien mit tubulären Leisten. ×13000

Eierstock des kastrierten Nagetiers wird durch gonadotrope Hormone seitens des Hypophysenvorderlappens stimuliert. Die Mechanismen des geschwulstigen Wachstums des Implantats wurden in zahlreichen Abhandlungen untersucht. Der alles beherrschende Faktor ist die Abwesenheit zirkulierenden Follikelhormons bis die Geschwulst die Autonomie erreicht hat und auch in kastrierte oder intakte Zweitwirte beiderlei Geschlechts verpflanzt werden kann. Östrogenbildung wurde histochemisch, histologisch und autoradiographisch in diesen Tumoren nachgewiesen. Aber auch im autonomen Stadium zeigen diese ursprünglich hyperplasiogenen Tumoren noch einen organoiden Aufbau und unterscheiden sich damit von dem anarchischen, infiltrativ destruktiven Wachstum mit Metastasierung eines echten Sarkoms oder Karzinoms.

Auch die durch Röntgenbestrahlung, Parabiose oder Teilkastration erzeugten Ovarialtumoren in Nagetieren benötigen zum Angehen und Wachstum die Stimulierung durch die FSH- und LH-Mehrsekretion. Auch das am häufigsten angewandte exogene Karzinogen DMBA wirkt in der Maus nur als kokarzinogener Faktor auf das Ovar: Tumoren entwickeln sich nicht, wenn ein funktionierendes Ovar wieder in das Tier eingepflanzt wird oder von der radiomimetischen Wirkung des DMBA geschützt worden ist. Teilkastration, Bestrahlung und DMBA zerstören die Follikel. Als Folge wuchern die Zellen der Membrana granulosa unter den luteinisierenden Stimuli des Hypophysenvorderlappens. Die spätere, an sich paradoxe Umwandlung in Granulosa-ähnliche Zellen ohne Luteinisierung wird als Dedifferenzierung der folgenden Zellgenerationen vorangegangenen Luteomzellen verstanden. In Ratten wirkt DMBA auf das Milzovar nur nach hoher und wiederholter Dosierung.

Sowohl lichtmikroskopisch wie auch ultrastrukturell zeigen die experimentellen Ovarialtumoren Übereinstimmung mit den Merkmalen der vom Stroma und Membrana granulosa sich herleitenden Zellen des normalen Nagetiereierstocks. Man sieht fibromyoblastenähnliche Elemente noch ohne Protein- oder Steroidsynthesezeichen. Mit der Luteinisierung nehmen dann lipidhaltige Vakuolen an Zahl zu. Das glatte endoplasmatische Retikulum tritt in den Vordergrund neben kristallinen Einschlüssen und vergrößerten Mitochondrien.

Summary

Experimental oncogenesis has not yet brought about a manageable model of the more frequent form of human ovarian malignancies, the carcinomas. So called functional tumors, e.g. luteomas, granulosa-cell tumors and granulosa-theca-cell tumors in contrast have been produced successfully and in considerable number since the inactivation of estrogen by the liver was discovered in 1934. An ovary implanted into the spleen of a castrated rodent is exposed to the uninhibited gonadotrophic growth-stimulus from the anterior pituitary gland. The conditions that would promote or prevent the development of these growths have been discussed in many papers. The overruling factor is the absence of any circulating estrogen until the growth has attained sufficient autonomy to grow independently without further gonadotrophic stimulation, allowing transplantation into castrated or intact secondary hosts of both sexes. Estrogen production has generally been proved in these tumors. But also at this stage the structure of these originally hyperplasiogenic tumors still does maintain an organoid pattern that distinguishes it from the dysregulatory anarchism, invasiveness or dissemination of a true sarcoma or carcinoma.

Ovarian tumors in rodents have also been produced by x-ray irradiation, parabiosis or partial castration; they all require the stimulation by uninhibited FSH and LH secretion in order to develop. Also the most frequently applied exogenic carcinogen DMBA acts in mice ovaries as a cocarcinogenic agent only: Tumors will not develop if a functioning ovary is reimplanted into the animal or has been protected from the radiomimetic action of the product. X-rays, DMBA and partial castration act by an initial destruction of follicles that is followed by the proliferation of stromal cells receptive to luteinizing stimuli from the anterior pituitary gland. The following paradoxical transformation into granulosa-like cells is understood as a proliferation of daughter-cells of dividing luteoma-cells. In rats, DMBA does only affect the splenic ovary after high and prolonged dosage.

Both by optical and electron-microscopy the experimentally produced functional ovary tumors resemble the morphology of the stroma and granulosa-derived cells of the normal ovary of the experimental rodent. One sees fibroblasts or fibromyoblast-like elements still without signs of protein-biosynthesis or steroid biosynthesis. Luteinizing changes go along with the appearance of lipoid containing vacuoles and increasing prominence of the agranulated endoplasmic reticulum. Crystalline inclusions may be found alongside of the activated Golgi-structures and swollen mitochondria with vesicular and tubular crests.

Literatur

1. Armuth V, Berenblum I (1979) Mechanism of ovarian carcinogenesis: Effect of 7,12-Dimethylbenz(α)anthracene administration on intrasplenic ovarian grafts in unilaterally ovariectomized C3HeB/Fe mice. JNCI 63:1047–1050
2. Bagheri SA, Boyer JL (1974) Peliosis hepatis associated with androgenic anabolic steroid therapy. A severe form of hepatic injury. Ann Intern Med 81:610–618
3. Bagwell JN, Chihal HJW, Peppler RD (1976) Fine structure of the corpus luteum of the autografted ovary in the rat. Cell Tissue Res 171:375–379
4. Bartók I, Mónus Z (1969) Peliosis hepatis. Neuere Beiträge zur Rolle hormonaler Faktoren. Zentralbl Allg Pathol 112:171–178
5. Biskind MS, Biskind GS (1944) Development of tumors in the rat ovary after transplantation into the spleen. Proc Soc Exp Biol Med 55:176–179
6. Brambell FWR, Parkes AS, Fielding U (1927) Changes in the ovary of the mouse following the exposure to X-rays. Proc Roy Soc Lond [Biol] 101:29, 95
7. Büngeler W, Dontenwill W (1959) Hormonell ausgelöste geschwulstartige Hyperplasien, hyperplasiogene Geschwülste und ihre Verhaltensweisen. Dtsch Med Wochenschr 84:1885–1894
8. Chopra S, Edelstein A, Koff RS, Zimelman AP, Lacson A, Neiman RS (1978) Peliosis hepatis in hematologic disease. J Am Med Wom Assoc 240:1153–1155
9. Deane HW, Fawcett DW (1956) Histochemical characteristics of intrasplenic ovarian transplants in gonadectomized rats. J Natl Cancer Inst 17:541–567
10. Dontenwill W, Squartini F (1966) Ovar. Tumoren II, Teil 13, Erzeugung von Krankheitszuständen durch das Experiment. Springer, Berlin Heidelberg New York, S 105–116

11. Furth J, Butterworth JS (1936) Neoplastic diseases occurring among mice subjected to general irradiation with X-rays. II Ovarian tumors and associated lesions. Am J Cancer 28:66
12. Gardner WU (1955) Development and growth of tumor in ovaries transplanted into the spleen. Cancer Res 15:109–117
13. Green JA (1957) Morphology, secretion and transplantability of 10 mouse ovarian neoplasms induced by intrasplenic ovarian grafting. Cancer Res 17:86–91
14. Hilfrich J (1973) A new model for inducing malignant ovarian tumors in rats. Br J Cancer 28:46–54
15. Hilfrich J, Mohr U (1972) Experimentelle Untersuchungen zur malignen Transformation sog. hyperplasiogener Ovargeschwülste (Milzovar) bei der Ratte. Verh Dtsch Ges Path (Tagung Graz) 56:532–535
16. Howell JS, Marchant June, Orr JW (1954) The induction of ovarian tumors with 9:10-Dimethyl-1:2-Benzanthracene. Br J Cancer 8:635–646
17. Ivankovic S (1969) Erzeugung von Genitalkrebs bei trächtigen Ratten. Arznm Forsch 19:1040–1041
18. Jull JW (1969) Mechanism of induction of ovarian tumors in the mouse by 7,12-Dimethylbenz(α)anthracene. VI. Effect of normal ovarian tissue on tumor development. JNCI 42:967–972
19. Klein M (1952) Ovarian tumorigenesis following intrasplenic transplantation of ovaries from weanling, young adult, and senile mice. JNCI 12:877–881
20. Krarup T (1969a) Oocyte destruction and ovarian tumorigenesis after direct application of a chemical carcinogen (9:10 DMBA) to the mouse ovary. Int J Cancer 4:61–75
21. Krarup T (1969b) Effect of 9,10 Dimethyl-1,2Benzanthracene on the mouse ovary. Ovarian tumorigenesis. Br J Cancer 24:168–186
22. Kuwahara I (1967) Experimental induction of ovarian tumors in mice treated with single administration of 7,12-Dimethylbenz(α)anthracene and its histopathological observation. Gan 58:253–266
23. Laffargue P, Adechy-Benkoël L (1972) Ultrastructure du corps jaune humain I. Ann Anat Pathol (Paris) 17:425–448
24. Li MH (1948) Malignant granulosa-cell tumor in an intrasplenic ovarian graft in a castrated male mouse. Am J Obstet Gynecol 55:316–320
25. Marchant J (1960) The development of ovarian tumors in ovaries grafted from mice pretreated with Dimethylbenzanthracene. Br J Cancer 14:514–518
26. Mardones E, Lipschutz A (1956) On the influence of cortisone on the evolution of tumoral growth in intrasplenic ovarian grafts in two strains of mice. Br J Cancer 10:517–526
27. McGiven AR (1970) Peliosis hepatis: case report and review of pathogenesis. J Pathol 101:283–285
28. Mühlbock O (1952) Neuere experimentelle Untersuchungen über die Genese der Ovarialtumoren, Geburtshilfe Frauenheilkd 12:289–301
29. Mühlbock O, Nie R van, Bosch L (1958) The production of oestrogenic hormones by granulosa cell tumors in mice. Ciba Found. Colloq Endocrinol 12:78–93
30. Myhre E (1964) Granulosacellesvulstenes histogenese. Nord Med 71:1–4
31. Ozols RF, Grotzinger KR, Young RC (1978) Murine ovarian cancer: A model for human disease. Proc Am Assoc Cancer Res 19:234
32. Schilling B v, Llombart Bosch A, Peydro-Olaya A (1979) Zum Einfluß des Dimethylbenzanthrazens (DMBA) auf Ovarialimplantate in der Milz kastrierter Ratten. Verh Dtsch Ges Pathol 63:667
33. Sekiya S, Endoh N, Kikiuczi Y et al. (1979) In vivo and in vitro studies of experimental ovarian adenocarcinoma in rats. Cancer 39:1108–1112
34. Silberberg M, Silberberg R, Leidler HV (1951) Effects of anterior hypophyseal transplants on intrasplenic ovarian grafts. Cancer Res 11:624–628
35. Vol'fson NI (1976) On the genesis of experimental granulosa-cell tumors of the ovary. Vopr Onkol 22:68–75

Neue Aspekte der Chemotherapie

Die Untersuchung von Tumorgewebe als Basis der Therapieplanung beim Ovarialkarzinom und ihre klinischen Konsequenzen

A. Pfleiderer, G. Teufel, W. Kleine, G. Meerpohl und M. Günther[1]

Eine Standardisierung der Therapie des Ovarialkarzinoms steht vor erheblichen Schwierigkeiten und führt immer wieder zu großen Enttäuschungen. Eine besonders große Vielfalt und das erfahrungsgemäß oft unerwartete Verhalten der malignen Tumoren des Ovars unter einer Standardtherapie zwingt zu einer Individualisierung der Behandlungsmaßnahmen. Den unterschiedlichen Verlauf der Erkrankung beim Ovarialkarzinom zeigen Krankengeschichten am besten.

Klinik des Ovarialkarzinoms und Krankheitsverlauf unter Standardtherapie

Fall 1: Die 44jährige Frau A. wurde im Juni 1979 wegen eines über das ganze Abdomen ausgedehnten Ovarialkarzinoms laparotomiert, und der Uterus, die Adnexe und das Netz entfernt. Bei der Operation blieb nur wenig Tumorgewebe zurück. Unter einer Chemotherapie mit Endoxan und 5-Fluorouracil fühlte sich die Patientin wohl, bis im März 1980 eine Pleurakarzinose auftrat. Mit Platinex, Adriblastin und Endoxan schien sich der Prozeß zunächst zu stabilisieren. Im Dezember 1980 kam es jedoch zu einer Progression des Pleuraergusses, und intraabdominal wurden rasch wachsende, große Tumoren tastbar. Trotz höherer Dosierung von Platinex und Endoxan war der Tumor intra abdomine so rasch progredient, daß diese Patientin im Mai 1981 verstarb.

Fall 2: Die 63jährige Patientin, Frau B., kam im Januar 1980 mit Ileusbeschwerden, einer ausgedehnten Pleura- und Peritonealkarzinose und großen verwachsenen Ovarialtumoren zur Aufnahme. Wegen des ausgedehnten Befundes war lediglich eine Netzteilresektion möglich. Unter Platinex, Adriblastin und Endoxan verschwand der Ileus, der Allgemeinzustand besserte sich, es kam zu einer Remission, und bei einer Relaparotomie im August 1980 konnten der Uterus, die Adnexe und das Netz mit wenigen Tumorresten entfernt werden. Die zytostatische Behandlung wurde noch 2 Monate fortgesetzt und anschließend eine Telekobaltbestrahlung des kleinen Beckens und der Paraaortalregion durchgeführt. Bei der letzten Kontrolluntersuchung im Januar 1982 war kein Hinweis auf ein Rezidiv gegeben.

Fall 3: Die damals 29jährige Frau C. kam im Oktober 1961 mit Aszites und massiver Peritonealkarzinose in die Klinik. Eine Inspektionslaparotomie ergab ein inoperables, seröses Ovarialkarzinom. Auf eine Endoxan-Dauerbehandlung und eine Großfeldbestrahlung mit nur 1500 RAD kam es zu einer Remission, so daß im Januar der Uterus und die Adnexe entfernt werden konnten und Tumorgewebe lediglich im Netz entlang des Querkolons zurückgelassen werden mußte. Bei der Netzresektion wenig später war kein Karzinom mehr zu finden. Wegen einer massiven Endoxanzystitis mußte 7 Monate später das Endoxan und damit jegliche Che-

1 Universitäts-Frauenklinik Freiburg, D-7800 Freiburg

motherapie abgesetzt werden. Unter einer konsequenten Therapie mit dem Gestagenpräparat Proluton Depot fühlte sich Frau C. wohl, bis im Januar 1970 bei der jetzt knapp 38jährigen Frau das Gestagen durch ein Östradiol-Gestagen-Sequenz-Präparat ersetzt wurde. Vier Monate später trat wieder Aszites auf, man konnte Tumoren im Abdomen tasten und bei einer Inspektionslaparotomie fand sich reichlich Tumorgewebe zwischen den Darmschlingen. Die erneute Endoxanbehandlung mußte wegen erheblicher Blasenblutungen schon nach 6 Wochen wieder abgebrochen werden, so daß als einzige Therapie jetzt das Gestagen Depostat gegeben wurde. Darunter kam es klinisch wieder zu einer Remission, die anhielt, bis im August 1973 die Depostat-Dosis wieder reduziert wurde: Palpatorisch und im Ultraschall fand sich ein Tumor in abdomine, der bei einer Erhöhung der Depostat-Dosis wieder verschwand. Die Gestagentherapie wurde deshalb unverändert bis April 1979 fortgesetzt, bis ein Astrozytom im Frontalhirn zur neurochirurgischen Intervention zwang. Die orale Therapie mit Clinovir 100 mußte nach 2 Monaten wegen Erbrechen abgesetzt werden. Seither war die Patientin ohne Gestagenbehandlung. Im Januar 1981 kam Frau C. erneut mit Aszites und einer Peritonealkarzinose zu uns. Wir konnten das Rezidiv eines hochdifferenzierten papillär-serösen Karzinoms laparoskopisch sichern und haben erneut mit Depostat begonnen.

Drei Ovarialkarzinome in weit ausgedehntem Stadium mit ganz verschiedenen Verläufen: Bei der ersten Patientin gelang die Operation primär. Trotz konsequenter Chemotherapie kam es aber zur nicht beeinflußbaren Progression. Bei der zweiten war der Tumor inoperabel, das Karzinom weiter ausgedehnt. Trotzdem trat unter einer ganz modernen Chemotherapie eine Totalremission ein. Die Patientin lebt rezidivfrei. Bei der dritten Patientin kam es unter einer niedrig dosierten Chemotherapie zur Remission. Sie konnte über 20 Jahre, entgegen allen Erfahrungen, trotz zahlreicher Rezidive ohne entscheidende Beschwerden, allein mit einer Gestagenbehandlung, am Leben erhalten werden. Für derart unterschiedliche Verläufe sind 4 Faktoren verantwortlich: 1) die Ausdehnung des Tumors, 2) seine Virulenz, 3) seine speziellen Sensibilitäten und 4) der Einfluß des Gesamtorganismus.

Die Erfassung der Ausdehnung des Tumors bei Therapiebeginn steht und fällt mit der Standardisierung und der Qualität der Erfassung der einzelnen Tumormetastasen im Rahmen der Primärdiagnostik und der Operation. Am schwierigsten erfaß- und standardisierbar und leider auch am wenigsten bekannt ist die Bedeutung des Organismus für das Wachstum des Tumors. Hier lassen sich höchstens das Alter und einige anamnestische Daten sicher erfassen. Über die viel beschworenen, aber bis heute kaum greifbaren immunologischen Parameter wissen wir jedoch fast nichts. Die Untersuchung des Tumorgewebes kann uns dagegen nicht nur über spezielle Sensibilitäten, sondern wahrscheinlich auch über die Virulenz des Tumors am meisten Auskunft geben. Sie wird so, zusammen mit der Erfassung der Ausdehnung, zur entscheidenden Basis für jede individuelle Therapie.

Morphologische Untersuchungen

Unsere eigenen Untersuchungen am Gewebe von Ovarialtumoren als Basis einer Therapieplanung haben sich auf 6 Parameter konzentriert: 1) den histologischen Typ, 2) den Differenzierungsgrad, 3) die Erfassung eines histochemischen Enzymmusters, 4) den Volm-Test, 5) den Steroidrezeptorstatus und 6) die Transplantation von Tumorgewebe auf die thymusaplastische Nacktmaus.

Der histologische Typ

Besonders viele und umfangreiche Daten sind über die Bedeutung des histologischen Typs für Verlauf und Prognose des Ovarialkarzinoms bekannt. Allerdings hat es erst eine Vereinheitlichung der Nomenklatur durch die FIGO und die WHO ermöglicht, hier zu größeren Zahlen und vergleichbaren Daten zu kommen. Über das international größte und homogenste Krankengut wird immer wieder aus dem Radiumhemmet von Oslo von Kolstad (1980) berichtet. Aus dieser Darstellung geht hervor, welche Bedeutung den verschiedenen histologischen Typen für die Prognose des Ovarialkarzinoms zukommt. Danach haben hellzellige, endometrioide und muzinöse Karzinome eine bessere Prognose als seröse und unklassifizierbare.

Tabelle 1. Ovarialkarzinom, Stadienverteilung und histologischer Typ. (Daten: Annual Report 1979, Vol. XVII)

	Stadium I [%]	Stadium II [%]	Stadium III [%]	Stadium IV [%]
Seröses Karzinom	48,3	52,9	51,9	45,1
Muzinöses Karzinom	23,5	11,1	10,5	7,6
Endometrioides und hellzelliges Karzinom	20,6	21,5	13,5	15,1
Unklassifizierbares Karzinom	7,6	14,4	24,1	34,5
Zahl	1199	1068	1719	830

Im neuesten, dem 17. Band des Annual Report von 1979, sind nach weitgehend einheitlichen Gesichtspunkten die Daten von 44 Kliniken aus der ganzen Welt zusammengestellt (Tabelle 1). Aus dieser Sammelstatistik über 4816 Fälle invasiver, epithelialer Ovarialkarzinome, die 1969–1972 behandelt worden waren, ergibt sich, daß die Verteilung der histologischen Typen auf die einzelnen Stadien unterschiedlich ist. Während zwar in allen Stadien etwa die Hälfte aller Karzinome dem serösen Typ zugerechnet wird, ist der muzinöse Typ bei auf das kleine Becken lokalisierten Karzinomen häufiger, das unklassifizierbare Karzinom dagegen bei den fortgeschrittenen Fällen. Auch endometrioide und hellzellige Karzinome scheinen unter den lokalisierten Karzinomen häufiger als unter den weiter ausgedehnten aufzutreten.

Bei 1199 Fällen, die als Stadium I gemeldet wurden, hat das muzinöse Karzinom mit einer Fünfjahresheilung von 77% die beste Prognose (Tabelle 2). Bekanntlich entspricht aber die Diagnose „Stadium I" beim Ovarialkarzinom in sehr vielen Fällen nicht der tatsächlichen Ausdehnung, da leider die diagnostischen Maßnahmen im Laufe der (ersten) Operation in sehr vielen Fällen ungenügend sind (Piver et al. 1978, u.a.). Die Erfassung einer Metastasierung ist wahrscheinlich bei muzinösen Karzinomen auch leichter möglich als bei anderen, insbesondere den unklassifizierbaren Karzinomen, da die muzinösen Karzinome eher lokalisiert zu wachsen scheinen und eher operabel sind.

Tabelle 2. Ovarialkarzinom, histologischer Typ und Prognose (Daten: Annual Report 1979, Vol. XVII)

	Stadium I		Stadium III	
	n	> 5 Jahre [%]	n	> 5 Jahre [%]
Seröses Karzinom	579	67,9	892	14,5
Muzinöses Karzinom	282	77,0	180	11,1
Endometrioides und hellzelliges Karzinom	247	63,6	232	7,8
Unklassifiziertes Karzinom und ohne Histologie	91	56,0	415	4,6

Betrachtet man die Fünfjahresheilung im Stadium III bei über 1700 Fällen, so scheint in diesem Stadium der seröse Typ vor dem muzinösen die beste Prognose zu haben. Allerdings sollte man sich auch hier wieder darüber klar werden, daß man bei einem muzinösen Karzinom im Stadium III eher einen Tumor findet, der sich primär radikal operieren (und eher heilen) läßt, während bei unklassifizierbaren Karzinomen die Zahl der Fälle sehr viel größer ist, bei denen man sich wegen absoluter Inoperabilität nur zu kleinen Eingriffen durchringen kann (Tabelle 3). Damit wird aber auch dem Histologen oft so wenig Gewebe zur Verfügung gestellt, daß eine sichere Klassifizierung unmöglich und damit häufiger die Diagnose „unklassifizierbares Karzinom" gestellt wird.

Wir haben hier an unserem Material zusammengestellt (Tabelle 3), wie häufig im Stadium III schon bei der ersten Laparotomie als Ausdruck besserer Operabilität der Uterus und beide Adnexe entfernt werden konnten. Bei uns waren die serösen und muzinösen Karzinome eher operabel als die unklassifizierbaren. Das gleiche gilt für die differenzierten gegenüber den undifferenzierten Karzinomen. So ist der histologische Typ nicht vom Ausbreitungsstadium und damit dem Wachstum innerhalb des Abdomens zu trennen.

Da es unser Ziel war, festzustellen, ob zwischen den einzelnen histologischen Typen Unterschiede in der Ansprechbarkeit auf eine Chemotherapie bestehen, haben

Tabelle 3. Beziehung des histologischen Typs und des Differenzierungsgrades zur Ausdehnung der ersten Laparotomie, Ovarialkarzinom Stadium III

	n=215 Hysterektomie bei Ersteingriff [%]
Seröses Karzinom (55%)	26
Muzinöses Karzinom (9%)	22
Endometrioides und hellzelliges Karzinom (21%)	21
Unklassifizierbares Karzinom (15%)	6
Hoch- und mitteldifferenziertes Karzinom (18%)	53
Entdifferenziert und unklassifizierbar (82%)	10

wir nur solche Fälle zusammengestellt, die primär nicht operabel, weit im Abdomen ausgedehnt waren und chemotherapeutisch behandelt wurden. In allen Fällen war eine Aussage über eine Remission relativ sicher möglich, da man Tumorgewebe gut tasten konnte. Dabei fanden wir zwischen serösen, endometrioiden und unklassifizierbaren Karzinomen keinen wesentlichen Unterschied (Tabelle 4) und nur bei der allerdings sehr kleinen Gruppe der muzinösen Karzinome ein schlechteres Ansprechen auf die Chemotherapie.

Tabelle 4. Histologischer Typ und Remission (Nur primär inoperable Ovarialkarzinome Stadium III und IV [Leber] mit Chemotherapie)

Histologischer Typ	N	Remissionsrate [%]
Serös	115	37
Muzinös	12	8
Endometrioid	31	42
Unklassifizierbar	69	39

Tabelle 5. Vergleich epitheliales Ovarialkarzinom und Granulosazelltumor. (Material der UFK Freiburg und Tübingen bis 1973)

	Vorkommen		> 3 Jahre lebend	
	Ovarialkarzinom %	Granulosazelltumor %	Ovarialkarzinom %	Granulosazelltumor %
I	8,9	59	89	92
II	28,3	19	57	57
III	40,5	20	16	25
IV	17,4	2	2	0
Ohne histologische Sicherung	4,7	0	0	0
Zahl		59		

Wahrscheinlich wird also die Prognose des Karzinoms durch den histologischen Typ dahingehend beeinflußt, daß unklassifizierbare Karzinome primär ausgedehnter, muzinöse primär lokalisierter wachsen. In ihrer Ansprechbarkeit auf eine Chemotherapie unterscheiden sie sich jedoch nur wenig, höchstens darin, daß muzinöse Karzinome schlechter anzusprechen scheinen.

Im allgemeinen nimmt unter den nichtepithelialen, malignen Ovarialtumoren der Granulosazelltumor eine gewisse Sonderstellung ein. 1973 haben wir das Material der Universitäts-Frauenklinik Tübingen und Freiburg zusammengestellt und es mit Ovarialkarzinomen aus den gleichen Kliniken verglichen (Tabelle 5) (Pfleiderer et al. 1976). Unter Berücksichtigung des Ausbreitungsstadiums entsprach die Dreijahresüberlebensrate der Granulosazelltumoren der der Ovarialkarzinome. Die Granulosazelltumoren zeichneten sich vor den Ovarialkarzinomen nur dadurch aus, daß mit fast 60% wesentlich mehr Fälle im Stadium I entdeckt werden. Zu ähnlichen Daten kamen jetzt auch Stenwig et al. (1979), die 78% im Stadium I und 4% im Stadium III mit einer Fünfjahresheilung von 22% fanden.

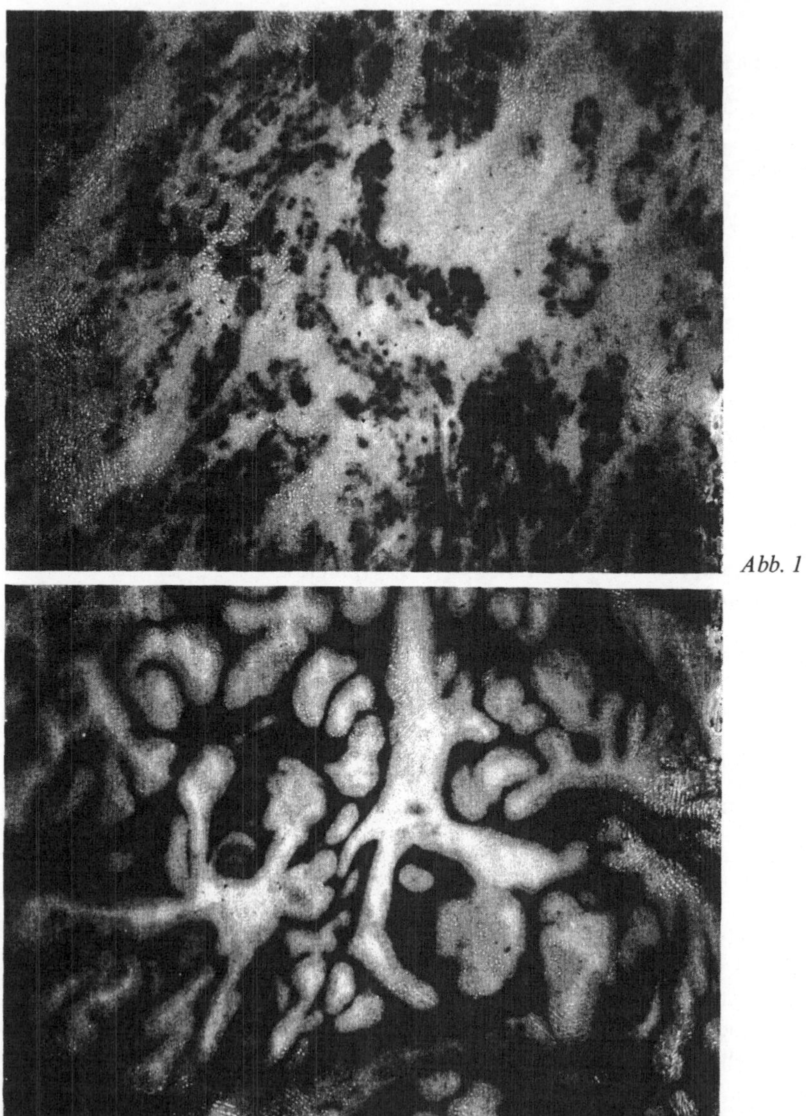

Abb. 1

Abb. 2

Abb. 1. Ovarialkarzinom: Tumorzellen mit positiver Reaktion auf alkalische Phosphatasen

Abb. 2. Ovarialkarzinom: Tumorzellen mit negativer, Bindegewebszellen mit positiver Reaktion auf unspezifische alkalische Phosphatasen

Differenzierungsgrad

In neuerer Zeit gewinnt das Grading wieder ein besonderes Gewicht (Barber et al. 1975; Day et al. 1975; Russell 1979; Ozols et al. 1969; Smith u. Day 1979). In allen Veröffentlichungen übereinstimmend ist die Prognose entscheidend vom Differenzierungsgrad abhängig. Eine gewisse Problematik ergibt sich allerdings beim Ovarialkarzinom dadurch, daß es schwierig ist, den Differenzierungsgrad seröser Karzinome festzulegen. Bis heute wechseln die Kriterien der Beurteilung des Differenzierungsgrades von Pathologe zu Pathologe so erheblich, daß viele auf eine solche Differenzierung sogar verzichten. Erst einheitliche Kriterien werden hier zu besseren Resultaten führen und es ermöglichen, die Daten verschiedener Kliniken miteinander zu vergleichen.

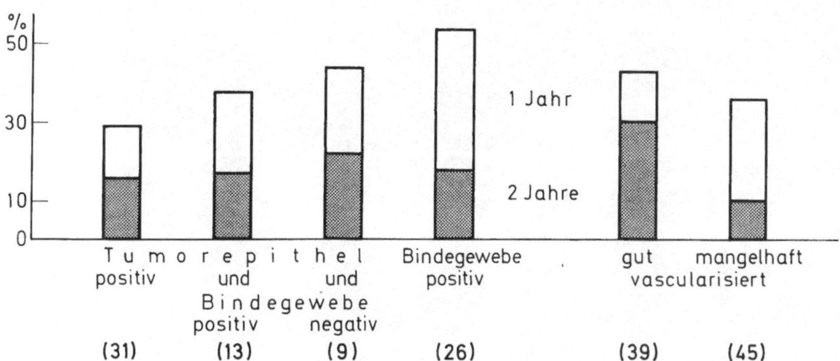

Abb. 3. Alkalische Phosphatase im Ovarialkarzinom, Überlebenszeit im Stadium III und IV

Was über histologische Typen ausgeführt wurde, gilt auch für den Differenzierungsgrad: Mit zunehmendem Ausbreitungsstadium steigt der Anteil der entdifferenzierten Karzinome (Smith u. Day 1979). So steht der Differenzierungsgrad ebenfalls in direkter Beziehung zur Ausdehnung des Tumors und ist damit ein Maßstab seiner Virulenz.

Histochemische Enzymverteilungsmuster

Vor etlichen Jahren sind wir der Frage nachgegangen, ob es mit enzymhistochemischen Methoden möglich wäre, nicht nur die einzelnen Ovarialkarzinome zu charakterisieren, sondern auch die Charakteristika dieser Enzymverteilungen für die Prognose des Ovarialkarzinoms heranzuziehen (Pfleiderer 1968; Pfleiderer et al. 1969, 1970; Pfleiderer et al. 1973).

So kann man Ovarialkarzinome, die sich durch eine positive Reaktion auf unspezifische alkalische Phosphatasen in den Tumorzellen auszeichnen (Abb. 1), von solchen unterscheiden, die in den Tumorzellen negativ, im Bindegewebe positiv reagieren (Abb. 2). Die Zusammenfassung einer Vielzahl von Fällen zeigt (Abb. 3), daß die Prognose mit zunehmender Reaktion im Bindegewebe besser wird. Das gleiche

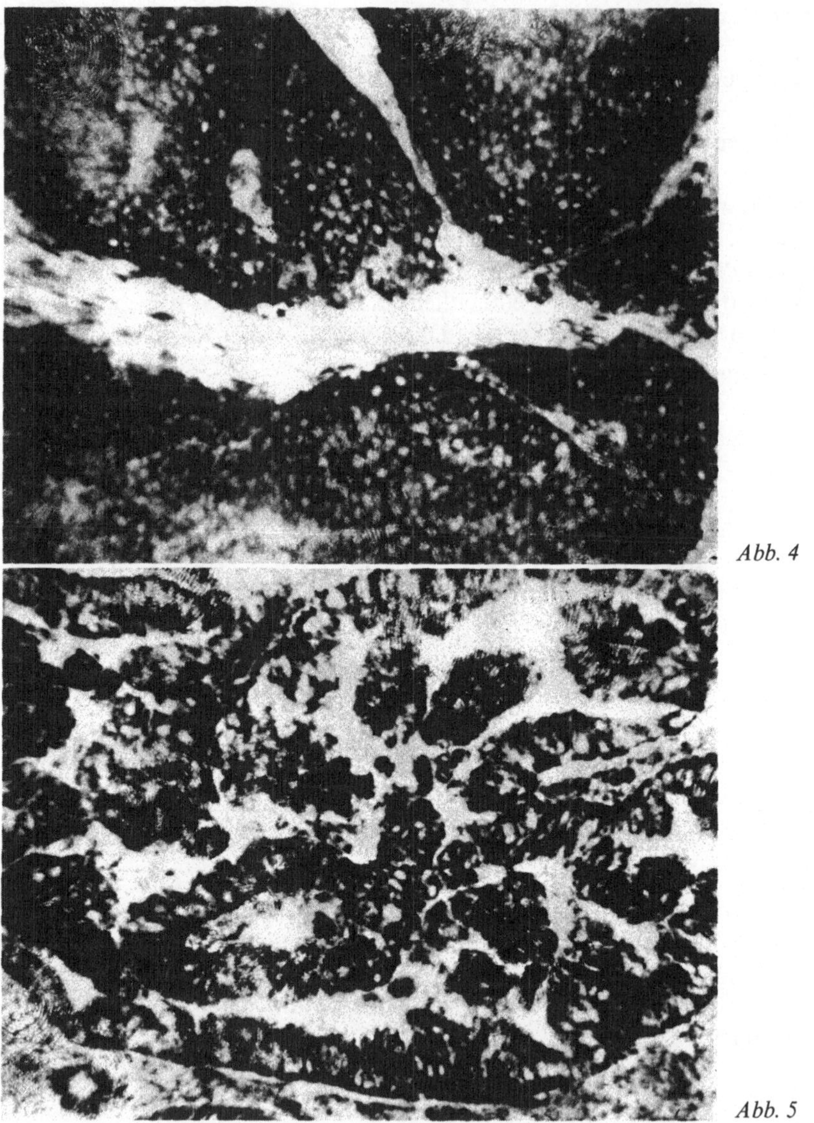

Abb. 4

Abb. 5

Abb. 4. Verteilung der Laktatdehydrogenase im Tumor: Relativ gleichmäßig, aber konzentriert auf die Randgebiete der großen Tumorareale

Abb. 5. Verteilung der Laktatdehydrogenase im Tumor: Konzentriert auf Einzelzellen oder Einzelzellkomplexe

scheint für die Vaskularisation zu gelten, die sich ebenfalls als ein Zeichen günstiger Prognose erweist (Pfleiderer u. Karzel 1970).

Als zweites Beispiel kann die Verteilung der Laktatdehydrogenase dienen, die sich einmal relativ gleichmäßig, aber konzentriert auf die Randgebiete der großen Tumorareale (Abb. 4), in anderen Fällen konzentriert auf Einzelzellen oder Einzelzellkomplexe findet (Abb. 5). Versucht man eine Aufteilung der Karzinome nach

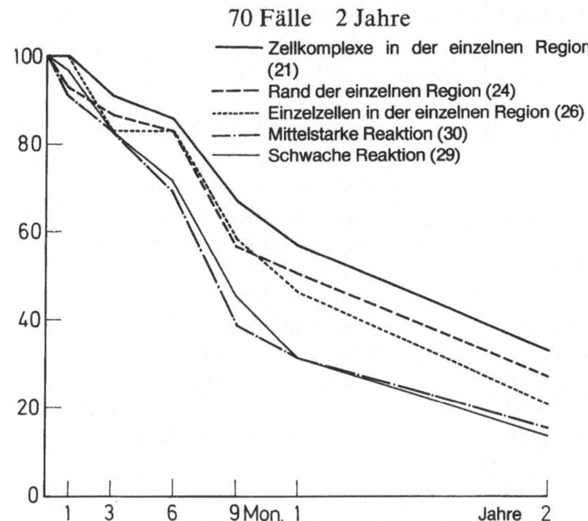

Abb. 6. Laktatdehydrogenaseverteilung im Tumor und Überlebensrate

solchen Enzymverteilungsmustern, so lassen sich gewisse Verteilungsmuster herausarbeiten und in ihrer prognostischen Bedeutung unterscheiden (Abb. 6) (Pfleiderer 1970).

Die Methode ist jedoch mühsam und hat letztlich nicht das gehalten, was wir erwartet haben, da die Befunde schlecht standardisierbar und kaum in Maß und Zahl auszudrücken waren, umfangreiche Gewebsuntersuchungen an vielen Stellen nötig machte und kein Vergleich mit dem Ursprungsgewebe des Karzinoms, dem Zölomepithel, möglich war.

Funktionelle und biochemische Untersuchungen

Alle diese klassischen morphologischen Methoden werden heute in zunehmendem Maße durch biochemische oder funktionelle Meßmethoden ergänzt und ersetzt.

Sensibilitätstest nach Volm

Von den heute viel diskutierten Methoden zur Tumortestung (Wright et al. 1957; Limburg u. Krahe 1964; Tanneberger u. Bacigalupo 1967; Wüst u. Matthes 1970; Mattern et al. 1972, 1975; Volm et al. 1974, 1979; Bastert 1976; Bastert et al. 1975, 1976; Possinger et al. 1976; Salmon et al. 1978; Teufel et al. 1979; Teufel 1979; KSST 1980) konnten wir im Rahmen einer kooperativen Studie (Tabelle 6) den Kurzzeittumortest nach Volm in seiner Anwendbarkeit, besonders beim Ovarialkarzinom, untersuchen (KSST 1980).

Bei diesem Test wird der Einbau von Nukleinsäurepräkursoren, Uridin bzw. Thymidin, sowie die Hemmung ihres Einbaus bei Tumorzellen durch Zytostatika gemessen. Beide Parameter korrelieren mit der Proliferation des Tumors (Volm et al. 1974, 1979). Nach den vorliegenden Erfahrungen lassen sich mit dem Kurzzeit-

Tabelle 6. An der Studie beteiligte Institutionen und Mitglieder

Kooperative Studie: Sensibilitätstestung von Tumoren (KSST)		
Heidelberg	Deutsches Krebsforschungszentrum	K. Goerttler, J. Mattern, M. Volm, K. Wayss, E. Weber
Frankfurt	Frauenklinik der Universität	G. Bastert, H. Schmidt-Matthiesen
Freiburg	Frauenklinik der Universität	A. Pfleiderer, G. Teufel
Hamburg	Frauenklinik der Universität	M. Albrecht, G. Trams
Heidelberg	Frauenklinik der Universität	M. Kaufmann, F. Kubli
Mainz	Frauenklinik der Universität	R. Kreienberg, F. Melchert
Tübingen	Frauenklinik der Universität	J. Neunhoeffer
Ulm	Frauenklinik der Universität	G. Geier, R. Schuhmann
Frankfurt	Zentr. der Biol. Chemie der Univ.	H. J. Hohorst
Münster	Medizinische Klinik der Universität	G. Segeth, G. Wüst
Heidelberg	Krankenhaus Rohrbach	P. Drings, M. Kleckow, I. Vogt-Moykopf

tumortest zytostatikaresistente Tumoren von wahrscheinlich zytostatikasensiblen trennen.

Das Prinzip der Methode besteht darin, daß frisches Tumorgewebe sofort mechanisch zerkleinert und zu einer Einzelzellsuspension aufgearbeitet wird (Tabelle 7). Die Suspension wird 2 h mit Adriamycin oder aktiviertem Endoxan (4-Hydroperoxycyclophosphamid) inkubiert. Anschließend werden die entsprechenden Nukleinsäurepräkursoren ^{3}H-Uridin (Adriamycin) oder ^{3}H-Thymidin (4-Hydroperoxycyclophosphamid) zugesetzt und eine weitere Stunde inkubiert. Dann wird der Versuch abgebrochen und der überschüssige Nukleotidpräkursor ausgewaschen. Die Einbaurate der Tumorzellen wird im Beta-Counter in CPM gemessen. Die Hemmung des ^{3}H-Uridineinbaus durch Adriamycin bzw. des ^{3}H-Thymidineinbaus durch 4-Hydroperoxycyclophosphamid wird in Prozent des Kontrollwertes der unbehandelten Tumorzellsuspension angegeben. Dadurch fallen evtl. Fehler durch einen unterschiedlichen Anteil toter Zellen, Unterschiede im Nukleotidpool und Laborunterschiede weg. Auch Zählfehler entfallen.

Tabelle 7. Prinzip der Sensibilitätstestung (Volm u. a., KSST)

→ Frisches Tumorgewebe

▼

→ Einzelzellsuspension

▼

2 h Inkubation mit Zytostatika
(z. B. Adriamycin, 4-Hydroperoxycyclophosphamid u. a.)

1 h Inkubation mit Nukleotid-Präkursoren
(z. B. ^{3}H-Thymidin, ^{3}H-Uridin)

→ Messung im Beta-Counter

→ Ergebnis: Einbaurate (in CPM)
Hemmung durch Zytostatika in % der Kontrolle

Die verschiedenen Tumoren sind durch unterschiedlich hohe Einbauraten gekennzeichnet (Tabelle 8). So weisen Ovarialkarzinome häufiger höhere Einbauraten auf als Korpus- und Zervixkarzinome. Hohe Einbauraten finden sich am häufigsten in Tumorzellen aus Aszites oder Pleuraergüssen. Das Gewebe gutartiger oder sog. Borderline-Tumoren des Ovars zeigt dagegen keine höheren Einbauraten. Das gleiche gilt für Korpus- und Zervixkarzinome (Teufel 1979).

Die Höhe des Einbaus von Uridin und Thymidin in Tumorzellen der Ovarialkarzinome steht in direkter Beziehung zur Hemmbarkeit durch Zytostatika einerseits und der klinischen Remissionsrate andererseits. Auch der autoradiographisch

Tabelle 8. Nukleotideinbau in Einzelzellsuspensionen (UFK Freiburg, G. Teufel 1979)

Tumor	n	^{3}H-Uridin	
		> 600 CPM [%]	> 1000 CMP [%]
Ovar Aszites/Pleura	36	56	36
Solider Tumor	103	30	18
Gutartiger/Borderline-Tumor	10	10	0
Corpus uteri	46	13	0
Cervix uteri	55	5	2

Tabelle 9. Beziehung: Einbauhemmung – Klinischer Verlauf (Ergebnisse KSST 1980)

System: Uridineinbau/Adriamycin 10^{-1} mg/ml
Getestet: Solides Tumorgewebe
62 inoperable Ovarialkarzinome Stadium III und IV
Therapie: Endoxan + 5-Fluoruracil

Hemmung in % der Kontrolle	Klinisch		
	Progression	No change	Remission
> 55% = resistent	21 (66%)	10 (31%)	1 (3%)
< 55% = sensibel	8 (27%)	6 (20%)	16 (53%)

ermittelte ^{3}H-Index und die Zahl der Mitosen im histologischen Präparat lassen sich mit dem Einbau korrelieren (Teufel 1979; Pfleiderer et al. 1979).

Hauptteil der Studie war die Testung von Tumorgewebe, das bei der ersten diagnostischen Laparotomie inoperabler, weit ausgedehnter Ovarialkarzinome gewonnen worden war. Der klinische Verlauf unter einer einheitlichen Therapie mit Endoxan und 5-Fluoruracil wurde abschließend mit dem Testergebnis verglichen (Tabelle 9) (KSST 1980; Kaufmann et al. 1979; Melchert et al. 1979; Pfleiderer u. KSST 1979; Teufel u. KSST, 1981). Die für die Klinik wichtige Voraussage einer Resistenz des Tumors gegen Zytostatika ist, nach unseren Erfahrungen, mit dem Adriamycin-Uridin-System am besten möglich. Die beste In-vivo/In-vitro-Korrelation ergibt sich bei einer Sensibilitätsgrenze von 55%, wobei ein Uridineinbau >55% des Kontrollwertes unter Adriamycin 10^{-2} mg/ml als Chemoresistenz bezeichnet wird. Von den 32 im Test resistenten Fällen zeigte nur eine Frau unter der Behandlung mit Endoxan und 5-Fluoruracil eine Remission, während 21 progredient waren und 10 ein No-change-Verhalten zeigten. No-change-Fälle haben 2 Aspekte: Einerseits kennen wir so langsam wachsende Tumoren, daß innerhalb einer Beobachtungszeit von 5 Monaten, bei der Schwierigkei solcher Beurteilungen beim Ovarialkarzinom, kein sicheres Wachstum registriert werden kann, andererseits gibt es zweifelsohne Fälle, bei denen jede entscheidende Verlangsamung des Tumorwachstums als Erfolg der Chemotherapie gewertet werden muß. So zeigten von 30 im Test sensiblen Fällen 16 eine Remission und 6 kein weiteres Wachstum (Tabelle 9).

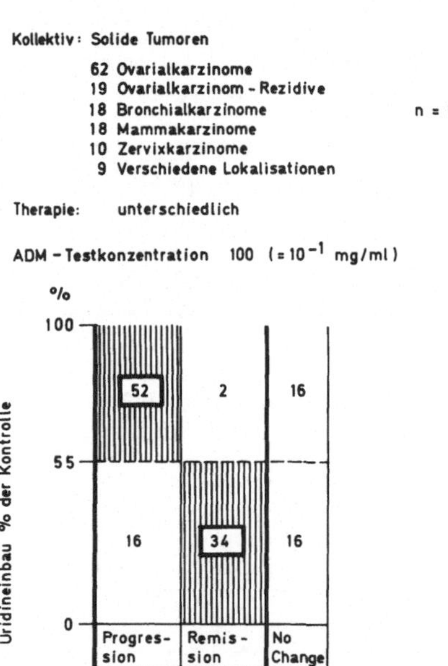

Abb. 7. Darstellung des Gesamtergebnisses der kooperativen Studie zur Sensibilitätstestung von Tumoren (KSST): In-vitro-/in-vivo-Korrelation des Verlaufs von 136 soliden Karzinomen verschiedener Lokalisation, unter unterschiedlicher Chemotherapie mit dem Ergebnis der Uridineinbauhemmung durch Adriamycin in der Konzentration 10^{-1} mg/ml in % der Kontrolle. Sensibilitätsgrenze 55% des Kontrollwertes

Faßt man alle Fälle zusammen, bei denen ein klinischer Verlauf mit dem Testergebnis verglichen werden konnte (Abb. 7), so ergibt sich das gleiche Resultat: Die *Resistenz* gegen alle bis dahin untersuchten Zytostatika bei den verschiedensten Karzinomen läßt sich mit hoher Sicherheit, die *Sensibilität* gegenüber Zytostatika nur in ca. 75% voraussagen (KSST 1980). Hier erhebt sich die Frage, ob es möglich ist, durch eine konsequentere, besser ausgewählte oder eine aggressivere Chemotherapie größere Erfolge zu erzielen.

Natürlich fragt man sich nach der praktischen Auswirkung dieser Sensibilitätstestung im klinischen Alltag. In der Universitäts-Frauenklinik Freiburg haben wir in den Jahren von 1975–1980 57 Ovarialkarzinome des Stadiums III getestet und primär behandelt. Bezeichnet man, wie dies in der Studie geschehen ist, alle die Untersuchungsproben, die auf unter 55% gehemmt werden, als „sensibel“, die anderen als „resistent“, so erwiesen sich in unserem Beobachtungsgut 31 als sensibel und 26 als resistent. Alle Patientinnen wurden in gleicher Weise mit Zytostatika behandelt. Die Sensiblen überlebten im Mittel 17,9, die Resistenten nur 8,8 Monate. Von den 31 Sensiblen lebten nach 1 Jahr noch 15, von den 26 Resistenten nur noch 7. Bis zum April 1981 waren von den Sensiblen noch 15 mit einer mittleren Überlebensdauer von 26,1 Monaten ohne Rezidiv, von den Resistenten nur 8 und zusätzlich nur 8,3 Monate lang am Leben, so daß hier wahrscheinlich bei der Mehrzahl der Fälle noch mit einem Rezidiv gerechnet werden kann (Tabelle 10). Diese Erfahrung zeigt, daß die Testaussage folgende Prognose erlaubt: Ovarialkarzinome mit hohem Uridineinbau bzw. starker Hemmbarkeit des Uridineinbaus durch Adriamycin, proliferieren wahrscheinlich rasch und sollten an sich schlechtere Überlebenschancen haben. Durch die Chemotherapie haben aber gerade sie bessere Aussichten auf Rezidivfreiheit und Überleben als die mit geringem Einbau und geringerer Proliferation.

Tabelle 10. Sensibilitätstestung nach Volm und klinischer Verlauf (UFK-Freiburg 1975 – 1980) (nach A. Pfleiderer, G. Teufel, M. Günther). Epitheliale Ovarialkarzinome Stadium III, Uridin-Einbauhemmung durch Adriamycin 10^{-1} mg/ml in % der Kontrolle

	Sensibel (< 55%)	Überlebens-zeit	Resistent (> 55%)	Überlebens-zeit
Zahl	31	17,9 Mo ± 15,8	26	8,8 Mo ± 8,8
> 1 Jahr lebend	15 (48%)		7 (27%)	
Progression/Rezidiv	16 (52%)	9,3 Mo ± 5,0	18 (69%)	9,0 Mo ± 8,9
Rezidivfrei	15 (48%)	26,1 Mo ± 19,0	8 (31%)	8,3 Mo ± 9,2

Neben grundsätzlichen Einwänden gegen die Volm-Methode (Seeber u. Schmidt 1977) sind einige Einschränkungen aufzuführen, die sich aus dem Ablauf der Studie ergaben. Dazu gehört, daß die Resistenzgrenze retrospektiv aufgrund der klinischen Erfahrung festgelegt wurde und daß der behandelnde Arzt, der auch das Ansprechen des Tumors zu beurteilen hatte, das Ergebnis der In-vitro-Testung kannte. Bei der schwerwiegenden Entscheidung, bei einem ausgedehnten Ovarialkarzinom auf eine Chemotherapie zu verzichten, und der Bedeutung, die sich daraus für die gesamte Chemotherapie ergibt, erscheint es nötig, die Testuntersuchung durch eine retrospektive Untersuchungsreihe an einer größeren Fallzahl noch einmal zu überprüfen. Eine erneute Studie zu diesem Problem, unterstützt vom BMFT, läuft deshalb im Mai 1981 an.

Erfahrungen und Ergebnisse mit einer modernen Kombinationschemotherapie des Ovarialkarzinoms

Erstes Ziel dieser Studie muß sein, an einem nicht bekannten Krankengut noch einmal zu überprüfen, ob sich die Aussage „Resistenz" für die gesamte Chemotherapie bestätigt und ob sich neuere Chemotherapieformen mit Adriamycin und Cis-Platin nur bei den sensiblen Karzinomen als wirksamer erweisen. Während mehrere Publikationen aus der neueren Zeit (Bruckner et al. 1979) zu beweisen scheinen, daß die Kombinationsbehandlung der Monotherapie mit einem Alkylans überlegen ist und Kombinationen mit Cis-Platin und Adriamycin wesentlich bessere Resultate bringen, zeigt ein Vergleich der Ergebnisse von Young et al. (1978) mit eigenen Erfahrungen (Pfleiderer, 1981) und Publikationen von Omura u.a. (1981) sowie von Klaasen et al. (1979), daß diese Aussage keinesfalls als gesichert gelten kann. Die hohen Remissionsraten, über die u.a. Bruckner et al. (1978), Ehrlich et al. (1979), Vogl et al. (1979), Alberts et al. (1979) berichtet haben, sind allerdings beeindruckend.

In dieser Studie sollen deshalb Endoxan allein mit einer Kombination von Endoxan und Cis-Platin (80–100 mg/m²) und einer solchen mit Adriamycin, Endoxan und Cis-Platin (50 mg/m²) verglichen werden (Tabelle 11).

Seit August 1979 haben wir 42mal bei einem ausgedehnten Ovarialkarzinom als Primärtherapie in über 230 Behandlungszyklen die Kombination Endoxan, Adriamycin und Cis-Platin eingesetzt. Dabei lief am 15. 4. 1981 bei 12 Patientinnen die Therapie noch. 5 von 42 hatten die Therapie wegen ihrer Nebenwirkungen abgebrochen, 3 sind interkurrent verstorben, keine von ihnen an einem Nierenversagen oder an einer Herzinsuffizienz. Von 21 Patientinnen, die mehr als 6 Therapiekurse erhalten hatten, leben 15 ohne Progression (Tabelle 12).

Bei 28 Patientinnen wurde die Behandlung wegen eines Stadiums III und IV in der Zeit zwischen 2. 8. 1979 und Dezember 1980 begonnen (Tabelle 13). Von diesen 28 Patientinnen zeigten 5 eine Vollremission, 10 eine Teilremission, 1 ein No-change und überraschenderweise nur 2 eine Progression. 9 Patientinnen leben ohne Progression mit primär so weitgehend entferntem Tumor, daß die Diagnose Remission nicht mehr gesichert werden kann. 5 Patientinnen sind verstorben, davon 2 interkurrent und 3 am Karzinom.

Tabelle 11. Kooperative Studie zur prospektiven Überprüfung der Volm-Testung

Ovarialkarzinome Stadium III und IV Primärtherapie Operation so radikal wie möglich	Testung nach Volm mit festgelegter Grenze Ergebnis verschlossen an die Zentrale	Randomisation unter Berücksichtigung des Stadiums, der Tumorresektion und der Klinik	Endoxan-PTT (hochdosiert) PTT-ADM-Endoxan Endoxan

Tabelle 12. Primärtherapie des Ovarialkarzinoms mit Cis-Platin (UFK-Freiburg i. Br., Stand 15. 4. 1981)

Zahl der Therapiezyklen	Fälle	Lebend ohne Progression	Mit Progression lebend	†	† intercurrent	Weitere Therapie abgelehnt	Therapie erst 1981 begonnen
– 3	13				2	2	9
4 – 5	8		2			3	3
6 – 10	21	15	2	3	1		
219 Zyklen							
PTT-ADM-CYT	42	15	4	3	3	5	12
12 Zyklen							
PTT-CYT hochdosiert							

Tabelle 13. Ovarialkarzinom Stadium III und IV, Primärtherapie mit PTT-ADM-CYT (UFK-Freiburg, Therapiebeginn 2. 8. 79 – 31. 12. 1980, Stand 15. 4. 81)

Zahl	Vollremission	Teilremission	Nicht beurteilbar, da Tumor entfernt, keine Progression	No change	Progression	† intercurrent
28	5	10	9	1	2	1

Tabelle 14. Ovarialkarzinom Stadium III und IV (UFK-Freiburg 1966 – 1980)

	n	† bis 4 Wochen [%]	> 6 Monate [%]	> 1 Jahr [%]	> 3 Jahre [%]	lebt noch [%]
Endoxan 1966 – 1971	95	12	65	33	2	0
Endoxan 1972 – 1975	66	9	67	36	15	9
Ifosfamid 1973 – 1974	21	19	62	38	19	5
Endoxan 5-Fu 1975 – 1979	103	12	61	46	20	22
Plat-ADM-End. ab 2. 8. 79	34	9	71	> 32	–	65

Vergleicht man dieses Resultat mit unseren bisherigen Erfahrungen, so ist ein vorsichtiger Optimismus erlaubt (Tabelle 15): Seit Anfang August 1979 behandeln wir mit der Kombination Platinex, Adriblastin und Endoxan. Bis Ende 1980 waren bei uns 34 Patientinnen mit einem Stadium III und IV, von denen allerdings nur 28 diese Kombination bekommen haben. Mit 71% (Tabelle 14) ist die Sechsmonateüberlebensrate recht gut. Da bei einer großen Zahl von Patientinnen der Therapiebeginn noch nicht 1 Jahr zurückliegt, ist die Zahl der Einjahresüberlebensrate noch geringer als in allen anderen Gruppen. Mit 65% leben aber heute noch so viele Patientinnen, die meisten von ihnen ohne Hinweis auf Tumorwachstum, daß eine Besserung des Ergebnisses erwartet werden kann. Die Übersicht zeigt auf der anderen Seite aber, daß wir weit davon entfernt sind, schon heute sagen zu können, daß die Kombinationstherapie mit Cis-Platin und Adriamycin allen anderen Therapien weit überlegen sei. Daraus ergibt sich, daß diese modernen Therapieformen in einer kooperativen Studie konsequent einer klassischen Therapie mit Endoxan gegenübergestellt werden müssen.

Weniger hoffnungsvoll hat sich bei uns der Einsatz von Cis-Platin und Adriamycin bei der Behandlung des trotz Chemotherapie mit Endoxan und 5-Fluorouracil progredienten oder rezidivierenden Ovarialkarzinoms erwiesen (Tabelle 15). Seit 1978 erhielten 39 solcher Patientinnen 169 Zyklen Platinex, Adriblastin und Endoxan und 6 Zyklen Endoxan und Platinex hoch dosiert. Dabei haben nur 3 Patientinnen, d.h. 8% eine Remission erlebt, die bis jetzt auch nur 2mal 4 Monate und 1mal 12 Monate anhält. Die mittlere Überlebenszeit beträgt 7,5 Monate. Sie ist bei unter der Chemotherapie progredienten Karzinomen mit 6,3 Monaten ungünstiger als bei Rezidiven nach Remission durch Chemotherapie mit fast 10 Monaten. Vergleicht man diese mit Platinex erzielten Ergebnisse mit denen, mit vorausgehenden Che-

Tabelle 15. Cis-Platin bei der Therapie des progredienten und rezidivierenden Ovarialkarzinoms. 39 Fälle, behandelt mit 169 Zyklen PTT-ADM-END und 6 Zyklen PTT-END hochdosiert, davon 3mal Remission (4/4/12 Monate)

Überlebenszeit	7,5 ± 5,4 Monate
26mal progredientes Karzinom	6,3 ± 4,6 Monate
13mal Rezidiv nach Remission	9,8 ± 6,4 Monate
24mal 3 oder mehr Zyklen PAC	8,8 ± 4,9 Monate

Tabelle 16. Sekundärtherapie bei progredientem oder rezidivierendem Ovarialkarzinom nach Operation und Endoxan oder Endoxan + 5-FU

Therapie	n	Mittlere Überlebenszeit (Monate)	† bis 1 Monat	> 1 J	80/81 noch lebend
Klassisch/nichts Endoxan/Gestagene	43	7,16	6	9	1
Ifosfamid	27	6,85	10	5	1
ADM-Mono	37	7,16	8	9	1
ADM-Kombination	29	8,93	4	6	7
PTT-ADM-CYT	22	8,45	2	8	7

motherapiemaßnahmen bei progredienten oder rezidivierenden Ovarialkarzinomen, so läßt sich leicht erkennen, daß wir hier noch nicht von Erfolgen sprechen können (Tabelle 16). Auch mit der Kombination Platinex/Adriamycin und Endoxan war es uns nicht möglich, bei einem unter der Chemotherapie progredienten Karzinom bessere Resultate zu erzielen als mit Adriamycinkombinationen.

Bestimmung des Steroidhormonrezeptorstatus

Eine Bestimmung der Hormonrezeptoren bei Ovarialkarzinomen liegt nahe, da sich diese Karzinome wie das des Endometriums vom Müller-Epithel ableiten und über günstige Erfolge einer Gestagentherapie auch beim Ovarialkarzinom berichtet wurde.

De Gregorio, Erz, Fuchs, Kleine sowie Teufel (Meerpohl et al., 1981) haben in den vergangenen Jahren bei 56 Ovarialkarzinomen Rezeptorbestimmungen nach der Charcoal-Methode ausgeführt. Dabei ergab sich, daß 15, d.h. ca. 27%, sowohl Östrogen- als auch Progesteronrezeptoren in einer Konzentration von mehr als 10 fmol enthielten (Tabelle 17).

Im allgemeinen gilt der Rezeptorgehalt als gutes Maß der Differenzierung und damit der Prognose. Beim Ovarialkarzinom läßt sich das nicht ohne weiteres bestätigen (Tabelle 18). Im Gegenteil, die rezeptorpositiven Ovarialkarzinome hatten sogar die schlechteste mittlere Überlebenszeit. Allerdings sind 3 dieser Frauen schon sehr früh interkurrent verstorben, so daß diesem Ergebnis keine endgültige Aussage zukommt. Faßt man andererseits die 25 Progesteronrezeptor-positiven Karzinome zusammen, so sind von diesen 3, von den 31 Progesteronrezeptor-negativen aber 11 am Karzinom verstorben.

Natürlich lag es nahe anzunehmen, daß es sich bei den rezeptorpositiven Ovarialkarzinomen um endometrioide Karzinome handelt. Zu unserer Überraschung war das nicht der Fall. Wir konnten im Vorkommen der Rezeptoren zu keinem der verschiedenen malignen Ovarialtumoren eine nachweisbare Korrelation finden. Selbst bei unklassifizierbaren Karzinomen waren Rezeptoren nachweisbar (Tabelle 19).

Tabelle 17. Die Bestimmung von Östrogen- und Progesteronrezeptoren in malignen Ovarialtumoren

Charcoal-Methode, + = > 10 fmol

Rezeptorstatus	ER + PgR +	ER∅ PgR +	ER + PgR∅	Er∅ PgR∅
Zahl	15	10	16	15

Tabelle 18. Hormonrezeptorstatus und Prognose des Ovarialmalignoms

Rezeptorstatus	ER + PgR +	ER∅ PgR +	ER + PgR∅	ER∅ PgR∅
Zahl	15	10	16	15
Lebt ohne Rezidiv	7	7	6	7
mit Rezidiv	2	1	4	2
Tod am Karzinom	3	0	6	5
interkurrent	3	2	0	1
Überleben in Monaten	7,3 ± 6,0	13,2 ± 11,6	10,4 ± 8,0	10,9 ± 8,7

Tabelle 19. Maligne Ovarialtumoren und Hormonrezeptorstatus

Rezeptorstatus	ER + PgR +	ER∅ PGR +	ER + PgR∅	ER∅ PgR∅
Zahl	15	10	16	15
Histologischer Typ				
Serös	10	4	12	7
Mucinös	1	2	2	1
Endometrioid	–	1	–	2
Hellzellig	–	–	2	–
Unklassifiziert	2	–	–	1
Granulosazelltumor	–	1	–	1
Keimzelltumor	1	1	–	1
Sarkom	–	–	–	1

Transplantation auf thymusaplastische nu/nu-Mäuse

Mit der thymusaplastischen Nacktmaus haben wir seit 1978 (Bastert, Fortmeyer und Schmidt-Matthiesen) ein Versuchstiermodell zur Verfügung, auf dem transplantierte Ovarialkarzinome erstaunlich gut wachsen (Teufel et al. 1981).

Kleine (1980), Kleine et al. (1979, 1980) und Schwörer (1979) haben bis Ende des Jahres 1980 von 118 Ovarialkarzinomen Tumorgewebe in die Milchleiste jeweils mehrerer Mäuse transplantiert. Dabei zeigte sich (Kleine et al., 1981); Teufel et al. 1981), daß die einzelnen Tumortransplantate auch auf verschiedenen Mäusen die gleichen Wachstumseigenschaften aufwiesen, daß aber diese Wachstumseigenschaften für jeden Tumor unterschiedlich waren (Teufel et al. 1981). 31% der transplantierten Ovarialkarzinome ließen innerhalb von 11 bis 13 Wochen kein oder fast kein Wachstum erkennen (Tabelle 20). Bei 29% war das Wachstum so gering, daß weder weitere Transplantationen noch Therapieversuche angestellt werden konnten. Bei 37% der Ovarialtumorfälle war jedoch das Wachstum so rasch, daß schon bald weitere Transplantationen möglich wurden (Tabelle 20). Insgesamt fällt also auf, wie unterschiedlich das auf jeweils verschiedenen Mäusen reproduzierbare Wachstum der Ovarialkarzinome auf der Maus ist.

Unterteilt man nach Ovarialkarzinomen, die kein oder nur ein geringes Wachstum zeigten, und solchen, die ein stärkeres Wachstum erkennen ließen und eine

Tabelle 20. Wachstum maligner Ovarialtumoren auf der nu/nu-Maus (UFK Freiburg 1978–1980)

Tumorgröße nach 11 – 13 Wochen in mm²		Zahl	[%]
Kein Wachstum	– 9	36	31
	10 – 25	34	29
	26 – 50	25	21
	51 – 100	9	
	101 –	10	16
Nicht beurteilbar		4	
Summe		118	

Tabelle 21. Wachstum des Tumortransplantats und Prognose des Ovarialmalignoms (UFK Freiburg 1978 – 1980)

	Kein Wachstum, in 12 Wochen < 25 mm², nicht passagierbar		Wachstum > 25 mm², 2. oder weitere Passagen	
Zahl	52	Δ Monate	49	Δ Monate
Lebt ohne Rezidiv	26 (50%)	11,5 ± 9,0	8 (16%)	9,4 ± 5,7
mit Rezidiv	8 (15%)	18,9 ± 8,9	9 (18%)	13,0 ± 9,5
Tod am Karzinom	14 (27%)	9,7 ± 8,5	29 (59%)	10,1 ± 7,1
interkurrent	4 (8%)	2,3 ± 2,9	3 (6%)	1,3 ± 2,3

Tabelle 22. Wachstum des Tumortransplantats und Prognose des Ovarialmalignoms

	Kein Wachstum, in 12 Wochen < 10 mm², nicht passagierbar	Sehr rasches Wachstum, in 12 Wochen > 70 mm², oder > 3 Passagen
Zahl	16	16
1. 4. 81 am Leben	9	0
Mittlere Überlebenszeit in Monaten	15,8 ± 15,0	10,9 ± 7,0

Tabelle 23. Wachstum des Tumortransplantats und Histologischer Typ (UFK Freiburg 1978 – 1980)

	Kein Wachstum, in 12 Wochen < 25 mm², nicht passagierbar	Wachstum > 25 mm², passagierbar
Zahl epitheliale Karzinome	49	48
Serös	30	30
Muzinös	7	1
Endometrioid	2	7
Hellzellig	1	0
Unklassifizierbar	2	5
Granulosazelltumor	3	1
Dysgerminom	1	0
Teratoma malignum	0	1
Karzinom im Dermoid	1	2
Sarkom	2	1

Passagierbarkeit ermöglichten, so ergaben sich überraschende Unterschiede (Tabelle 21): Während von den 52 nicht oder langsam auf der Maus wachsenden Ovarialkarzinomen noch 26 Patientinnen ohne Rezidiv leben, sind es von den 49 rasch wachsenden nur 8. Auch von den mit Rezidiv Lebenden ist die mittlere Überlebenszeit bei den rasch wachsenden geringer als bei den langsam wachsenden.

Greift man nur solche Karzinome heraus, die in den Jahren 1978 und 1979 transplantiert wurden, also eine Beobachtungszeit der Patientin über mindestens 16 Monate ermöglichen, und stellt zusätzlich nur solche ohne Wachstum den besonders rasch (> 70 mm² in 12 Wochen) wachsenden gegenüber, so sind das jeweils 16 Fälle in beiden Gruppen (Tabelle 22). Von den 16 Patientinnen mit auf der Maus nicht oder langsam wachsenden Karzinomen waren am 1. 4. 1981 noch 9 mit einer mittleren Überlebenszeit von jetzt schon 15,8 Monaten am Leben. Von den 16 Frauen, deren Transplantate ein extrem rasches Wachstum zeigten, lebt heute dagegen keine mehr. Ihre mittlere Überlebenszeit liegt mit 10,9 Monaten schon jetzt eindeutig niedriger.

Natürlich lag es nahe, das Wachstum des Tumortransplantats nach den verschiedenen histologischen Typen zu analysieren. Dabei fanden sich nur relativ geringe Unterschiede (Tabelle 23). Bemerkenswert ist trotzdem, daß muzinöse Karzinome auf der Maus in der Regel nicht oder sehr langsam, endometrioide dagegen meist rasch wachsen. Das gleiche gilt für unklassifizierbare Karzinome. Bei den sog. seltenen malignen Ovarialtumoren ist die Fallzahl noch zu gering, um hier Aussagen zu machen, wenn auch eine gewisse Tendenz mit den allgemeinen klinischen Erfahrungen übereinzustimmen scheint.

Interessant ist, daß sich bisher zwischen dem Wachstum auf der Maus und dem Ergebnis des Volm-Tests im Uridin-Adriamycin-System keine Beziehung feststellen ließ (Tabelle 24). Diese Erfahrung weist darauf hin, daß der Faktor Hemmbarkeit des Uridineinbaus und damit wohl die Proliferationsrate für das Wachstum auf der Maus nicht so entscheidend verantwortlich sein kann, wie man das anzunehmen geneigt ist.

Auch zwischen dem Hormonrezeptorstatus und dem Wachstum auf der Maus ergaben sich keine eindeutigen Beziehungen, wenn auch eine gewisse Tendenz nicht zu übersehen ist. (Tabelle 25). So scheinen Karzinome mit Östrogen- und besonders mit Progesteronrezeptoren schlechter, solche ohne Östrogen- und Gestagenrezeptoren besser auf der Maus zu wachsen.

Tabelle 24. Wachstum des Transplantats und Ergebnis der Volm-Testung

	Kein Wachstum	Wachstum $> 25\ mm^2$
Resistent	15	20
Sensibel	16	16

Tabelle 25. Wachstum des Tumortransplantats und Hormonrezeptorstatus 1978 – 1980

	kein/schlechtes Wachstum	eindeutiges Wachstum
	31	21
ER+ PgR+	10	5
ERø PgR+	5	2
ER+ PgRø	9	6
ERø PgRø	7	8

Tabelle 26. Endometriumkarzinom, klinischer Verlauf und Wachstum auf der nu/nu-Maus

	n	lebend		lebend →		†
		> 6 Mo	> 1 Jahr	ohne Rezidiv	mit Rezidiv	
Kein Wachstum						
Wenig Wachstum	25	20	14	22	0	3
Gutes Wachstum	16	6	6	4	4	8

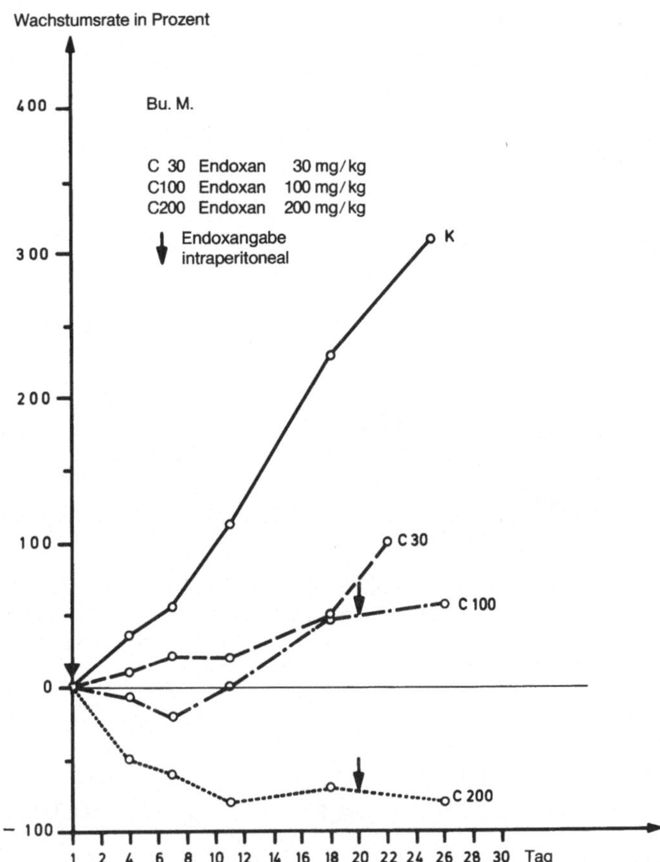

Abb. 8. Einfluß verschiedener Dosen von Cyclophosphamid (Endoxan®) auf das Wachstum eines Ovarialkarzinoms, transplantiert auf die nu/nu-Maus. Ausgang 100 mm^2 große Tumoren: Der Erfolg der Zytostatikatherapie ist dosisabhängig. Auch bei niedriger Dosis zeigt sich ein Erfolg (Kleine et al. 1980)

Alles das weist darauf hin, daß zwischen dem Wachstum des Tumors auf der Maus und dem klinischen Verlauf des Karzinoms bei der Patientin eine auffallende Beziehung besteht, die sich weder allein mit dem histologischen Typ, noch mit der Hemmbarkeit des Uridineinbaus und damit möglicherweise der Proliferation, noch mit dem Rezeptorstatus eindeutig erfassen läßt.

In diesem Zusammenhang verdient Erwähnung, daß für das Endometriumkarzinom ähnliche Gesichtspunkte zu gelten scheinen (Tabelle 26). So haben Kleine und Teufel auch hier entsprechende Beziehungen feststellen können (Pfleiderer, 1981). Während von 25 Endometriumkarzinomen, deren Transplantat auf der Maus kaum ein Wachstum zeigte, nur 3 Patientinnen gestorben waren, waren von den 16 mit raschem Wachstum auf der Maus bei Abschluß der Untersuchung nur noch 4 rezidivfrei und 8 schon tot.

Unabhängig von dieser Korrelation ermöglicht die Transplantation auf die Maus verschiedene Therapieversuche am Transplantat. Dazu gehören die Möglich-

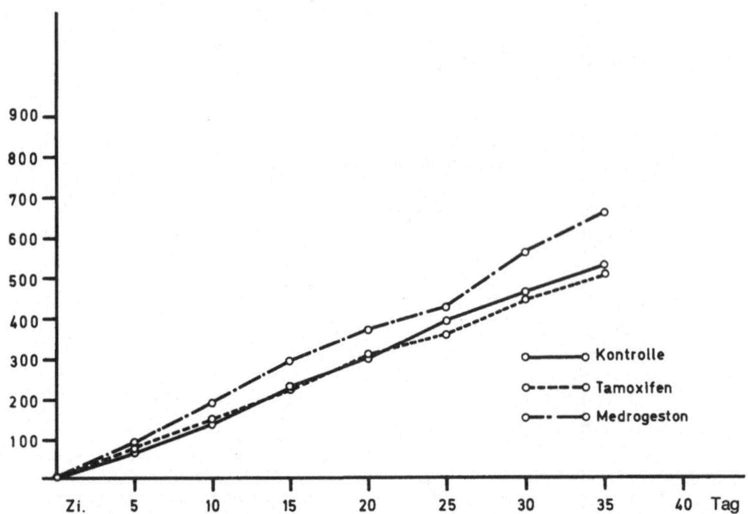

Abb. 9. Einfluß einer Hormontherapie auf das Wachstum eines Östrogen- und Progesteronrezeptor-positiven Ovarialkarzinoms, transplantiert auf die nu/nu-Maus. Ausgang 100 mm² große Tumoren. Weder das Antiöstrogen Tamoxifen noch das Gestagen Medrogeston beeinflussen das Wachstum dieses Tumors (Kleine et al. 1981)

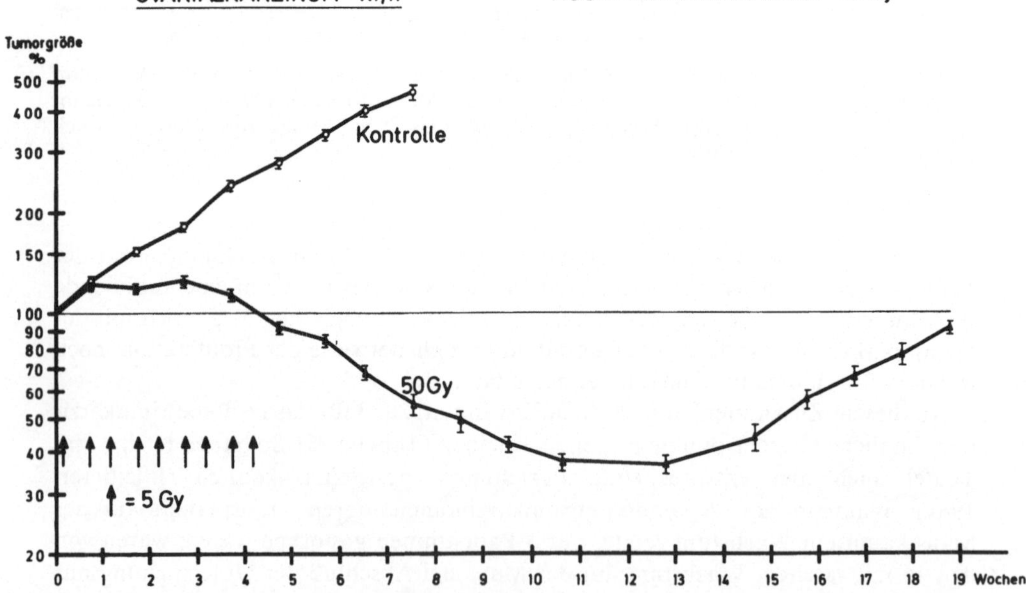

Abb. 10. Einfluß einer Hochvoltbestrahlung mit 50 GY auf ein Ovarialkarzinom, transplantiert auf die nu/nu-Maus: Unter einer Dosis von 50 GY bildet sich der Tumor zurück, ohne ganz zu verschwinden. Nach 12 Wochen setzt ein erneutes Wachstum ein (Kleine et al. 1981)

keiten, verschiedene Zytostatikakombinationen und Hormonpräparate, aber auch den Erfolg einer Strahlentherapie zu vergleichen und auszutesten. So läßt sich z.B. zeigen, daß der Erfolg einer Chemotherapie von der Dosis abhängt (Abb. 8) (Kleine et al. 1980, 1981). Interessant sind die Beobachtungen von Kleine et al. (1981). daß bei einem steroidrezeptorpositiven Ovarialkarzinom (Abb. 9) weder mit Medrogeston noch mit Tamoxifen eine signifikante Verlangsamung des Tumorwachstums zu erzielen war. Das könnte damit erklärt werden, daß bei Ovarialkarzinomen in der Mehrzahl der Fälle das Vorkommen von Östrogen- und Gestagenrezeptoren in der Tumorzelle nicht mit der Proteinsynthese und damit der Zellproliferation so gekoppelt ist, wie dies bei Mamma- und Endometriumkarzinomen bekannt ist. Schließlich lassen sich auch am Transplantat die typischen Bedingungen einer Strahlentherapie simulieren. Kleine, Stange, Wrzodek und Ladner (Kleine 1980, 1981) haben neben anderen Karzinomen auch auf die Maus transplantierte Ovarialkarzinome einer Telekobaltbestrahlung unterzogen. Bei einer Bestrahlung des Tumors mit 50 GY (Abb. 10) findet sich in dem angeführten Beispiel eine Tumorregression, die aber nur von vorübergehender Dauer ist und schließlich zum Rezidiv führt. Andere Ovarialkarzinome verhalten sich anders: Beobachtet wurde eine Ausheilung, aber auch eine raschere Progression.

So eröffnet die Transplantation und die Untersuchung menschlichen Tumorgewebes auf der thymusaplastischen Nacktmaus verschiedene Möglichkeiten, von denen schon der Vergleich des Wachstums des Transplantats mit dem klinischen Verlauf Bedeutung hat. Daneben besteht die Möglichkeit einer vergleichenden Testung von Zytostatikakombinationen, die Untersuchung neuer Zytostatika und die einer Strahlenwirkung sowie die Untersuchung des Hormoneinflusses bei bekanntem Rezeptorgehalt. Nachteilig sind jedoch die aufwendige Tierhaltung und Tierzucht sowie die Tatsache, daß erst nach 12–14 Wochen Dauer erste Ergebnisse vorliegen können. Ein Routinetest auf eine Zytostatikasensitivität aller Ovarialkarzinome verbietet sich schon wegen der Unterschiedlichkeit des Tumorwachstums. Schließlich sind es Probleme der Vergleichbarkeit der Dosis bei Maus und Mensch, die bis heute nicht befriedigend gelöst sind.

Zusammenfassung

Trotz konsequenter Therapie zeichnen sich Ovarialkarzinome durch sehr unterschiedliche Verläufe aus. Neben dem Stadium und der Beobachtung des Gesamtorganismus kommt der Untersuchung von Tumorgewebe als Basis der Therapieplanung besondere Bedeutung zu. Sie hat sich bis jetzt vorwiegend auf morphologische Parameter gestützt. Hier verdienen neben dem histologischen Typ ganz besonders der Differenzierungsgrad Beachtung. So stehen muzinöse und unklassifizierbare Karzinome zum Stadium und damit der Prognose in Beziehung. Für den Differenzierungsgrad gelten noch strengere Beziehungen zu Stadium und Prognose. Beim histochemischen Enzymmuster verdient neben der Gleichmäßigkeit der Enzymverteilung der Vergleich der Reaktion im Tumor- und Bindegewebe besondere Beachtung.

Von den „funktionellen Parametern" ermöglicht die Sensibilitätstestung nach Volm die Erkennung einer proliferationsabhängigen Chemoresistenz. Zur Überprüfung dieser Methode ist eine neue kooperative Studie angelaufen. Dabei werden moderne aggressive Zytostatikakombinationen einer konservativen Chemotherapie gegenübergestellt. Über erste Ergebnisse einer Kombinationschemotherapie mit Cis-Platin, Adriamycin und Endoxan bei 42 Primärfällen eines Stadiums III und IV und 39 Rezidivfällen wird berichtet.

Mit der Bestimmung des Hormonrezeptorstatus konnten wir bisher bei Ovarialkarzinomen weder zur Prognose noch zum histologischen Typ eine eindeutige Korrelation finden. Neue Aspekte ergibt die Beobachtung des Tumorwachstums auf der Nacktmaus. Es scheint möglich, besonders maligne Tumoren frühzeitig zu erkennen. Ob und inwieweit sich aber die Therapieversuche an solchen Karzinomen dann auf die Patientinnen übertragen lassen, wissen wir bis heute nicht.

Literatur

Alberts DS, Hilgers RD, Noon TE, Martimbeau PW, Rivkin S (1979) Combination chemotherapie for alkylator – resistant ovarian carcinom: A prelimenary report of a Southwest oncology group trial. Cancer Treat Rep 63:301–305

Annual Report on the Results of Treatment in gynecological Cancer (1979) Vol XVII

Barber HRK, Sommers SC, Snyder R, Kwon TH (1975) Histologic and nuclear grading and stromal reactions as indices for prognosis in ovarian cancer. J Obstet Gynecol 121:795–807

Bastert G (1976) Heterotransplantation menschlicher Tumoren, vorzugsweise Mammakarzinome, auf thymusaplastische nu/nu-Mäuse. Ein wissenschaftliches und klinisches Testmodell Habilitationsschrift, Universität Frankfurt

Bastert G, Schmidt-Matthiesen H, Voelcker G, Peter G, Hohorst HJ (1975) In vitro Sensibilitätstestung von Tumoren gegenüber aktiviertem Cyclophosphamid (4-Hydroxyclophosphamid). Kurzzeitinkubation von Originaltumorzellen und ^{3}H-Uridin bzw. ^{3}H-Thymidineinbau. Z Krebsforsch 84:37–47

Bastert G, Voelker G, Peter G, Schmidt-Matthiesen H, Hohorst HJ (1976) Zum Problem der in vitro Sensiblitätstestung von Tumoren gegen Cyclophosphamid. ^{3}H-Uridineinbau in RNS menschlicher Tumorzellen nach Inkubation mit 4-Hydroperoxycyclophosphamid. Z Krebsforsch 85:299–307

Bruckner HW, Cohen CJ, Wallach RC (1978) Treatment of advanced ovarian cancer with cis-dichlorediamine-platinum (Poor-risk patients with intensive prior therapy). Cancer Treat Rep 62:555–558

Bruckner HW, Pango M, Falkson G et al. (1979) Controlled prospective trial of combination chemotherapy with cyclophosphamide, adriamycin, and 5-fluoro-uracil for the treatment of advanced ovarian cancer: a prelimenary report. Cancer Treat Rep 63:297–299

Day TG Jr, Gallager HS, Rutledge FN (1975) Epithelial carcinoma of the ovary prognostic importance of histologic grade. Natl Cancer Inst Monogr 42:15–21

Ehrlich CE, Einhorn L, Williams SD, Morgan J (1979) Chemotherapy for stage III–IV epithelial ovarian cancer with cis-Dichlorodiammineplatinum II, Adriamycin, and cyclophosphamide. A prelimenary report. Cancer Treat Rep 63:281–288

Klaassen D, Goldenberg (1977) Trial of combination versus single drug sequential chemotherapy in advanced ovarian cancer. Proc Am Soc Clin Oncol 18:357–361

Kleine W (1980) Das Modell der thymusaplastischen Nacktmaus und seine klinische Relevanz. 3. Sitzung der Freiburger Medizinischen Gesellschaft im Sommersemester 1980 am 3. 6. 1980

Kleine W, Teufel G, Pfleiderer A (1979) Xenotransplantation menschlicher Ovarialkarzinome auf nu/nu-Mäuse. (Vortrag 87) Tagung der Nordwestdeutschen Gesellschaft für Gynäkologie in Hamburg, 23.–25. 11. 1979

Kleine W, Teufel G, Pfleiderer A (1980) Thymusaplastische Nacktmäuse: Ein tierexperimentelles Modell zum Vergleich verschiedener Therapieformen bei individuellen menschlichen Karzinomen (Vortrag). Deutscher Krebskongreß, 11. März 1980, München

Kleine W, Wrzodek W, Schwantes H, Teufel G, Ladner HA, Pfleiderer A (1981) Experimentelle Strahlentherapie gynäkologischer Karzinome auf der nu/nu-Maus. Arch Gynecol 232:304–305

Kleine W, Teufel G, Schwörer D, Pfleiderer A (1981a) Experimental chemotherapy of human malignant ovarian carcinomas xenotransplantat in nude mice. In: Bastert GBA (ed) Thymusaplastic nude mice and rats in clinical oncology, Fischer, Stuttgart New York, pp 62ff.

Kleine W, Fuchs A, Niederstadt T, Teufel G, Pfleiderer A (1981b) Experimental hormonal treatment of human ovarian carcinomas xenotransplantet in nude mice. In: Bastert GBA et al. (eds) Thymusaplastic nude mice and rats in clinical oncology. Fischer, Stuttgart New York, pp 70ff.

Kleine W, Wrzodek W, Stange S (1981c) Hochvoltstrahlung xenotransplantierter menschlicher Ovarial-Endometrium- und Zervixkarzinome. In: Wannenmacher M, Schreiber, Ladner H-A (Hrsg) Kombinierte chirurgische und radiologische Therapie maligner Tumoren. Urban & Schwarzenberg, München. S 289–295

Kolstadt P (1980) Prognostic indicators and staging. In: Newman, Ford, Jordan (eds) Ovarian cancer. Pergamon, Oxford, pp 67–78

KSST (1980) Sensibilitätstestung menschlicher Tumoren gegenüber Zytostatika mit einem in vitro-Kurzzeittest. Kooperative Studie für Sensibilitätstestung von Tumoren. Dtsch Med Wochenschr 105: 1 105:1493–1496

Limburg H, Krahe M (1964) Die Züchtung von menschlichem Krebsgewebe in der Gewebekultur und seine Sensibilitätstestung gegen neue Zytostatika. Dtsch Med Wochenschr 89:1938–1946

Mattern J, Kaufmann M, Volm M, Schütze U, Wayss K, Goerttler K, Tasca C (1972) Zur Sensibilitätstestung maligner menschlicher Tumoren gegenüber Zytostatika. Klin Wochenschr 50:196–198

Mattern J, Kaufmann M, Hinderer H, Wayss K, Volm M (1975) Sensitivity tests of tumors to cytostatic agents. II. Investigation on human tumors. Z Krebsforsch 83:97–104

Meerpohl HG, Kleine W, Teufel G, Erz K-H, Bührer S, Pfleiderer A (1981) Steroidhormonrezeptoren bei Ovarialkarzinomen. Arch Gynecol 232:262–263

Omura GA (1981) GOG protocol 22. In: Gynecologic oncology group. Statistical report Miami, january 8–10, 1981, pp 31–40

Ozols RF, Garvin AJ, Costa I, Simon RM, Young RC (1969) Histologic grade in advanced ovarian cancer. Cancer Treat Rep 63:255–263

Pfleiderer A (1970) Histochemical enzyme pattern of ovarian carcinoma as a hint at prognosis and its change after chemotherapy. VIth World Congress Obstet Gynecol, New York, 13. 4. 1970

Pfleiderer A (1981) Die Kombination von Operation und Strahlentherapie aus der Sicht des Operateurs beim Endometrium- und Ovarialkarzinom. In: Wannenmacher M et al (Hrsg) Kombinierte chirurgische und radiologische Therapie maligner Tumoren. Urban & Schwarzenberg, München, S 259–270

Pfleiderer A (1981) Die Therapie des Ovarialkarzinoms. Arch Gynecol 232:200–268

Pfleiderer A, KSST (1980) Is chemosensitivity-testing worth-while? Report of a cooperative study. (Gynecology and Obstetric International Congress Ser 512 FIGO World Congress Tokyo 1979) Excerpta Med 1143–1147

Pfleiderer A, KSST (im Druck) Testung der Tumorsensibilität gegen Zytostatika. Vortrag München 21. 3. 1980. Urban & Schwarzenberg, München

Pfleiderer A, Kidess E, Jung G (1970) Klinische Bedeutung des Vorkommens und der Verteilung von Aminopeptidasen im Ovarialkarzinom. Untersuchungen mit biochemischer und histochemischer Methodik. Arch Gynaekol 209:121–135

Pfleiderer A, Karzel M, Morlok KF, Schaal R (1973) Neue Methoden zur Beurteilung der Wirkung von Zytostatika beim Ovarialkarzinom. II. Planimetrische Vermessung enzym-histochemisch gefärbter Gewebeschnitte. In: König PA, Pfleiderer A Jr (Hrsg) Neue Aspekte in Diagnose und Therapie des Genitalkarzinoms der Frau. Enke, Stuttgart, S 75–81

Pfleiderer A, Wipprecht KG, Ritzmann H, Tan TH (1976) Die Potenz der malignen Entartung der Ovarialtumoren. Fortschr Med 94:81–88

Pfleiderer A, Kleine W, Teufel G, Fuchs A (1979) Ovarian tumors. Morphology, kinetics, hormonal receptors, and transplantation on nude mice. A comparison. Precongr Education Lecture Tokyo 24/10/79

Pfleiderer A Jr (1976) Vorkommen und Verteilung von Lactat-Dehydrogenase (LDH) und sog. Leucinaminopeptidase beim Ovarialkarzinom. Histochemische Untersuchungen. Vortrag V. Akad. Tagg. Deutschspr. Doz. für Geburtshilfe und Gynäkologie, Graz 1968. Thieme, Stuttgart, S 357

Pfleiderer A Jr, Karzel M (1971) Histochemie der unspezifischen Phosphatasen im Ovarialkarzinom und ihre Beziehung zur Klinik. Arch Gynaekol 211:335–336

Pfleiderer A Jr, Kidess E, Jung G (1969) Klinik und Pathologie der Lactatdehydrogenase im Ovarialkarzinom. Z Krebsforsch 72:329–340

Piver MS, Barlow JJ, Shashikant BL (1978) Incidence of subclinical metastasis in stage I and II ovarian carcinoma. Obstet Gynecol 52:100–104

Possinger K, Hartenstein R, Ehrhart H (1976) Resistenztestung von menschlichen Tumoren gegenüber Zytostatika. Klin Wochenschr 54:349–355

Russell P (1979) The pathological assessment of ovarian neoplasms. I: Introduction to the common "epithelial" tumours and analysis of benign "epithelial" tumours. Pathology 11:5–26

Salmon SE, Hamburger AW, Soehnlein B, Durie BG, Alberts DS, Moon TE (1978) Quantitation of differential sensitivity of human tumour stem cells to anticancer drugs. N Engl J Med 298:1321–1327

Schwörer D (1979) Wachstum und Chemotherapie menschlicher, maligner Ovarialtumoren nach Heterotransplantation auf thymusaplastische nu/nu-Mäuse, Inaugural-Dissertation

Seeber S, Schmidt CG (1977) Zum Problem der prätherapeutischen Sensibilitätsbestimmung von Tumoren durch Inkorporationsstudien in vitro. Klin Wochenschr 55:1127–1136

Smith JP, Day TG Jr (1979) Review of ovarian cancer at the University of Texas systems. Cancer Center, M.D. Anderson hospital and tumour institute. Am J Obstet Gynecol 135:984–993

Stenwig J, Hazekamp JT, Beecham JB (1979) Granulosa cell tumours of the ovary: a clinicopathological study of 118 cases with long-term follow up. Gynecol Oncol 7:136–152

Tanneberger S, Bacigalupo G (1967) Die Benutzung von Zellkulturen zur Ermittlung der Sensibilität menschlicher Tumoren gegenüber Zytostatika. Dtsch Gesundheitswes 22:11–15

Teufel G (1979) Proliferation von Karzinomen des weiblichen Genitale und ihre Bedeutung für die zytostatische Therapie. Habilitationsschrift, Universität Freiburg

Teufel G, KSST (1981) Sensibilitätstestung von Ovarialkarzinomen gegen Zytostatika. Ergebnisse der kooperativen Studiengruppe zur Sensibilitätstestung von Tumoren. Vortrag Deutsche Gesellschaft in Hamburg 1980. Arch Gynecol 232:258–260

Teufel G, Pfleiderer A, Doerjer O, Weigand J (1977) Untersuchungen über den Einbau von Nucleotidpraecursoren in Einzelzellsuspensionen von Ovarial- und Zervixkarzinomen unter dem Einfluß von Zytostatika. Arch Gynaekol 223:163–172

Teufel G, Kleine W, Günther M, Pfleiderer A (1981) Growth of human ovarian carcinomas in thymusaplastic nude mice. In: Bastert GBA (ed) Thymusaplastic nude mice and rats in clinical oncology. Fischer, Stuttgart New York

Vogl SE, Berenzweig M, Kaplan BH, Moukhtar M, Bulkin W (1979) The CHAD and HAD regimens in advanced ovarian cancer: Combination chemotherapy including cyclophosphamide, hexamethylmelamine, adriamycin and cis-dichlorodiammineplatinum II. Cancer Treat Rep 63:311–317

Volm M, Kaufmann K, Wayss K, Goerttler K, Mattern J (1974) Gezielte Tumorchemotherapie durch Onkobiogramme. Dtsch Med Wochenschr 99:38–43

Volm M, Wayss K, Kaufmann M, Mattern J (1979) Pretherapeutic detection of tumour resistance and the results of tumour therapy. Eur J Cancer 15:983–994

Wright JC, Cobb JP, Gumport SL, Safadi D, Walker GD, Golomb FM (1957) Investigation of the relation between clinical and tissue-culture. Response to chemotherapeutic agents on human cancer. N Engl J Med 257:1207–1211

Wüst GP, Matthes KJ (1970) In-vitro-Messung des Einbaus von ^{3}H-Thymidin im Jensen-Sarkom unter Zytostatikaeinwirkung mit Hilfe der Flüssigkeits-Szintillationsspektrometrie. Z Krebsforsch 73:204–214

Young RC, Chabner BA, Hubbard SP, Canellos GP, DeVita VT (1978) Advanced ovarian adenocarcinoma. A prospective clinical trial of melphalan (L-PAM) versus combination chemotherapy. N Engl J Med 299:1261–1266

Gegenwärtiger Stand der Therapie des Ovarialkarzinoms

F. Kubli[1]

Die Heilungsergebnisse beim Ovarialkarzinom sind nach wie vor schlecht, bedingt in erster Linie durch die hohe Zahl forgeschrittener, zur Behandlung kommender Karzinome und durch deren begrenzte therapeutische Beeinflußbarkeit (Abb. 1). Die Fünfjahresergebnisse für das Stadium III liegen auch in hochqualifizierten Zentren bei etwa 15%, die Zehnjahresergebnisse bei etwa 12% [15] (Abb. 1).

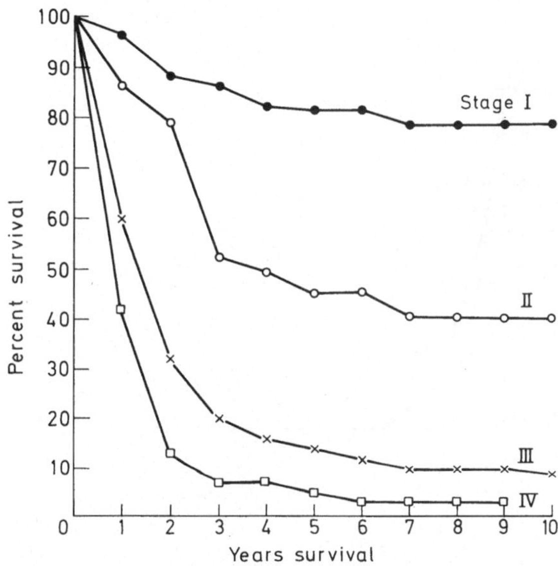

Abb. 1. Fünfjahres- und Zehnjahresüberlebensraten bei epithelialen Ovarialkarzinomen in Abhängigkeit vom Stadium zum Zeitpunkt der Primärbehandlung. (Nach Smith [15])

Mit der Einführung der Chemotherapie ließen sich Remissionen in eindrucksvoller Häufigkeit, Heilungen aber leider unverändert nur selten erzielen. Dies führte zu dem etwas resignierten Statement von Lewis u. Blessing [8], wonach „for ovarian cancer seemingly everything works, but practically nothing succeeds".

Trotzdem ist in die therapeutische Landschaft in jüngerer Zeit etwas Bewegung gekommen. Die entscheidenden Impulse gingen dabei von den großen, vorwiegend angelsächsischen oder skandinavischen Zentren aus, die praktisch als einzige über

---

1 Universitäts-Frauenklinik, Voßstraße 9, D-6900 Heidelberg

ein ausreichend großes Beobachtungsgut bei diesem heterogenen Krankheitsbild verfügen. Im Folgenden sollen der gegenwärtige Stand und die Tendenzen in der Behandlung des Ovarialkarzinoms kurz zusammengefaßt werden unter ausschließlicher Berücksichtigung der invasiven epithelialen Karzinome.

Prognostisch wichtige Variablen (Tabelle 1)

Die Prognose wird entscheidend durch einige wenige Variablen beeinflußt. Eine davon ist bekanntlich die Ausdehnung – das *Stadium* – des Turmos zum Zeitpunkt des Therapiebeginns; die Verhältnisse sind in Abb. 1 dargestellt. Ebenso wichtig ist der *Differenzierungsgrad* (Grading) des Tumors. Gut differenzierte Tumoren haben eine gute, schlecht differenzierte eine schlechte Prognose [2, 6, 15]. Rutledge [12] fand

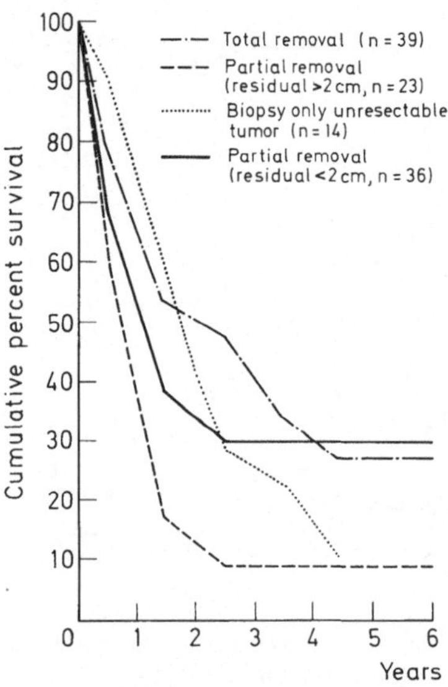

Abb. 2. Überlebensraten nach Second-look-Operationen in Abhängigkeit von der dabei im Abdomen verbliebenen Tumorlast. (Nach Schwartz u. Smith [13])

den Differenzierungsgrad wichtiger als das klinische Stadium, wobei allerdings eine Interdependenz insofern besteht, als bei fortgeschrittenen Stadien vorwiegend entdifferenzierte Tumoren zu finden sind [6, 15].

Ein weiterer prognostisch relevanter Faktor ist das Alter der Patientin. Die Daten von Kolstad [6] zeigen, daß die Prognose bei jüngeren Frauen deutlich besser ist (Tabelle 2).

Eine entscheidende Variable bildet schließlich die *Tumorlast*, die bei Abschluß der primären chirurgischen Therapie im Abdomen zurückbleibt. Tendenzmäßig

Tabelle 1. Ovarialkarzinom. Für die Prognose entscheidende Variablen

Prognose abhängig von
1) Alter der Patientin
2) Tumorstadium
3) Tumorgrading (Differenzierung)
4) Maximaler Durchmesser von zurückgelassenen Tumormassen (bezogen auf den größten einzelnen Knoten): Grenze bei 1 – 2 cm

Tabelle 2. Ovarialkarzinom. Abhängigkeit der Prognose vom Alter der Patientin. (Nach Kolstad [6])

252 Stage III epithelial carcinomas			
Age	Survival > 2 years		
	No.	Percent	Total No.
< 50	27	38.0	71
> 50	40	16.5	181

Tabelle 3. Ovarialkarzinom. Abhängigkeit der Prognose von der Größe der nach chirurgischer Primärbehandlung im Abdomen zurückgebliebenen Tumormasse (Durchmesser des größten zurückgebliebenen Knotens). (Nach Smith [15])

Tumor Size	No. of Patients	Percent Survival	
		2-year	5-year
none	31	80	63
0 – 1 cm	84	70	41
1 – 2 cm	46	49	15
3 – 6 cm	144	28	8
7 – 9 cm	36	16	0
> 10 cm	273	16	3

gleiche Ergebnisse von verschiedenen Zentren [2, 4, 14, 15] weisen darauf hin, daß der Größe der einzelnen zurückbleibenden Tumorknoten die entscheidende Bedeutung zukommt, wobei ein Durchmesser von 1–2 cm die kritische Grenze darstellt (Tabelle 3). Ähnliches trifft für die Situation bei der Second-look-Operation (Abb. 2) [13] zu.

Zusammenfassend sind demnach das Alter der Patientin, Stadium, Differenzierungsgrad und maximale Größe der im Abdomen zurückbleibenden Tumorknoten die prognostisch entscheidenden Variablen (Tabelle 1).

Chirurgische Therapie

Das chirurgische Vorgehen ist z. Zt. determiniert einerseits durch die prognostische Bedeutung der nach der Primärbehandlung zurückbleibenden Tumorlast und andererseits durch die Erkenntnis, daß die Ausdehnung der Karzinome auch intraoperativ häufig unrichtig eingeschätzt wird. Es besteht daher allgemein die Tendenz zu *möglichst großer Radikalität*, wobei aber verstümmelnde Operationen, d.h. praktisch Anus praeter oder supravesikale Harnableitung, beim Primäreingriff zumindest nach Möglichkeit vermieden werden. Die Standardtherapie besteht aus der *Hysterektomie mit Adnexen und Resektion des großen Netzes.* Zusätzlich ist – wenn nicht das Abdomen makroskopisch durch ausgedehnte Tumormassen gefüllt ist – ein intensives *intraoperatives Staging* mit multiplen Biopsien erforderlich. Dabei sind sämtliche aspektmäßig verdächtigen Bereiche im gesamten Bauchraum zu biopsieren. Auch bei makroskopisch unverdächtigem Aspekt werden multiple Probeentnahmen aus dem Peritoneum des kleinen Beckens, des Dünndarms, des Dünndarmmesenteriums, des Peritoneum parietale besonders in den parakolischen Räumen beiderseits, von den paraaortalen Lymphknoten, der Leber und schließlich auch dem Diaphragma gefordert. Nach Smith liegt dabei die Zahl der notwendigen einzelnen Biopsien zwischen 20 und 30 [15].

Finden sich im Abdomen große Tumormassen, die nicht radikal entfernbar sind, wird größtmögliche Tumorresektion bereits bei der Primäroperation angestrebt, und zwar eine Reduktion vor allem der großen Tumormassen mit Durchmesser über 2 cm [2, 4, 14, 15].

Dieses chirurgische Vorgehen ist wesentlich radikaler, auch zeitraubend und potentiell gefährlicher als das allgemein beim Ovarialkarzinom bisher Geübte. Daher empfiehlt der Ausschuß Onkologie der Deutschen Gesellschaft für Gynäkologie und Geburtshilfe auch die Überweisung von Verdachtsfällen zur Primärtherapie an onkologische Zentren [1].

Der typische und vollständige Eingriff ist im wesentlichen nur von einem medianen Längsschnitt, der bis über den Nabel reicht, durchzuführen [1]. Bei Tumoren im kleinen Becken, deren Dignität präoperativ unklar ist, dürfte sich unter diesem Aspekt eine direkt präoperativ durchgeführte Laparoskopie zur Beantwortung der einfachen Frage, ob von einem Querschnitt operiert werden kann oder ob ein Längsschnitt notwendig ist, lohnen. Findet sich ein Ovarialkarzinom als Überraschungsbefund in einem durch tiefen Querschnitt eröffneten Abdomen, sind die laparoskopischen Instrumente für die Biopsieentnahmen im Oberbauch hilfreich.

Second-look-Operationen

Die geplante Zweitoperation wurde vor Jahren vorwiegend mit therapeutischer Zielrichtung eingeführt, verlor dann aber wegen der eher zweifelhaften Ergebnisse an Bedeutung. Zur Zeit erlebt die Second-look-Operation wieder eine Renaissance. Dabei ist die Zielrichtung heute vorwiegend und in erster Linie diagnostisch zur Überprüfung klinischer Vollremissionen. Technisch gelten dabei dieselben Richtlinien wie beim Primäreingriff: Multiple Biopsien sind notwendig bei noch vorhandenen minimalen Tumormassen oder bei makroskopischer Tumorfreiheit – in dem bisher größten Beobachtungsgut von Schwartz u. Smith [13] war in 19 von 142 Fällen der Tumornachweis intraoperativ nur histologisch zu erbringen.

Das therapeutische Potential der Second-look-Operation dürfte geringer sein; es wird aber auf jeden Fall eine Tumorreduktion analog derjenigen beim Primäreingriff angestrebt. Von 128 Patientinnen in dem oben angeführten Beobachtungsgut von Schwartz u. Smith [13], bei denen noch Tumor zum Zeitpunkt des Zweiteingriffs vorgefunden war, hatten 7 bisher eine Fünfjahresheilung, also etwa 5%. Mit der wichtigste Grund allerdings für die Second-look-Operation ist das Bestreben, bei echter, auch histologischer Vollremission die potentiell gefährliche Chemotherapie rechtzeitig und motiviert beenden zu können.

Strahlentherapie

Die Strahlentherapie wird in der Behandlung der epithelialen Ovarialtumoren nach wie vor uneinheitlich beurteilt. Es besteht aber weitgehende Einigkeit darüber, daß i. allg. eine lediglich lokale, d. h. auf das Becken beschränkte radiologische Therapie nicht sinnvoll ist [16], es sei denn in Kombination mit Chemotherapie. Entsprechend der biologischen Verhaltensweise des Ovarialkarzinoms ist, wenn überhaupt, in der Regel eine Bestrahlung des *gesamten Abdomens*, und zwar entweder nach der Großfeldtechnik oder der Moving-Strip-Technik anzustreben, wobei relativ niedrige Dosen (nach Bush 22 Gy) [2] appliziert werden. Die Ergebnisse sind widersprüchlich. Nach Kolstad et al. [7] sind im Stadium III die Ergebnisse identisch mit denen einer zytotoxischen Monotherapie, bei allerdings ausgeprägteren Nebenwirkungen. Bush [2] hingegen findet die Strahlentherapie im Stadium III bei „minimal residual disease" der Chemotherapie überlegen, während für Smith et al. [15] genau das Gegenteil gilt.

Nicht indiziert – und darüber besteht wieder Einigkeit – ist die Bestrahlung, wenn die residuellen Tumormassen im Durchmesser 2 cm überschreiten und generalisiert im Abdomen vorhanden sind [16].

Auch die *intraperitoneale Instillation* radioaktiver Substanzen wird heute noch kontrovers beurteilt. Zwar wird über gute Ergebnisse, vor allem bei den Stadien I und IIc und bei Kapselruptur berichtet [7, 11], doch wurden auch in den neueren Behandlungsserien z. T. noch massive lokale Nebenwirkungen (Adhäsionen und Fibrose des Darms) beobachtet [7, 11]. Es ist aber denkbar, daß bei verbesserter Technik und reduzierter Dosis diese Art der lokalen Strahlentherapie wenigstens einen umschriebenen Anwendungsbereich beibehält oder wieder erhalten wird.

Chemotherapie

Die Chemotherapie hat bekanntlich eine beeindruckende Zahl von *Remissionen* bewirkt, doch blieben echte Heilungen über 5 Jahre bis heute leider nach wie vor die Ausnahme. Mit *Monotherapie* liegen die Remissionen um 30% [9]. Unter relativ

Tabelle 4. Gegenwärtig verwendete aggressive Kombinationschemotherapien. (Nach Wiltshaw [19])

"Code Name"	Drug doses in mg/m²					Ref.
	Cisplat	Adria	HMM	Cyclo	Chlor	
PAC-I	50	50	–	750	–	Ehrlich
PAC-V	100[a]	50	–	750	–	Ehrlich
CHAD	50	25	150 × 14	600	–	Vogl
Pt+Ad	50	50	–	–	–	Bruckner
B	20	–	–	–	5 × 7	Wiltshaw
C	20	50	–	–	5 × 7	Wiltshaw
Plat Mid	50	–	–	–	–	Bruckner

[a] Cisplatin given as 20 mg/m² daily × 5. HMM and chlorambucil given daily for 14 and 7 days respectively

Tabelle 5. Ergebnisse und Nebenwirkungen aggressiver Kombinationschemotherapie. (Nach Wiltshaw [19])

"Code Name"	No. Cases	% Resp.		% Tumor < 3 cm	% Toxicity			Hair loss	No. deaths	Price/ course (£)
		RR	CR		% WBC < 1,000	Pl < 50,000	Hb < 9.5 g			
PAC-I	18	61	39	40	39	28	89	+	2	146
PAC-V	17	76	35	37	65	30	82	+	1	261
CHAD	26	90	48	30	0	11	42	±	0	122
Pt+Ad	18	66	?	?	?	?	?	+	1	172
B	46	52	28	0	0	0	3	0	0	34
C	39	54	28	0	3	3	5	+	2	120
Pt Mid	17	35	?	?	?	?	?	0	0	86

standardisierten Versuchsbedingungen ergaben sich am M.D. Anderson folgende Remissionshäufigkeiten:

Alkeran 32%, 5-Fluoruracil 12%, Hexamethylmelamin (HMMA) 27% und Adriblastin schließlich 28% [12].

Demgegenüber scheinen Remissionen mit *aggressiver Kombinationstherapie* [10, 19, 20] mit neueren Medikamenten, insbesondere Cis-Platin deutlich häufiger zu sein (Tabelle 4 und 5) und bei 50% und darüber zu liegen [10, 19]. Dabei sind vor allem erfolgversprechend Kombinationen von Alkylantien, HMMA, Cis-Platin und evtl. auch Adriblastin. Die Toxizität dieser Kombinationen und z.T. auch der einzelnen Medikamente ist allerdings exzessiv. Dabei muß festgehalten werden, daß eine Überlegenheit dieser aggressiven Kombinationstherapie heute bezüglich Langzeitergebnisse, d.h. echter Heilungen und unter Berücksichtigung der Lebensqualität gegenüber der Monotherapie noch nicht bewiesen ist. In randomisierten Studien sind durchwegs noch Gruppen mit Monotherapie erlaubt und wohl auch angezeigt. Die Vermutung, daß eine Langzeitchemotherapie einen *kanzerogenen Effekt* haben kann, hat sich leider auch in der Therapie des Ovarialkarzinoms bestätigt. Schwartz u. Smith [13] berichten über 4 Fälle von Leukämie bei 30 Patientinnen mit mehr als 16 Alkeran-Stößen. Gegen diesen Hintergrund ist bei Vollremissionen eine histologische Klärung anzustreben und bei histologisch nachgewiesener Remission die Chemotherapie abzusetzen.

Mögliches therapeutisches Vorgehen

Zusammenfassend läßt sich nach dem Gesagten folgendes therapeutisches Vorgehen skizzieren (Tabelle 6).

1) Gut differenzierte Tumoren des Stadium I a und I b werden mit abdomineller Hysterektomie mit den Adnexen und Netzresektion behandelt, wobei das intraoperative Staging mit Biopsie obligatorisch sein sollte. Fällt dieses negativ aus, ist eine Zusatztherapie nicht notwendig.

2) Weiter fortgeschrittene, aber nach wie vor auf das kleine Becken beschränkte Tumoren (Stadium II), die radikal durch abdominale Hysterektomie mit Adnexen ohne makroskopische Tumorresidien saniert werden können, bedürfen einer *adjuvanten Therapie*. Dabei kommen in Frage eine Chemotherapie, evtl. (im Stadium II b) kombiniert mit einer auf das kleine Becken lokalisierten Strahlentherapie. Alternativ sind allerdings auch Strahlentherapie über das ganze Abdomen in Form von Moving-Strip oder Großfeldbestrahlung oder auch Radiogoldinstillation möglich. Die letztere Maßnahme erscheint sinnvoll bei den Stadien I c, II c und intraoperativer Kapselruptur.

Eine klare Überlegenheit der Chemotherapie über die Strahlentherapie oder umgekehrt erscheint in dem adjuvanten Therapiebereich nicht erwiesen, wobei aus

Tabelle 6. Mögliches therapeutisches Vorgehen

1) – Stadium I a (und I b?), gut differenziert
Abd. Hyst. + Adnexe + Netzresektion
Intraoperatives Staging
Keine Zusatztherapie

2) – Stadien I a und b, schlecht differenziert
– Stadien I c, II a – c
Radikal operiert ohne makroskopische Tumorresiduen
Adjuvante Therapie:
- Chemotherapie (+ Rx lokal)
- Rx (gesamtes Abdomen)
- Radiogold (+ Rx lokal)

3) – Stadien III und IV
– Nicht radikal operierbare Stadien II
Maximal mögliche Tumorreduktion
a) Verbleibende Tumorreste ≧ 2 cm: Aggressive Chemotherapie
b) Verbleibende Tumorreste < 2 cm: Aggressive Chemotherapie, Rx (gesamtes Abdomen)

4) – Second Look Operationen
Diagnostisch nach klinisch kompletter Remission
Therapeutisch-diagnostisch bei Persistenz

der Sicht des Chirurgen und im Hinblick auf einen möglichen Zweit- und Dritteingriff allerdings die Tendenz besteht, der Chemotherapie gegenüber der radiologischen Behandlung den Vorzug zu geben.

3) Bei den intraperitoneal disseminierten Stadien III und IV ist möglichst die radikale Sanierung oder doch wenigstens Tumorreduktion anzustreben. Resultiert diese in lediglich minimalen makroskopisch verbliebenen Tumorresten, so ist als Zusatzbehandlung alternativ eine aggressive Chemotherapie oder aber auch eine Bestrahlung des ganzen Abdomens möglich, wobei wiederum unklar ist, welche Therapie der anderen deutlich überlegen ist. Hingegen besteht Einigkeit darüber, daß bei größeren im Abdomen verbleibenden Tumormassen lediglich eine Chemotherapie in Frage kommt. Dabei besteht heute die Tendenz zur aggressiven Kombinationschemotherapie, doch ist alternativ auch eine Monotherapie mit Alkylanzien möglich.

4) Second-look-Operationen dürften die Regel werden, und zwar in diagnostischer Intention nach klinisch kompletter Remission und mit therapeutisch-diagnostischer Zielsetzung bei Tumorpersistenz, wobei dann einer Tumortestung [5, 17] und evtl. auch Hormonrezeptortestung [8] eine gewisse Bedeutung zukommen.

Zusammenfassung

Die therapeutische Situation bei den epithelialen Ovarialkarzinomen ist z.Zt. charakterisiert durch:

1) Tendenz zur Radikalisierung des chirurgischen Vorgehens, wobei die Verminderung der Tumorlast und die bioptische intraoperative Stadieneinteilung (Staging) beim Primäreingriff im Vordergrund stehen;
2) eine Tendenz zu aggressiver Kombinationschemotherapie, wobei deren Überlegenheit gegenüber der Monotherapie bisher nur für Remissionen, nicht aber für Heilungsziffern erwiesen ist;
3) die Second-look-Operation als integraler Teil eines Behandlungsplans vor allem bei Voll- und Teilremissionen und
4) eine unklare Situation bezüglich der Bedeutung der Strahlentherapie in Situationen mit „minimal residual disease“.

Literatur

1. Ausschuß Onkologie der Deutschen Gesellschaft Gynäkologie, Geburtshilfe (1981) Zur gegenwärtigen Situation der Diagnostik und Therapie des Ovarialcarcinoms. Mitt Dtsch Ges Gynaekol Geburtshilfe 5: III
2. Bush RS, Dembo AJ (1980) Current status of treatment for patients with ovarian cancer. In: Newman CE, Ford CHJ, Jordan IA (eds) Ovarian Cancer. Pergamon, Oxford New York
3. Editorial (1980) Management of advanced ovarian cancer. Lancet II: 1010
4. Griffith CT, Parker LM, Fuller AF (1979) Role of cytoreductive surgical treatment in the management of advanced ovarian. Cancer Treat Rep 63: 235

5. Kaufmann M (1980) Clinical application of in vitro chemosensitivity testing. In: Newman CE, Ford CHJ, Jordan IA (eds) Ovarian Cancer. Pergamon, Oxford New York
6. Kolstad P (1980) Prognostic indicators and staging. In: Newman CE, Ford CHJ, Jordan IA (eds) Ovarian Cancer. Pergamon, Oxford New York
7. Kolstad P, Davy M, Hoeg K (1977) Individualized treatment of ovarian cancer. Am J Obstet Gynecol 128:617
8. Lewis GC, Blessing J (1977) Ovarian Cancer: use of multiple modality programs involving surgery, radiation therapy and chemotherapy. Cancer 40:588
9. Lewis B, Young R (1980) Adjuvant and first line chemotherapy for ovarian cancer. In: Newman CE, Ford CHJ, Jordan IA (eds) Ovarian Cancer. Pergamon, Oxford New York
10. Lewis B, Young R (1980) Ovarian Cancer – Future approuches to the development of treatment. In: Newman CE, Ford CHJ, Jordan IA (eds) Ovarian Cancer. Pergamon, Oxford New York
11. Pezner RD, Stevens K, Tong D, Allen CV (1978) Limited epithelial carcinoma of the ovary treated with curative intent by the intraperitoneal instillation of radiocolloids. Cancer 42:2563
12. Rutledge F (1980) Das Ovarialcarcinom. Referat, Fortbildungskurs der I. Frauenklinik der Universität München, 21./22. 3. 1980
13. Schwartz PE, Smith JP (1980) Second look operations in ovarian cancer. Am J Obstet Gynecol 138:1124
14. Smith JP (1978) Treatment of ovarian cancer. Adv Chemother Japan Sci Soc Press, Tokyo/Univ. Park Press, Baltimore
15. Smith JP (198) Surgery for ovarian cancer. In: Newman CE, Ford CHJ, Jordan IA (eds) Ovarian Cancer. Pergamon, Oxford New York
16. Schüren E von der, Bojärt W, Gonzalez D (1980) Role of radiotherapy in the treatment of ovarian cancer. In: Newman CE, Ford CHJ, Jordan JA (eds) Ovarian Cancer. Pergamon, Oxford New York
17. Volm M, Wayss K, Kaufmann M, Mattern J (1979) Therapeutic detection of tumour resistance and the results of tumour chemotherapy. Eur J Cancer 15:983
18. Welander C, Kjorstat E, Kolstad P (1978) Postoperative indication and chemotherapy in patients with advanced ovarian cancer. Acta Obstet Gynecol Scand 57:161
19. Wiltshaw E (1980) Cis-platinum in adenocarcinom of the ovary: A critical review. In: Newman CE, Ford CHJ, Jordan JA (eds) Ovarian Cancer. Pergamon, Oxford New York
20. Young RC, Chabner BA et al. (1978) Advanced ovarian adenocarcinoma: a prospective clinical trial of melphalan versus combination chemotherapy. N Engl J Med 299:1261

Klinische Anwendbarkeit der histologischen Klassifikation

S. SIEVERS [1]

Die malignen Ovarialbildungen sind so vielfältig, daß die Ovarialtumoren auch dann nicht als Einheit betrachtet werden können, wenn es um therapeutische Maßnahmen geht. Aus diesem Grunde gilt es, Selektionskriterien zu schaffen, die eine individuelle Therapie ermöglichen.

Mit der Aufstellung von international geltenden Stadieneinteilungen nach FIGO und UICC ist ein großer, aber noch nicht ausreichender Schritt in diese Richtung getan.

Tabelle 1. Verteilung der histopathologischen Befunde

Histopathologische Diagnose		Patienten
Gruppe 1 =	Vom Deckepithel ausgehende Tumoren	95
Gruppe 2 =	Von abwegig diff. Coelomepithel ausgehende Tumoren	57
Gruppe 3 =	Von der Keimleiste ausgehende Tumoren	23
Gruppe 4 =	Von den Keimzellen ausgehende Tumoren	14
Gruppe 5 =	Genetisch unklare Tumoren	31
Gruppe 6 =	Metastatische Tumoren	?
Insgesamt		220

Durch die histologische Klassifikation der Ovarialtumoren nach Dallenbach-Hellweg haben wir weitere Informationen über das Ovarialkarzinom auch hinsichtlich der Prognose und damit der Therapie erwartet. So konnten die histologischen Befunde von 220 Patientinnen mit einem Ovarialkarzinom nach dem Schema von Frau Dallenbach-Hellweg wie folgt aufgeteilt werden (Tabelle 1).

Die Patientinnen der Gruppe 6 mit metastatischen Tumoren bleiben bei unseren Betrachtungen unberücksichtigt, da sie zur Behandlung in die dem Primärtumor entsprechende Fachklinik verlegt werden.

1 Frauenklinik im Klinikum Mannheim der Universität Heidelberg, D-6800 Mannheim

Gegenüberstellung von Alter und histopathologischem Befund

Das Durchschnittsalter der Patientinnen betrug bei Therapiebeginn 57,2 Jahre; die älteste Patientin war 87 Jahre, die jüngste 16 Jahre alt. Insgesamt waren 92% der beobachteten Fälle 40 Jahre und älter.

Vor dem 30. Lebensjahr traten nur die von den Keimzellen ausgehenden Tumoren auf. Die genetisch unklaren Tumoren sind relativ gleichmäßig in jedem Alter über 30 Jahre zu finden. Lediglich die Tumoren, die von der Keimleiste und vom Deckepithel ausgehen, finden sich gehäuft ab dem 4. Lebensjahrzehnt.

Die Gruppe 2 wurde bei der weiteren Beurteilung mit der Gruppe 4 zusammengefaßt, einerseits wegen der nahezu analogen klinischen Parameter, andererseits zur gemeinsamen Erfassung aller mucinösen Karzinome als der in Gruppe 2 – alternativ Gruppe 4 – häufigsten Tumorform.

Ausdehnung des Primärtumors und des histologischen Befundes

Betrachtet man die Ausdehnung (T-Stadium) des Primärtumors in Abhängigkeit vom histopathologischen Befund, so zeigt sich, daß der Prozentsatz bei Tumoren, die bei Therapiebeginn auf nur ein oder beide Ovarien beschränkt waren, am höchsten bei der Gruppe 3 war (61%).

Tabelle 2. Ausdehnung des Primärtumors und histopathologischer Befund

Histopathologie-Gruppe	T-Werte [%]		
	T_1	T_2 u. T_3	T_4
1	15	30	55
3	61	9	30
4	48	18	34
5	16	20	64

Ganz anders ist die Situation bei der Gruppe 5 mit den genetisch unklaren Tumoren (16%). In 64% der Fälle hat der Tumor bei Therapiebeginn bereits auf die Umgebung übergegriffen. Auch die Gruppe 1 zeigt ähnliche Verhältnisse (Tabelle 2).

Es scheint somit so zu sein, daß sowohl die genetisch unklaren Tumoren als auch die Tumoren, die vom Deckepithel ausgehen, ein viel schnelleres Wachstum auf die Umgebung zeigen, als die Tumoren, die von den Keimzellen oder der Keimleiste ausgehen.

Die Metastasierung ist bei Therapiebeginn ebenfalls in Abhängigkeit vom histopathologischen Befund unterschiedlich weit fortgeschritten. Hier zeigen die Tumoren der Gruppe 3 und 4 die geringste Metastasierung. Auch die Tumoren, die vom

Tabelle 3. Metastasierung und histopathologischer Befund

Histopathologie-Gruppe	Metastasierung [%]		
	Keine	M_{1A}, M_{1B}, M_{1C}	M_X
1	60	33	7
3	65	25	10
4	73	19	8
5	30	63	7

Deckepithel ausgehen, sind relativ günstig. Nur die Tumoren der Gruppe 5 wiesen bei Therapiebeginn eine erhebliche, nachgewiesene Metastasierung auf (63%) (Tabelle 3).

Die Tumoren, die von den Keimzellen und von der Keimleiste ausgehen, sind somit zu den therapeutisch günstigeren Tumoren zu zählen, denn in 84% bzw. 82% der Fälle konnte durch eine Operation eine Verkleinerung der Tumormassen erreicht werden. Bei den genetisch unklaren Tumoren fanden bei 48% nur diagnostische Maßnahmen wie Probelaparotomien, hintere Kolpotomie, Laparoskopien statt.

Es kann also festgestellt werden, daß die nach Dallenbach-Hellweg gebildeten histopathologischen Gruppen bei Therapiebeginn klinisch sinnvoll sind. Die Unterschiede in den einzelnen Gruppen sind statistisch signifikant, sowohl in der Ausdehnung des Tumors als auch im Vorhandensein von Metastasen.

Ist diese Einteilung auch sinnvoll hinsichtlich der Prognose?

Es ist zu vermuten, daß die Überlebensrate der Patientinnen mit einem Ovarialkarzinom von der Ausdehnung des Primärtumors bei Therapiebeginn abhängt.

Tatsächlich sinkt die Überlebensrate deutlich von T_1 nach T_4. Während nach 2 Jahren noch 75% der Patientinnen mit einem Tumorstadium T_1 (unabhängig vom

Tabelle 4. „Geschätzte" Überlebensrate in Abhängigkeit vom Tumorstadium bei Therapiebeginn

Tumorstadium	Kontrollzeitraum in Monaten	
	24 [%]	60 [%]
T_1	75	66
T_2	69	14
T_3	27	20
T_4	25	10
T_X	21	18

Tabelle 5. „Geschätzte" Überlebensrate in Abhängigkeit von der Tumorausdehnung bei Therapiebeginn

Ausmaß der Metastasierung	Kontrollzeitraum in Monaten	
	24 [%]	60 [%]
M_0	68	52
M_{1A}	13	0
M_{1B}	15	2
M_{1C}	0	0
M_X	47	40

histologischen Befund) leben, sind es im Stadium T_4 nur noch 25%. Nach 5 Jahren leben noch 66% der Patienten mit einem Stadium T_1 (Tabelle 4).

Auch das Ausmaß der Metastasierung ist bei der Beurteilung der Prognose von Bedeutung. Nach 2 Jahren leben noch 68% der Patientinnen, bei denen keine Metastasen bei Therapiebeginn diagnostiziert wurden. Dagegen lebten noch 13% der Patienten in einem Stadium M_{1a} und 0 Patientinnen mit einem Stadium M_{1c}. Nach 5 Jahren leben nur noch Patientinnen, die bei Therapiebeginn keine Metastasen aufwiesen (Tabelle 5). Diese Ergebnisse sind natürlich nicht ohne Einfluß auf die Beurteilung der Überlebensrate in Abhängigkeit der verschiedenen histologischen Tumoren, denn die Gruppen weisen bei Therapiebeginn unterschiedliche Ausbreitungen auf. Nach 2 Jahren zeichnen sich deutlich die relativ guten Überlebenschancen der Patientinnen mit den von den Keimzellen ausgehenden Tumoren gegenüber denen mit genetisch unklaren Tumoren ab. Auch nach 5 Jahren hat sich das Bild nicht verändert (Tabelle 6).

Tabelle 6. „Geschätzte" Überlebensrate in Abhängigkeit vom histopathologischen Befund

Histopathologie-Gruppe	Kontrollzeitraum in Monaten	
	24 [%]	60 [%]
Gruppe 1	48	29
Gruppe 3	53	41
Gruppe 4	63	41
Gruppe 5	26	14

Überlebensrate in Abhängigkeit der Histologiegruppen unter Ausschluß des TNM-Systems

Es stellt sich nun die weitere Frage, ob diese unterschiedlichen Überlebensraten nur deshalb zustandekommen, weil bei Therapiebeginn in den einzelnen Histologiegruppen unterschiedliche T- bzw. M-Stadien festgestellt wurden, oder ob auch die Histologiegruppen unter Ausschaltung des Einflusses der T- bzw. M-Stadien prognostisch bedeutungsvoll sind.

Aus diesem Grunde wurde die Überlebensrate in den einzelnen T-Stadien den histopathologischen Befunden gegenübergestellt. Es zeigt sich dabei, daß auch bei dieser Abhängigkeitsprüfung deutliche Unterschiede in den Überlebensraten vorkommen, die nicht so groß sind wie unter Berücksichtigung des TNM-Stadiums. Da die Fallzahlen bei dieser Aufteilung jedoch so klein werden, ist eine statistisch gesicherte Aussage nicht mehr möglich. Folgende Tendenzen sind jedoch deutlich zu erkennen: Die schlechteste Prognose haben die genetisch unklaren Tumoren, es folgen dann die vom Deckepithel abstammenden Malignome. Die besten Überlebenschancen haben Patientinnen mit einem Tumor, der vom Keimepithel abstammt.

Die Prognose eines malignen Ovarialtumors hängt damit bei Tumoren gleicher Histologie vom Stadium und bei Tumoren gleichen Stadiums auch noch vom histopathologischen Befund ab.

Bei der prognostischen Beurteilung wie auch bei der Therapieplanung des Einzelfalles ist es daher notwendig, beide Parameter, Tumorstadium und histopathologischen Befund, zu berücksichtigen.

Abschließend kann festgestellt werden, daß die angewandte histologische Einteilung der Ovarialkarzinome nach Dallenbach-Hellweg klinisch gerechtfertigt ist und sich praktisch auch durchführen läßt, da der erfahrene Pathologe die histologische Zuordnung sehr gut vornehmen kann.

Sachverzeichnis

Die *kursiven* Seitenzahlen verweisen auf die Seiten, auf denen das betreffende Stichwort ausführlich behandelt wird

Subject Index

Page numbers *in italics* refer to the principle discussion of each subject

Topics on Cancer Chemotherapy

Proceedings of the International Symposium on Adriamycin and Other Drugs in Antitumor Chemotherapy
Editors: Wu Huanxin, Shen Jiaxiang, F. B. Nicolis, Lin Changxiao, Huang Liang, Fang Gang, Song Shaozhang, Wang Dechang, C. Praga, G. Beretta
1981. 100 figures, 157 tables. XII, 435 pages
Cloth DM 67,50
ISBN 3-540-10997-8
Distribution rights for the People's Republic of China: China Academic Publishers

Die Dermatologische Indikation zur Interruptio

Herausgeber: H.-J. Bandmann
Unter Mitarbeit von M. v. Ingersleben
1980. 14 Abbildungen, 13 Tabellen.
IV, 52 Seiten (Der Hautarzt/Supplementum 4)
DM 28,–
ISBN 3-540-09888-7

Endocrine Treatment of Breast Cancer

A New Approach

Editors: B. Henningsen, F. Linder, C. Steichele
1980. 76 figures, 81 tables. XIX, 225 pages
(Recent Results in Cancer Research, Volume 71)
Cloth DM 80,–
ISBN 3-540-09781-3

P. J. Keller

Hormonal Disorders in Gynecology

Translated from the German by T. C. Telger
1981. 89 figures, 9 tables. IX, 113 pages
DM 28,–
ISBN 3-540-10341-4

Klinische Onkologie

Leitfaden für Studenten und Ärzte
Herausgegeben unter der Aufsicht und Mitwirkung der UICC
1982. 31 Abbildungen. XV, 314 Seiten
DM 39,–
ISBN 3-540-10896-3

U. Lorenz

Antepartale Lungenreifebestimmung durch Fruchtwasseranalyse

1982. 46 Abbildungen, etwa 12 Tabellen.
VIII, 86 Seiten
DM 40,–
ISBN 3-540-11088-7

P. Mauvais-Jarvis, F. Kuttenn, I. Mowszowicz

Hirsutism

1981. 32 figures, 10 tables. XI, 116 pages
(Monographs on Endocrinology, Volume 19)
Cloth DM 68,–
ISBN 3-540-10509-3

Proteins and Steroids in Early Pregnancy

Editors: H. M. Beier, P. Karlson
With the collaboration of numerous experts
1981. 153 figures. XI, 346 pages
Cloth DM 82,–
ISBN 3-540-10457-7

W. E. Stewart II

The Interferon System

2nd, enlarged edition. 1981. 23 figures.
XII, 493 pages
DM 98,–
ISBN 3-540-81634-8

Springer-Verlag
Berlin
Heidelberg
New York

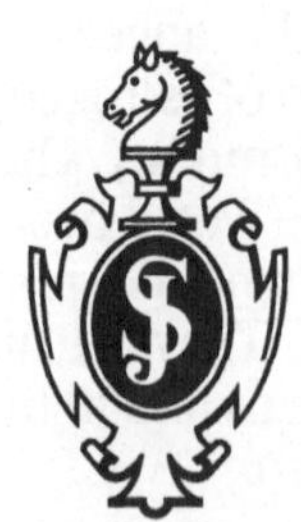